PUSHING THE LIMITS!

Total Body Strength With No Equipment

By Al Kavadlo

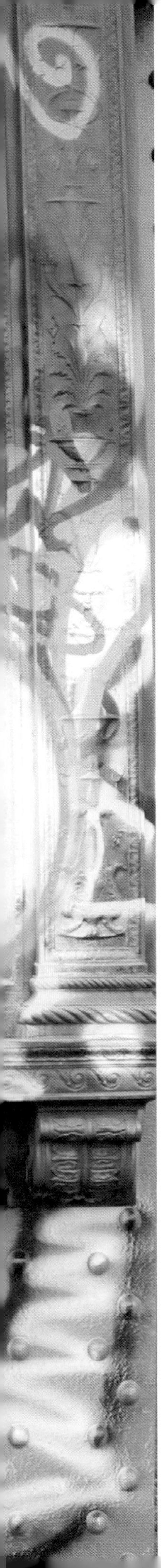

PUSHING THE LIMITS!

By Al Kavadlo

A Dragon Door Publications, Inc production

Published in the United States by: Dragon Door Publications, Inc
5 East County Rd B, #3 • Little Canada, MN 55117
Tel: (651) 487-2180 • Fax: (651) 487-3954
Credit card orders: 1-800-899-5111 • Email: support@dragondoor.com • Website: www.dragondoor.com

ISBN 10: 0-938045-86-5 ISBN 13: 978-0-938045-86-1

This edition first published in May, 2013
Printed in China

Book design and cover by Derek Brigham • www.dbrigham.com • (763) 208-3069 • bigd@dbrigham.com

Photos by Colleen Leung and Jordan Perlson
Additional Photos: Magnus Unnar, Trevor Reid, Kartik Tamhane, Abdiel Munoz, Danny Kavadlo
Cover Photo: Magnus Unnar
Back Cover Photo: Jordan Perlson
Models: Al Kavadlo, Danny Kavadlo, Adrienne Harvey, Lauren Sison, Kristin Leung, Meng He, Jasmine Brooks
Illustration by Billy Hongkong (www.BillyHongkong.net)

—Table of Contents—

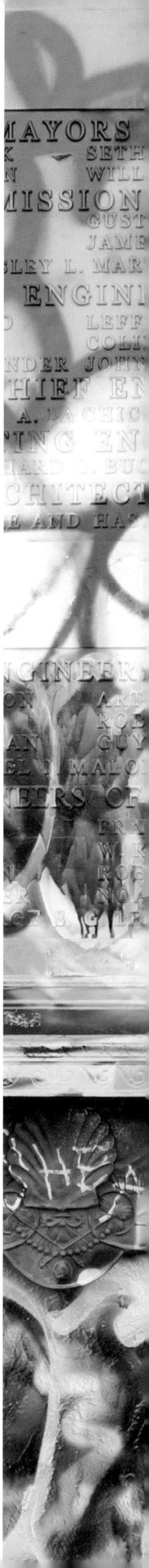

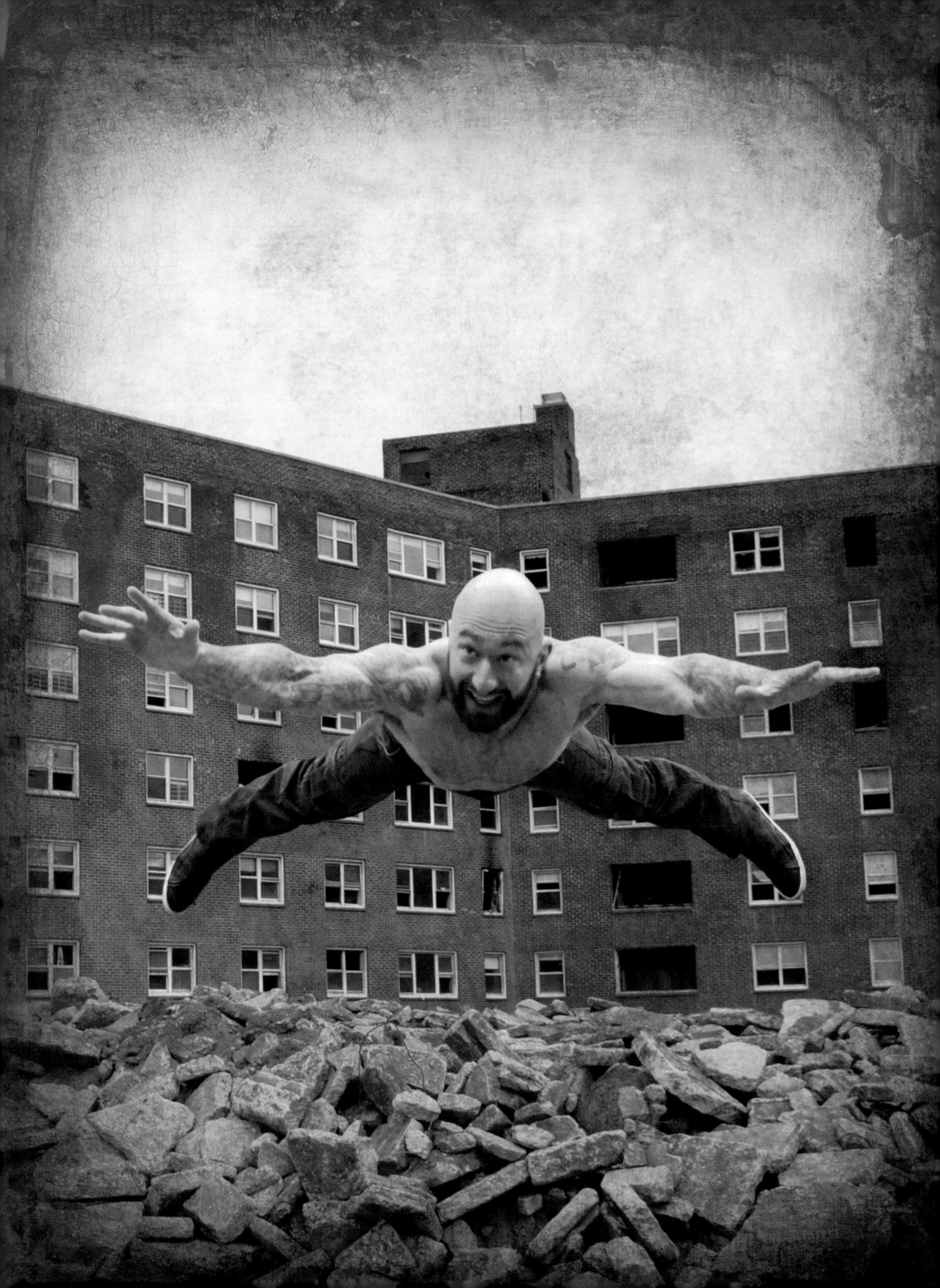

FOREWORD:

By Jason Ferruggia

I'm kind of jealous. I know I shouldn't be but I am. I wish I had authored a book that was this badass and visually stunning.

About a year ago my good friend Derek Brigham (who did the amazing job with the layout and design of ***Pushing the Limits!***) emailed me to tell me I had to check out a new project he worked on. It was a book called ***Raising The Bar*** by Al Kavadlo.

I came to find that like me, Al is an East Coaster, covered in tattoos with a love for old school professional wrestling and bodyweight training. Immediately I was interested. What I didn't know at the time was that Al did a lot of his workouts in the exact same park I once lived across the street from and spent several months training at.

It was the spring of 2005. For the previous ten years I'd been running my own hardcore training center in New Jersey called Renegade Gym. Even though New York City was only a half hour away I'd never spent more than 24 hours there. I was too busy coaching for twelve hours a day on the gym floor. But that was about to change. A few things happened with my business that made it possible for me to do something I'd always wanted to do- move into New York City. I sold my house in the suburbs and relocated to the East Village; 1st and Avenue A to be exact.

After finding a gym to train clients I was faced with the even more difficult challenge of finding a place to train myself. I always kept Renegade stocked with the best and most unique equipment available so I'd become spoiled. An average public gym with a bunch of machines and testosterone sapping music wasn't going to cut it. I had to look elsewhere. Little did I know when I found my apartment, that Tompkins Square Park, which was right across the street, would later become famous on YouTube as the home to some of the most impressive masters of bodyweight strength training the world has ever seen.

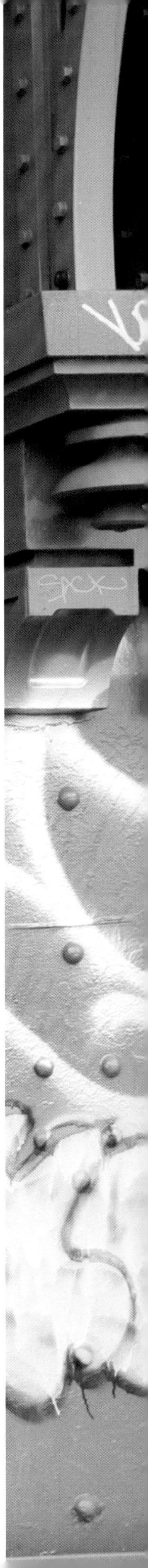

PUSHING THE LIMITS!

One day, after growing tired of checking out one chrome and fern place after another I decided to go train in the park. Bodyweight exercises had always been a staple in my programs but never the main focus. At the very least I figured I could make do on them for a while. When I got to Tompkins I started doing the basics like chins and dips. There were a few other guys at the park doing the same. After thirty minutes or so I was about to head back to my apartment when four guys started warming up on the bar.

These dudes were ripped and jacked. They moved with effortless ease and were doing things I'd never seen before. I decided to extend my workout so I could hang around and watch. By the time this mind-blowing display was over I was convinced that I wouldn't be heading back inside to the gym anytime soon.

Since the day I started training back in the late 80's I was always a fan of guys like Arnold and Bill Kazmaier. My workouts were largely influenced by Iron Game legends such as John McCallum, Ed Coan, Arthur Saxon and Dorian Yates. That meant that loading up a bar and hoisting heavy weight was a mainstay in all of my programs.

We had a few big barbell lifts each week and the rest of the program was made up of dumbbells, strongman and bodyweight exercises. I'd always admired the physiques of male gymnasts and was inspired by their training. That's why we always did tons of dips, chins, inverted rows, glute ham raises, pushups and single leg squat variations. But I'd never forgone the barbell completely. The bodyweight exercises were thought of simply as "assistance work." Chins and dips were the potatoes and veggies. Squats or bench presses were the steak.

Until that day in Tompkins Square Park.

I'd suffered my fair share of injuries over the years and decided I could use a break. I was living in a new city so it seemed like a good time for a completely new style of training. I decided I'd train outside for the entire summer. Give it a solid twelve-week run where I didn't touch a weight and see what would happen. Every day I went across the street and trained alongside guys who would later become legends on YouTube. I pushed myself to get better, to try new variations of exercises, to keep getting stronger. And I loved every minute of it.

By the time Fall rolled around I'd improved dramatically on all bodyweight exercises and shockingly, was able to run faster and jump higher than ever before. I didn't gain much size but it was the summer and I wasn't really eating for that goal. However, I certainly didn't lose any, as I'd always feared. If anything I was carrying the exact same amount of muscle and noticeably less bodyfat.

At that point I was 100% convinced that anyone could get strong, ripped and jacked on nothing but bodyweight training. The added bonus is that it doesn't beat you up like traditional barbell work does.

PUSHING THE LIMITS!

Even my guys who are obsessed with pushing up their squats and bench presses know that we use exercises like chin ups and pushups as a measuring stick. If your numbers on the barbell lifts are going up but your performance on bodyweight exercises is going down that means you aren't gaining true functional strength; you're simply gaining bodyfat and improving your leverages.

So you could say that bodyweight training keeps you honest.

Pushing the Limits! is the book I wish I had when I first started working out. Knowing Al's secrets and various progressions would have saved me years of wasted time, frustration and injuries. As awesome as ***Raising the Bar*** was I think Al has taken it to another level with ***Pushing the Limits!*** The variations of The Big Three and progressions Al lays out will keep you busy for years.

I love the fact that Al stresses slowly working your way through one level to the next and explains how connective tissue doesn't adapt as quickly as muscles do. In the instant gratification world we live in this is critically important. To remain injury free and able to train long into the future you absolutely have to heed his words and deliberately work your way through each step without ever trying to rush them.

A lot of times people see certain bodyweight exercises performed and think they're too easy so they disregard their effectiveness. This won't be the case when you work up to the hardest progressions Al has in store for you. Even the strongest lifters will be challenged to the max. Other times people see advanced bodyweight exercises and think that there's no way they'd ever be able to perform such a circus trick. That's simply because they don't know the proper steps to take to get there.

Al will teach you those in ***Pushing the Limits!***, and a few months from now you'll be doing things you never would have dreamed possible. You also look, feel and perform a whole lot better than you do right now.

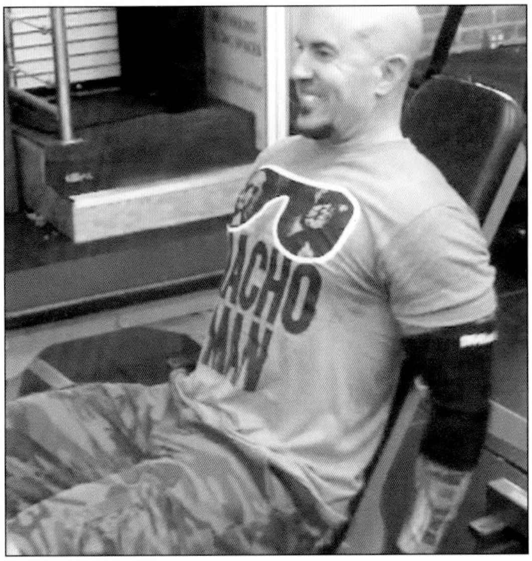

In strength,

Jason Ferruggia

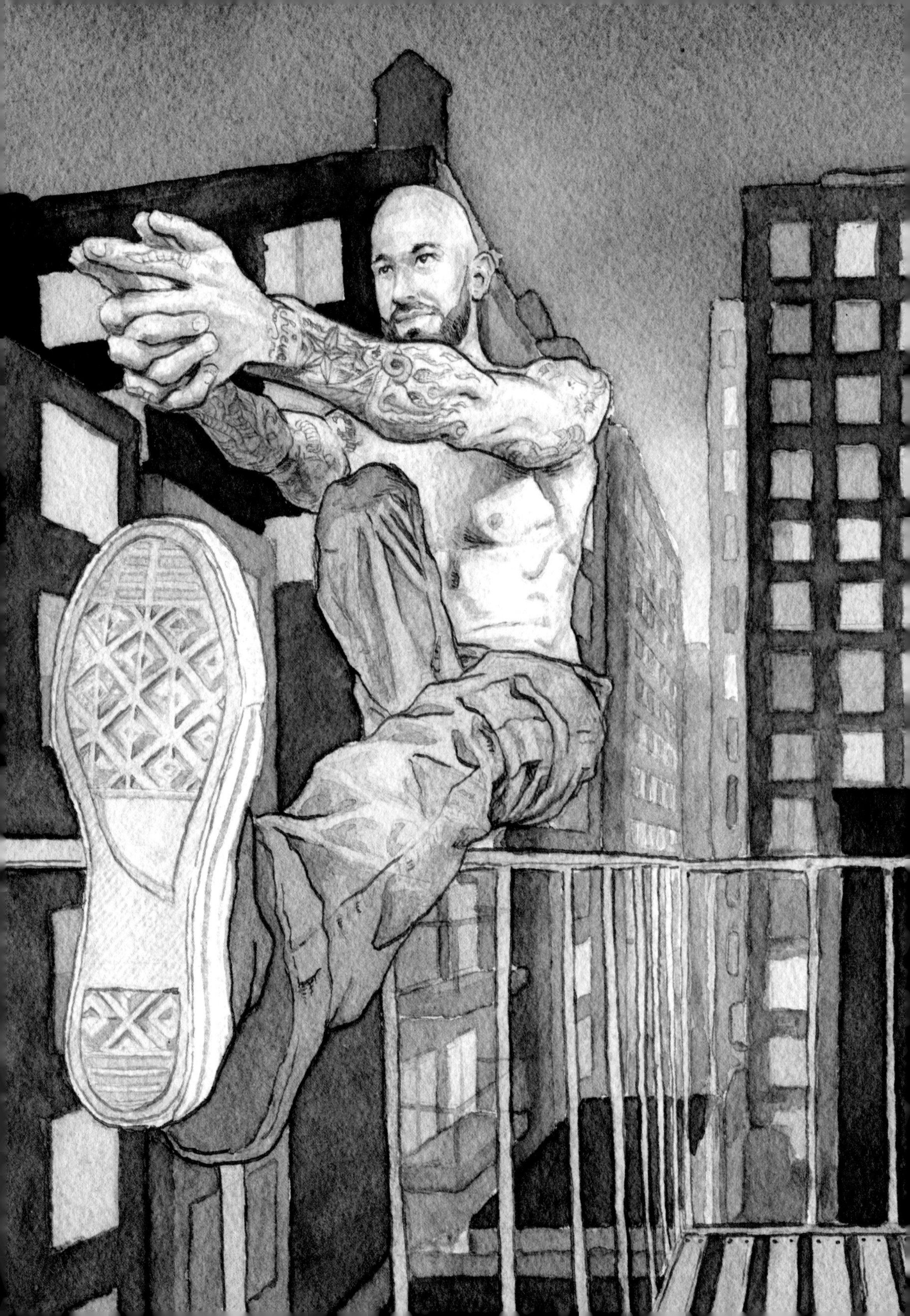

"Only those
who will risk
going too far
can possibly find out
how far one can go."

–T.S. Eliot

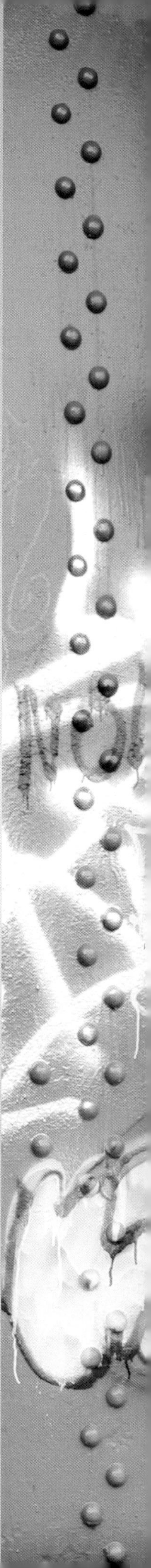

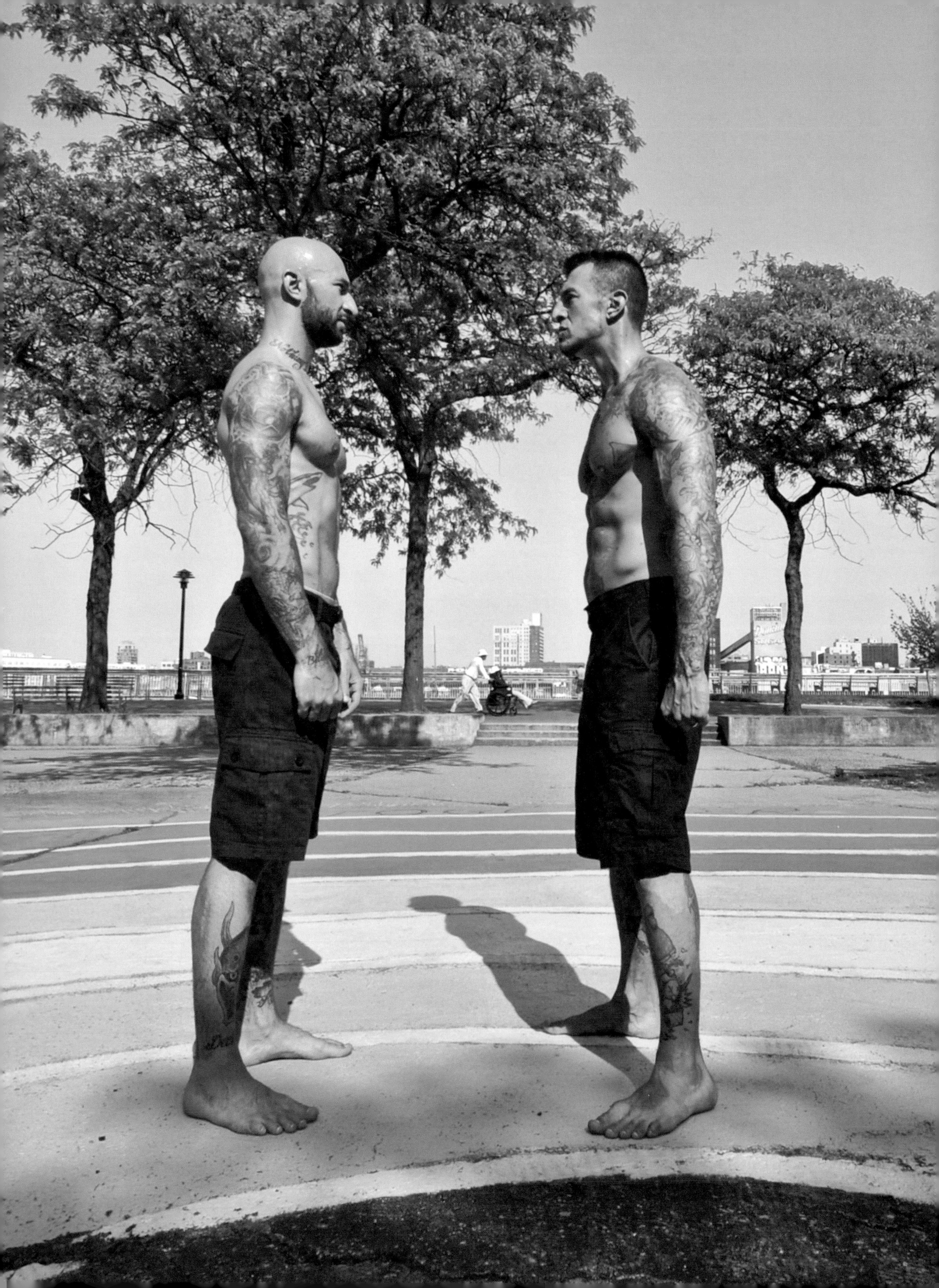

INTRODUCTION:

Wrestling With Fitness

As a kid, I was a huge pro wrestling fan. There is just something magical about watching larger-than-life musclemen kick the crap out of each other (or at least pretend to in a way that's convincing enough for a child to accept). As a result, I idolized guys like Hulk Hogan, "Macho Man" Randy Savage and "Mr. Perfect" Curt Hennig. Even once I figured out that pro wrestling was staged, I still admired these men for their strength, power and charisma. Of course I wanted to be just like them!

For me, it was never a question of trying to motivate myself to work out, it was only a question of trying to convince my mother that I could do so without getting hurt or stunting my growth — that old wives' tale is still so pervasive.

When I was around eleven years old, we made a deal that I would be allowed to start lifting weights when I turned thirteen. In fact, my parents even agreed to buy me a weight set, a bench and a pull-up bar for my thirteenth birthday. Since I had older brothers, we already had a rusty old barbell and a couple of dumbbells lying around in the basement that had been passed down from one of my uncles. I'm don't remember them really getting much use, though. Besides, I wanted to get my own set of weights! I knew very little about strength training at the time, and like most people I was convinced that a skinny kid like me would need to lift weights in order to get big and strong.

Big? Maybe.

Strong? Not so much.

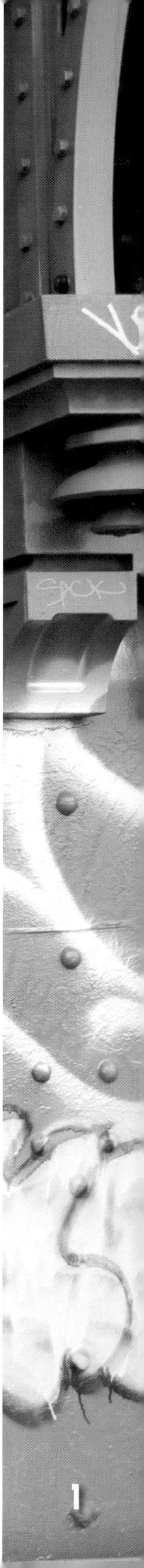

Growing Pains

I waited for my thirteenth birthday with great anticipation. I probably nagged my mom about the weights every day for the next two years. She didn't budge though. I had to wait it out for what seemed like an eternity. At the time I hated it, but in retrospect making me wait was one of the best things my mother ever did for me.

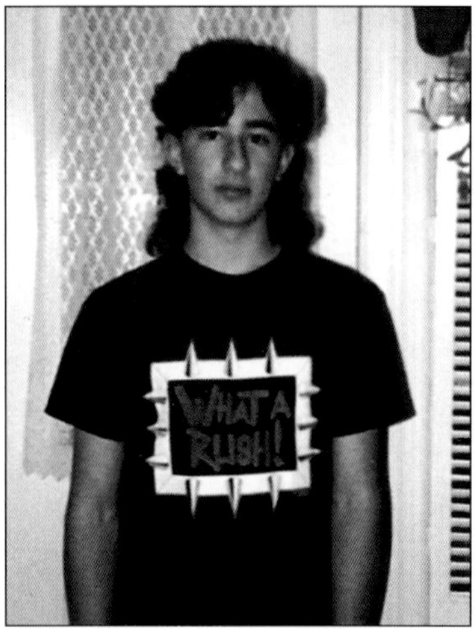

By age 13, I was already my full height of 5'11" – but I barely weighed 130 pounds!

I went through a growth spurt when I was 12 and by the time I turned 13 I was already my full height of 5'11" — but I barely weighed 130 pounds! It was finally time to put some muscle on this frame. (At least we didn't have to worry about working out stunting my growth anymore.)

Since I was really into the idea of getting huge and muscular like my wrestling idols, over the years I dedicated myself to bodybuilding and tried every (legal) supplement I could find in an attempt to make that happen. Though weight training was a lot of fun, I never got quite as jacked as those guys. No matter how much I tried and how many supplements I ate, it never seemed enough. Years later, when I decided to pursue a career as a personal trainer, I was concerned that my lack of mass would hurt my chances. After all, most of the trainers I saw at gyms back then were a lot bigger and stronger looking than I was.

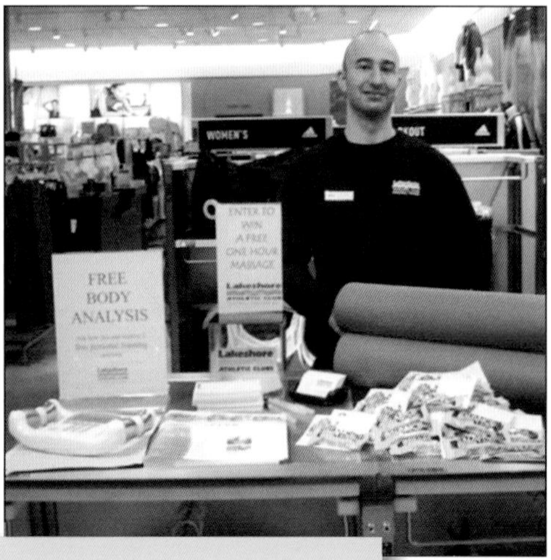

My first year as a trainer. Gotta pay your dues before you pay the rent.

Turns out I wound up doing pretty good as a trainer in spite of not being as huge as the Macho Man. In fact, a few years into my career, I abandoned the idea of building mass altogether, instead choosing to focus on having fun with my training. By that time I had bulked up to 190 pounds but I didn't feel as good as I thought I would. Bodybuilding made me stiff and slow. I could leg press almost half a ton but couldn't do a back bridge, a handstand push-up or even run a respectable mile. I always had stomach aches from drinking protein powder and eating excessively in an attempt to build mass. Eventually my objectives changed from lifting heavy and getting as huge as possible to feeling good, enjoying life and performing better. I've found that pursuing bodyweight training allows me to do those things more than bodybuilding-style weight training ever did.

Jacked Or Ripped

Different people naturally have different body types. While nobody can gain muscle without some effort, some people can put on bulk easier than others. As much as I desperately wanted to get as big as possible when I was younger, I was fighting my body type. Though I didn't want to accept this truth in my formative years, genetics is an undeniable factor in how our bodies look. Just like I can't do much to change having been born with brown eyes, I've also always had small wrists, narrow hips and narrow shoulders. These bony reference marks are good ways of measuring a person's frame. Frame size and body fat percentage are two very different things, however. You can't just look at the size of someone's body, as most people are carrying more fat than you might realize.

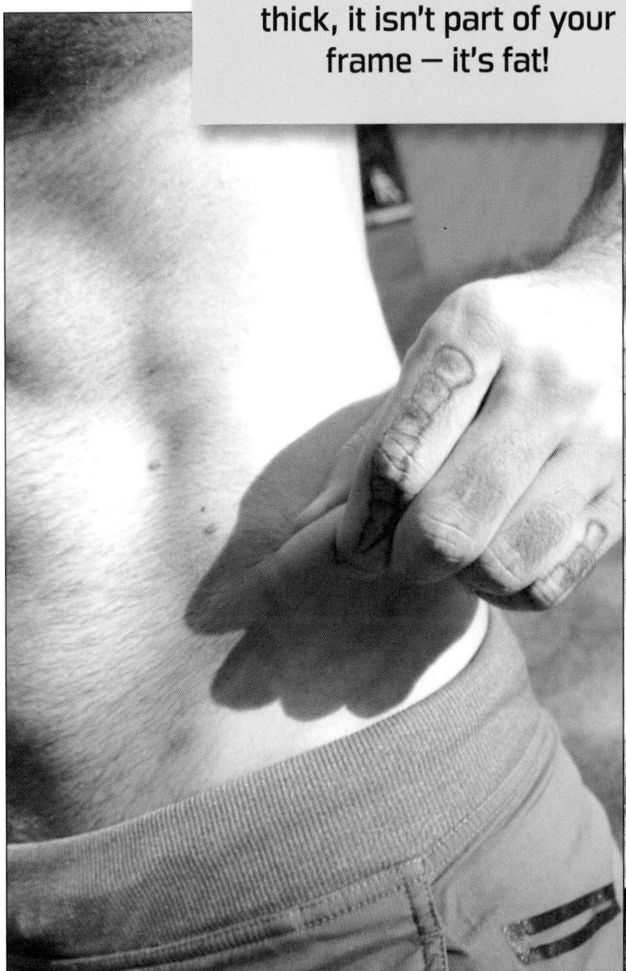

If you are having a hard time finding your wrist bones, shoulder blades and/or hip bones, it means you are carrying a lot of excess body fat. Someone can have a large frame but still be lean while another person with a small frame may still be fat (Arnold Schwarzenegger and Danny DeVito in *Twins* come to mind).

If you want to test the size of your frame, locate any of those areas and give a good hard squeeze. Try to grab as much of your flesh as you can. If you get a hold of anything more than a few centimeters thick, it isn't part of your frame — it's fat!

If you get a hold of anything more than a few centimeters thick, it isn't part of your frame – it's fat!

"Lean" On Me

People who practice calisthenics come in all different shapes and sizes; some are big and some are small. The one thing that all the advanced practitioners have in common, however, is that they are all relatively *lean*. Calisthenics is about building strength relative to your size. Performing bodyweight exercises will gradually shape your body to its most functionally efficient natural state by building muscle and shedding fat to accommodate the specific demands of the training.

Because I have a lanky frame, I'm still fairly small and light for how much muscle I am carrying. Obviously the 13 year old me was way too skinny for his frame at 130 lbs. but

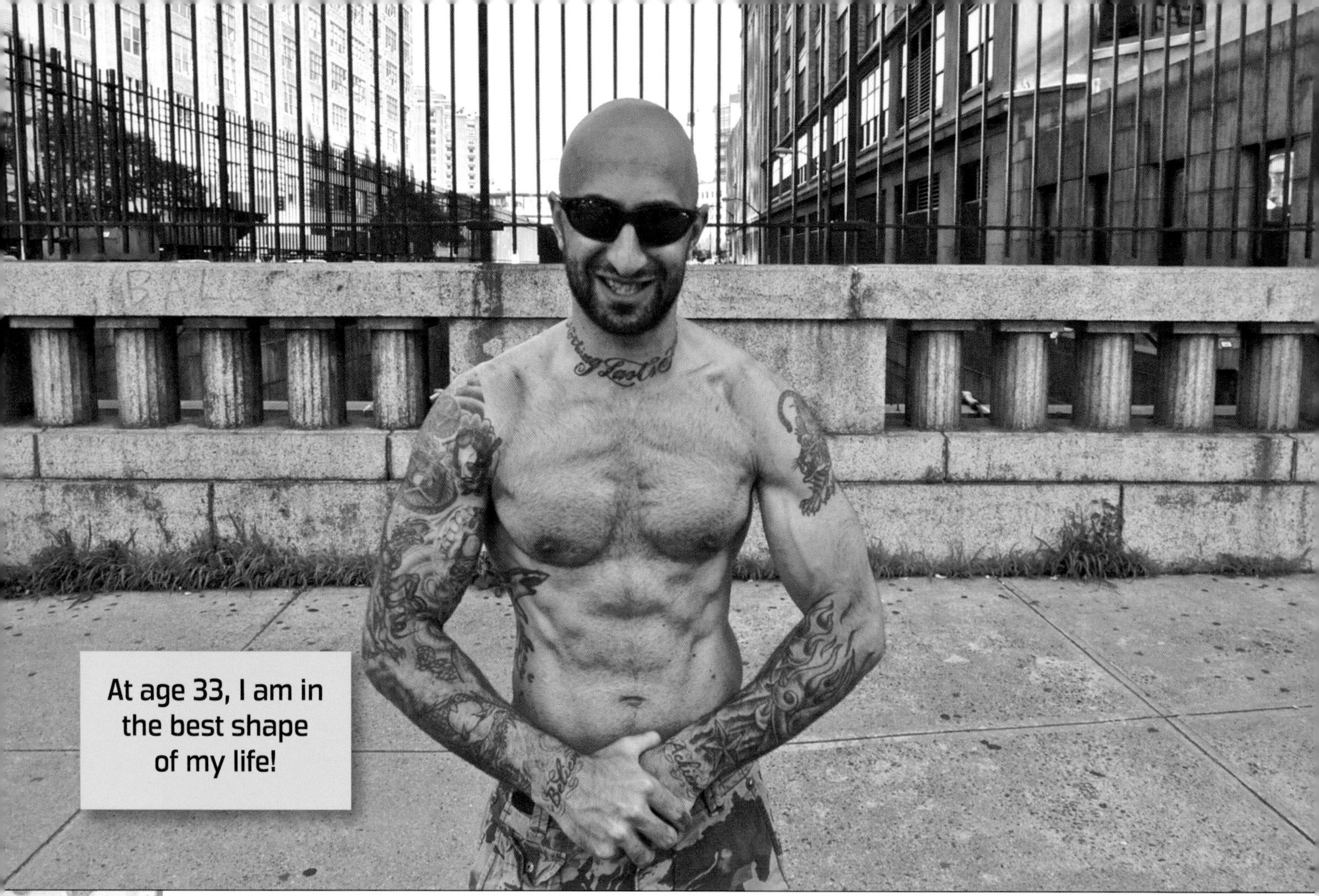

At age 33, I am in the best shape of my life!

the 190-pound me at age 25 was too big! Now at age 33, I am a lean, mean 160 lbs. I'm pound-for-pound stronger than I've ever been and I feel the best that I ever have.

People are sometimes surprised to find out how light I am. I meet lots of athletic guys with less muscle than I have who still outweigh me by ten or twenty pounds. The reason I am light in spite of having a lot of muscle is that I have practically no fat on my little frame! Many people are carrying a lot more excess weight than they realize. A man who is my height doesn't need to weigh anywhere near 200 pounds to look strong and muscular.

Beginners and intermediates can experience muscle growth from calisthenics training, but at a certain point the body will level off size-wise. There is only so far that you can go naturally where aesthetics are concerned, however strength gains can continue indefinitely. Since a large part of strength actually happens in your brain, there is seemingly no limit to how strong one can become. Your muscles can only get so big, but the brain has an amazing way of learning and reinforcing movement patterns that goes beyond the physical playing field, and into the neurological. Strength isn't all about muscles — it's about knowing how to use your muscles.

Besides, if you could continue to keep getting bigger forever from bodyweight training, I'd finally be the size of Hulk Hogan by now!

Ironically, many of the wrestlers I looked up to as a kid wound up with serious health problems (or worse) as they got older. By eating clean, staying supplement free and training for fun and functionality, I'm hoping to avoid those pitfalls.

Total Body Strength

If you've spent much time in a commercial gym, you've probably noticed most of the people in the strength training areas using weights and/or machines to try to work each body part separately from the others. Though performing isolation movements is a cornerstone of bodybuilding training, in calisthenics the opposite approach is more effective.

I want you to use every muscle in your body for every rep of every exercise.

Sure, a push-up places more emphasis on the upper-body, while squats are more of a leg workout, but the rest of the body must support what those muscles are doing. There is no such thing as a true isolation exercise. If you're going to work towards a one arm push-up or pistol squat, you need to understand the concept of total body tension from the get go. It is the key to performing advanced calisthenics with power, grace and control. I want to help you bring awareness to how your muscles are interconnected and use them together to be as efficient as possible in your movement.

I want you to use every muscle in your body for every rep of every exercise.

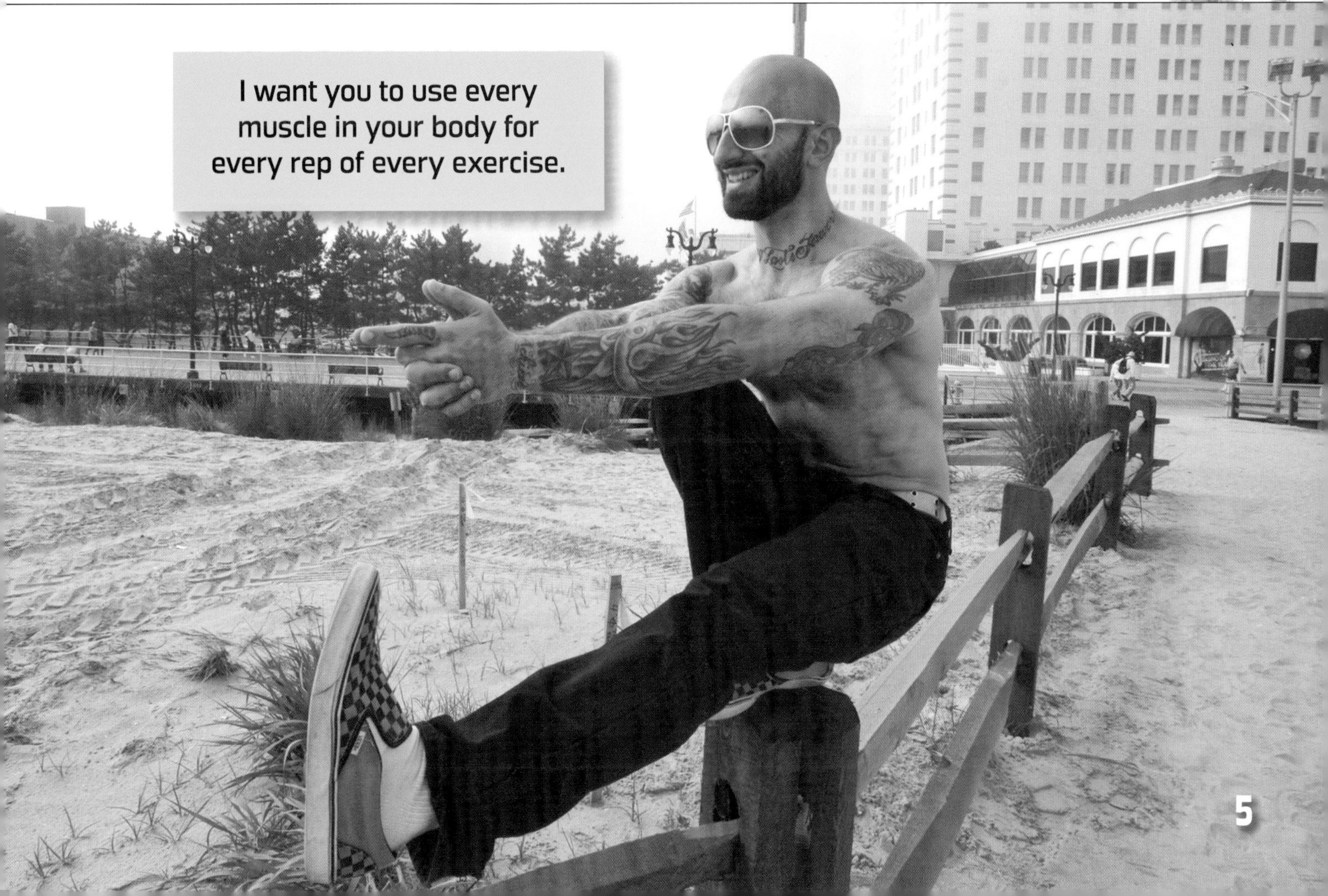

For The Ladies

There are a lot of misconceptions about women and strength training. For starters, a lot of women are unnecessarily concerned about gaining mass, but without testosterone supplementation, it is very unlikely to happen. The women you see in bodybuilding magazines have worked very hard to achieve that aesthetic — they want to look that way! It's a bit insulting to all their hard work when weak, chubby women say things like "I can't do squats or my legs will get huge!"

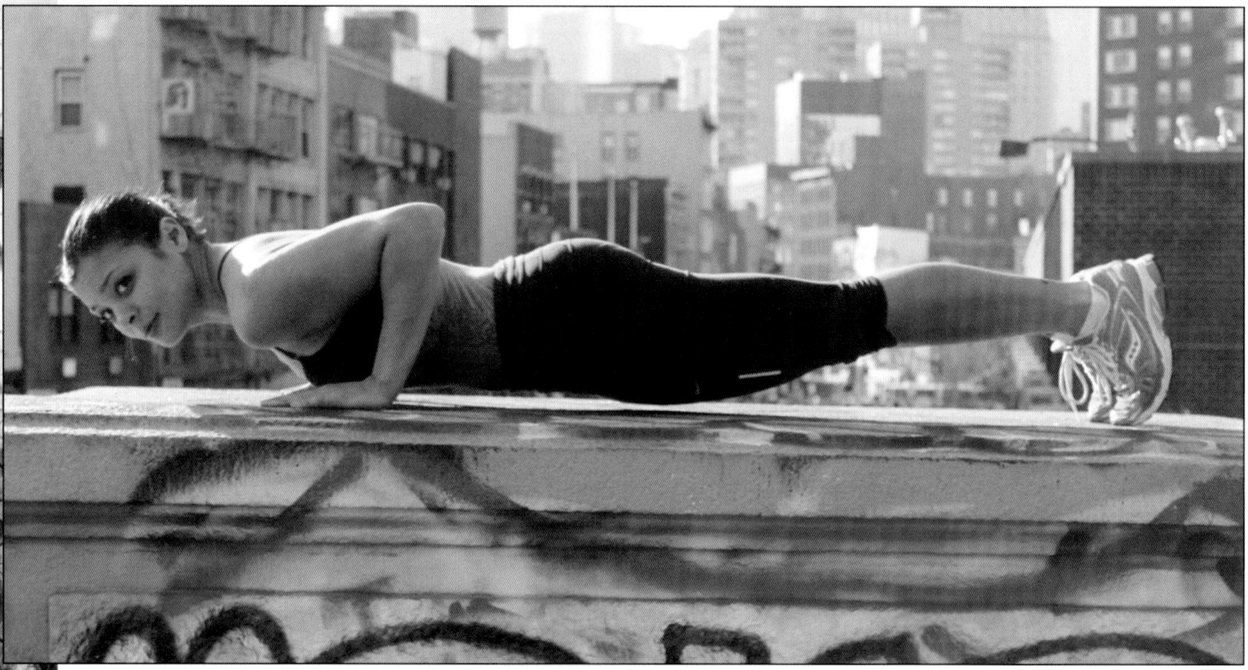

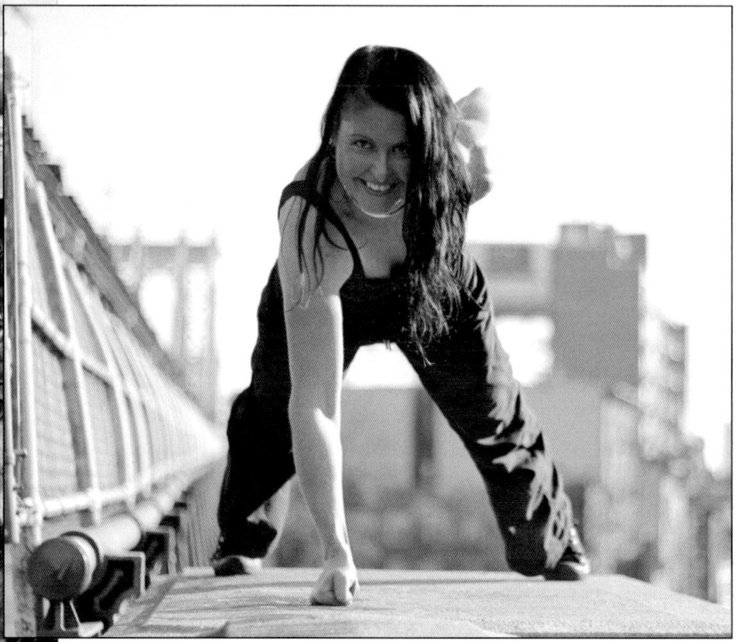

In reality, push-ups and squats are the two best exercises for strengthening and toning the parts of the body my female clients tend to be most concerned with: the backs of the arms, the thighs and of course, the butt. Women who consistently practice calisthenics usually wind up with lean, toned physiques — not huge, rippling muscles like bodybuilders.

Remember, nobody ever got big muscles by accident. Even for most men, it takes years of hard work and boatloads of discipline to gain any significant amount of mass. Many people have gotten big by accident — but just not their muscles! Don't kid yourself about your muscle-to-fat ratio. Bodyweight exercises will not add any significant amount of bulk to a woman's frame.

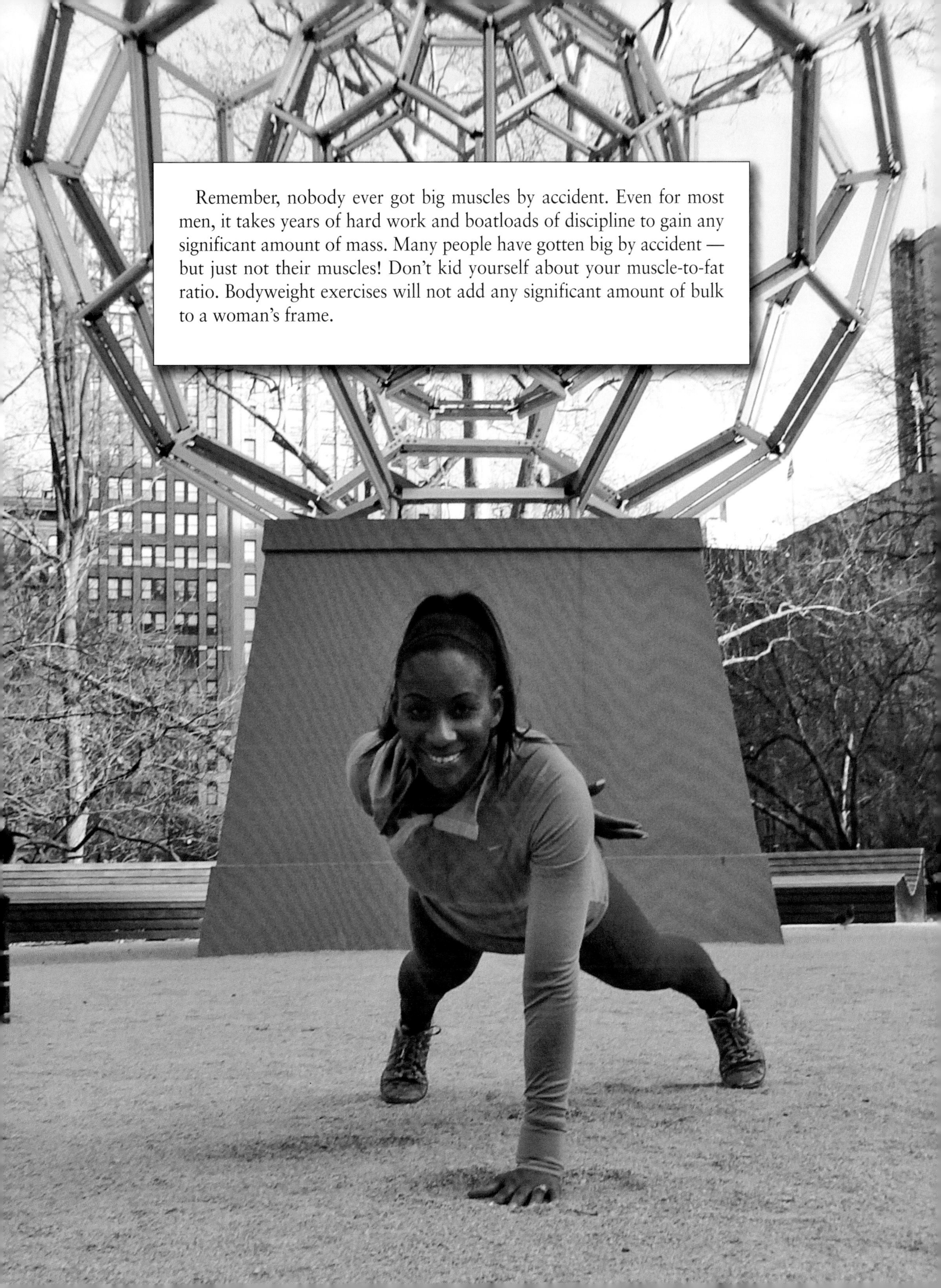

The Big Three

In my last book, ***Raising The Bar: The Definitive Guide to Pull-up Bar Calisthenics***, I broke down pretty much everything there is to do using my favorite piece of workout equipment, the pull-up bar. In this one, I'll show you all the essential moves for strength training with no equipment at all. All you need to start building strength right now is the floor you are standing on. And if you don't have any floor, well, then you've got much bigger problems!

In ***Raising The Bar***, I told you there are basically only three exercises to do on the bar and everything else is just a combination or variation of those moves. Though there are more than three types of exercises to do on the floor, I've chosen to focus this book on the three that I deem most essential: **push-ups**, **squats**, and **inversions**. While you can build a strong, aesthetically appealing body with just these exercises, the ultimate bodyweight strength training program combines elements from both books.

Don't get me wrong, you will work every muscle in your body by following the advice in this book; the lats and biceps work as stabilizer muscles during push-ups (especially one arm push-ups) and all of your back muscles do a considerable amount of work during bridges. Heck, you can even get your lats firing during pistol squats if you focus on keeping your chest upright, but there's simply no substitute for pull-ups.

Now that we've got that out of the way, let's start ***Pushing The Limits***!

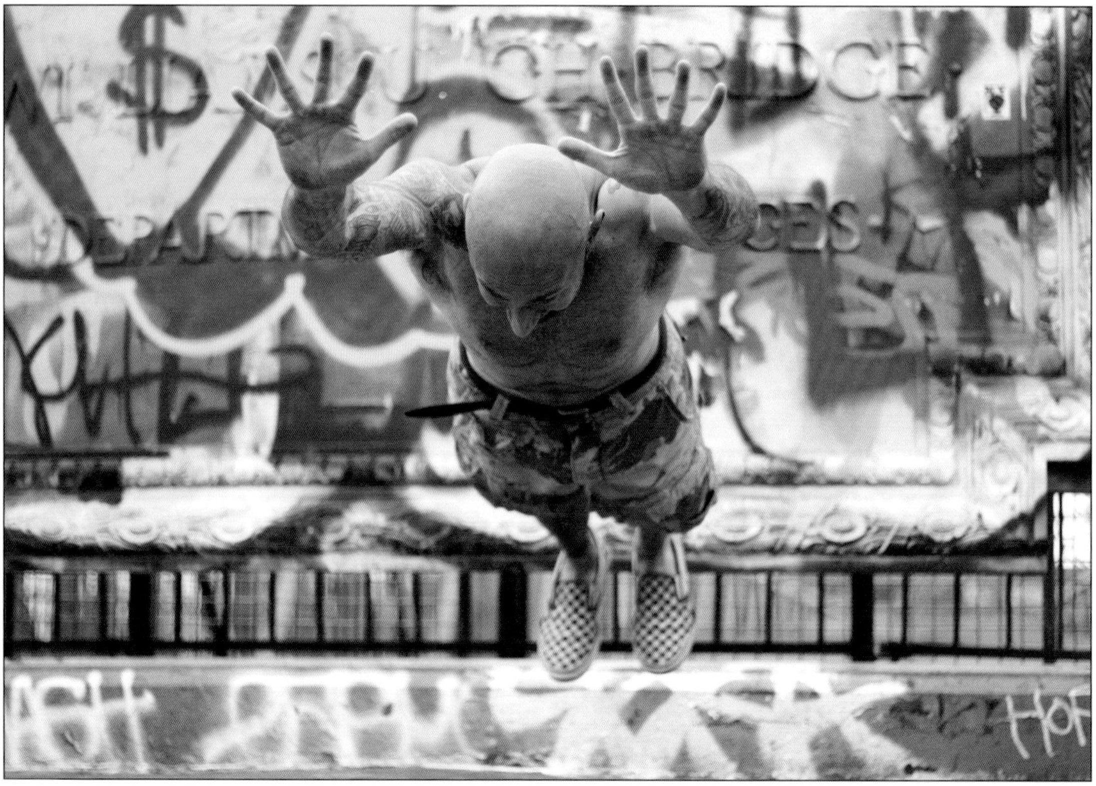

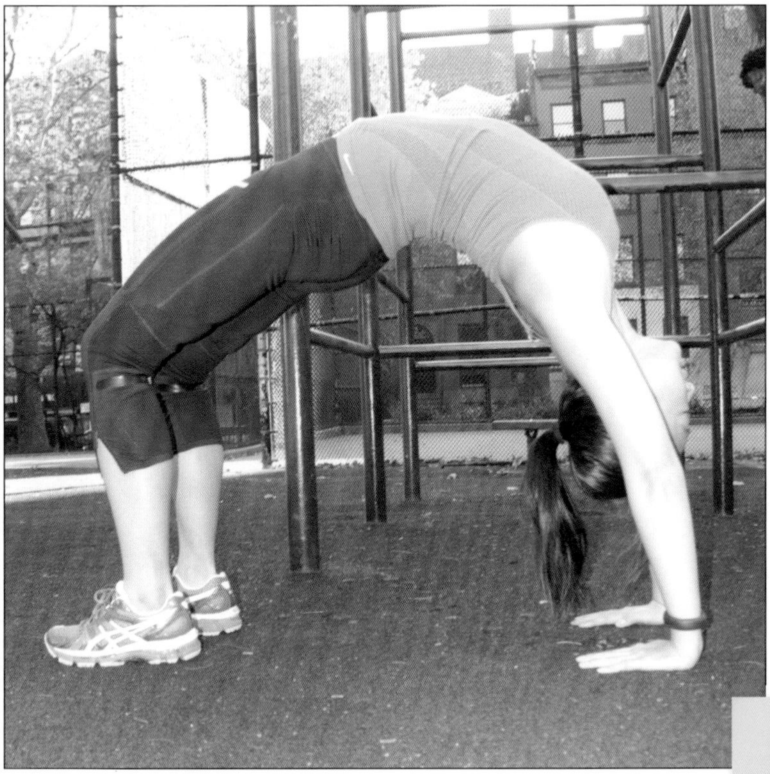

I've chosen to focus this book on the three floor exercises that I deem most essential: push-ups, squats, and inversions.

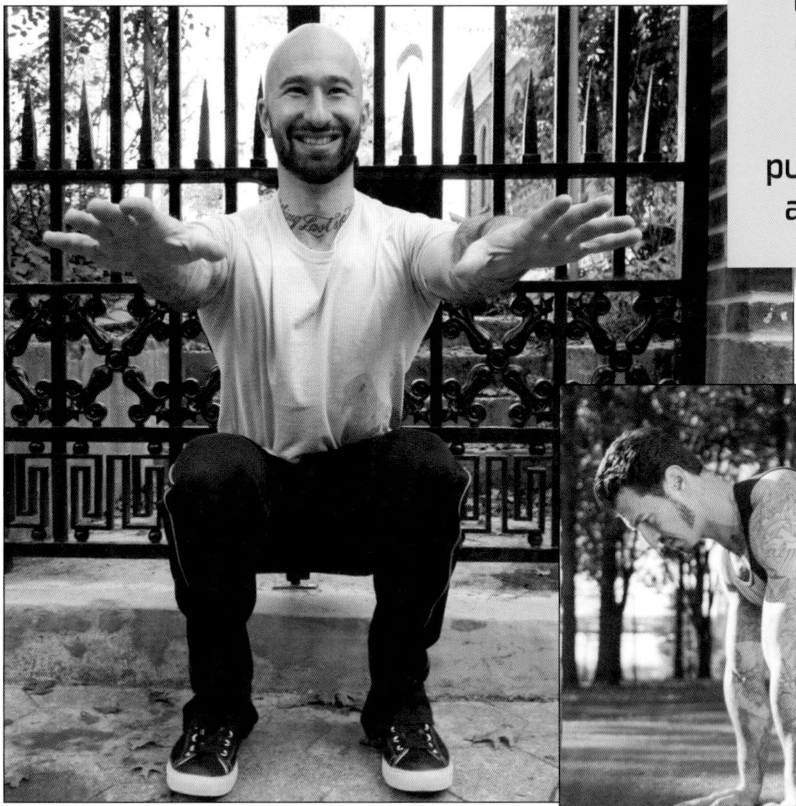

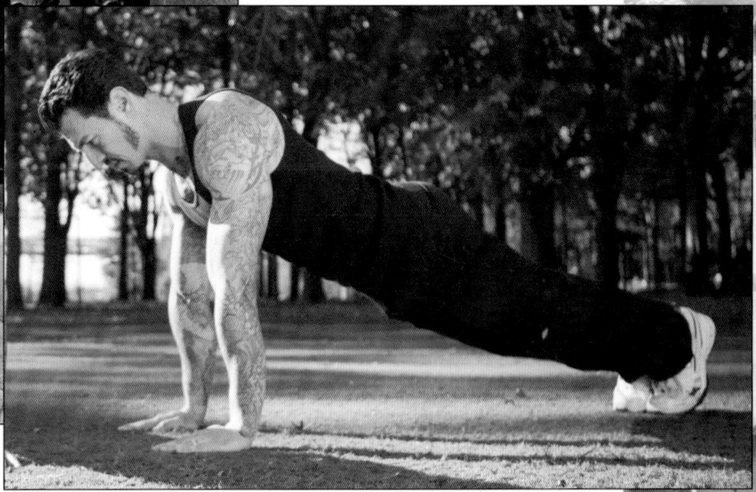

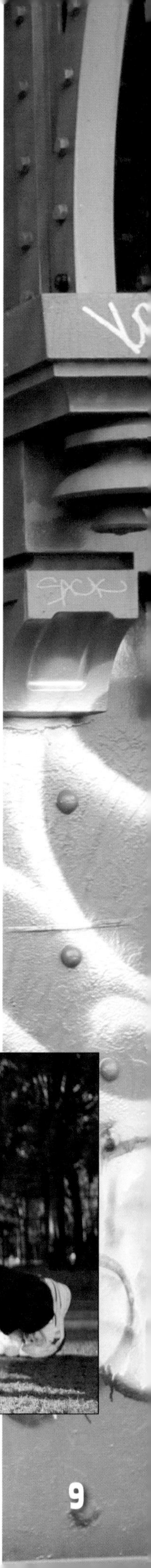

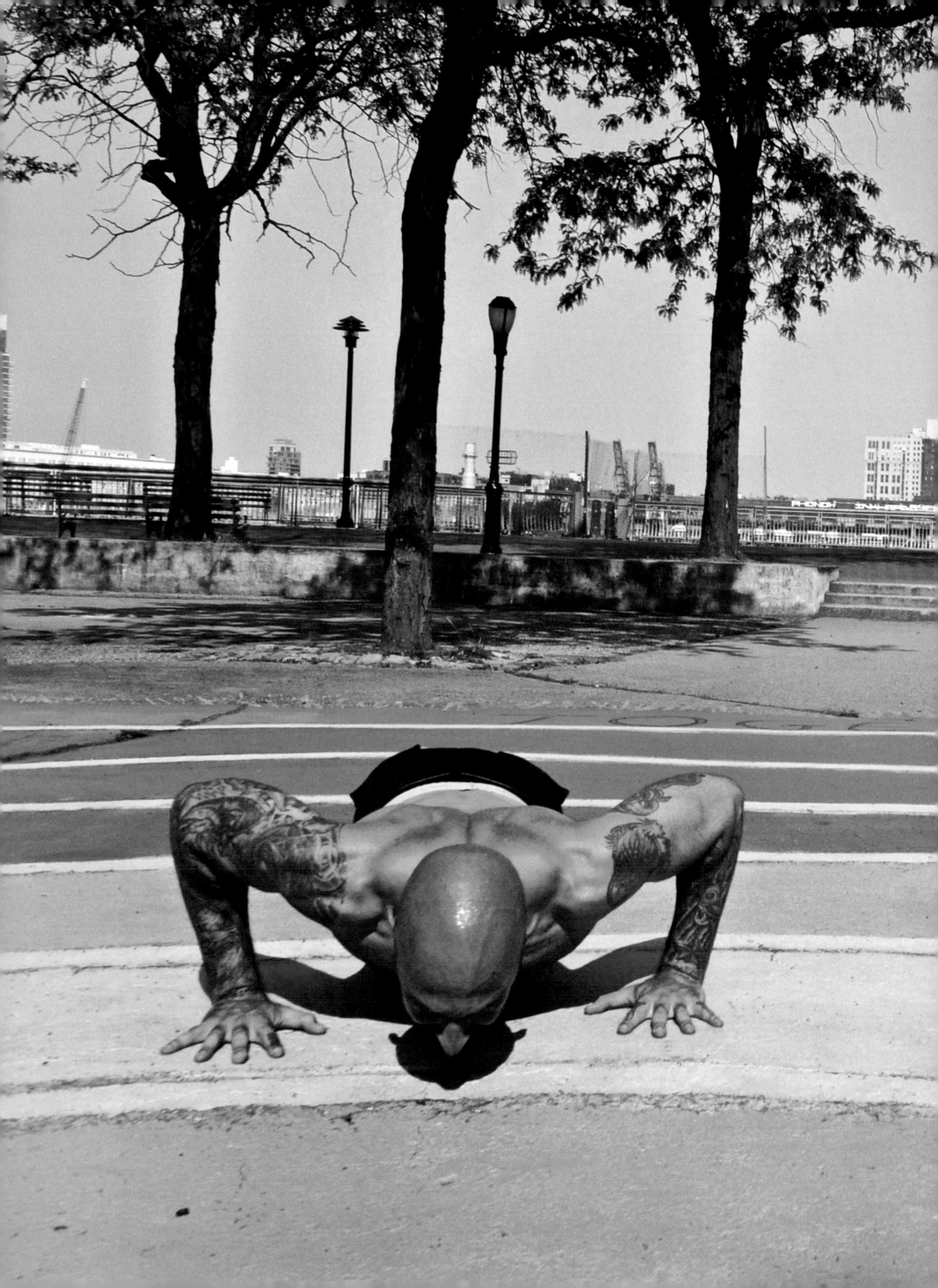

Chapter One:

Progressing to Proper Push-ups

The push-up is about as close to a perfect exercise as you can get. Push-ups require no equipment (even pull-ups require a bar) and they can be modified in an infinite number of ways. While I couldn't possibly go over every single type of push-up that's ever been done, I've chosen to focus on those I feel are most worthwhile. But first things first, you've got to master the basic version — which might be a hard enough task on its own!

The initial step towards doing a proper push-up is learning how to stand up straight. Seriously. It's amazing how many people can't even do that. Understanding proper spinal alignment is essential for implementing safe and effective push-up technique.

The three biggest problems I see when observing push-up form in new clients are a forward tilted head, shrugged shoulders and an overly-arched lower back — the same symptoms of poor posture that plague people while standing. Bringing your awareness to these things while you are upright will make the transition to practicing proper push-ups much easier. Knowing how to fix one will almost automatically wind up fixing the other.

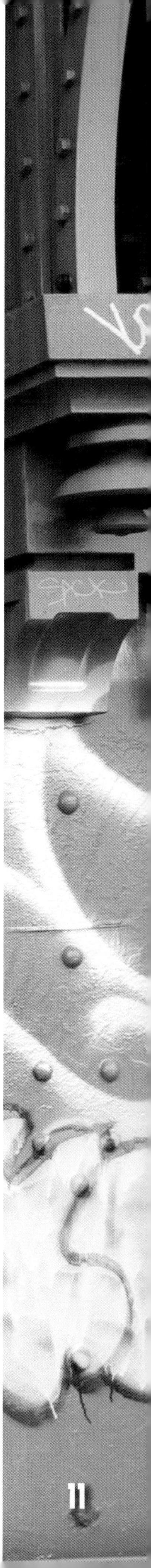

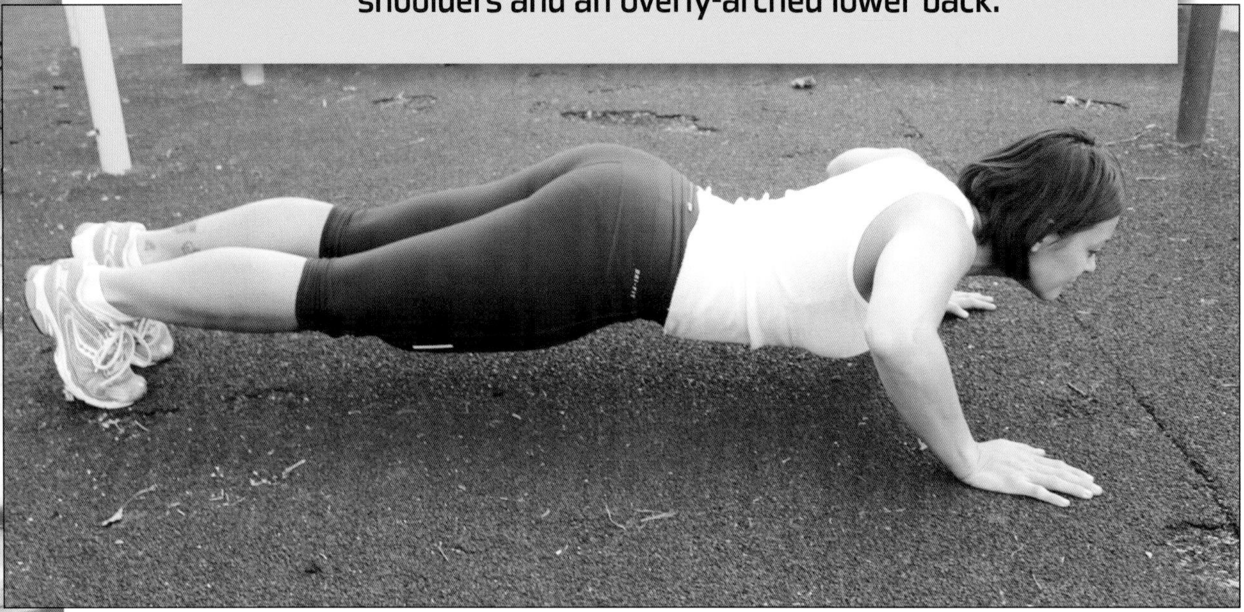

The three biggest problems I see when observing push-up form in new clients are a forward tilted head, shrugged shoulders and an overly-arched lower back.

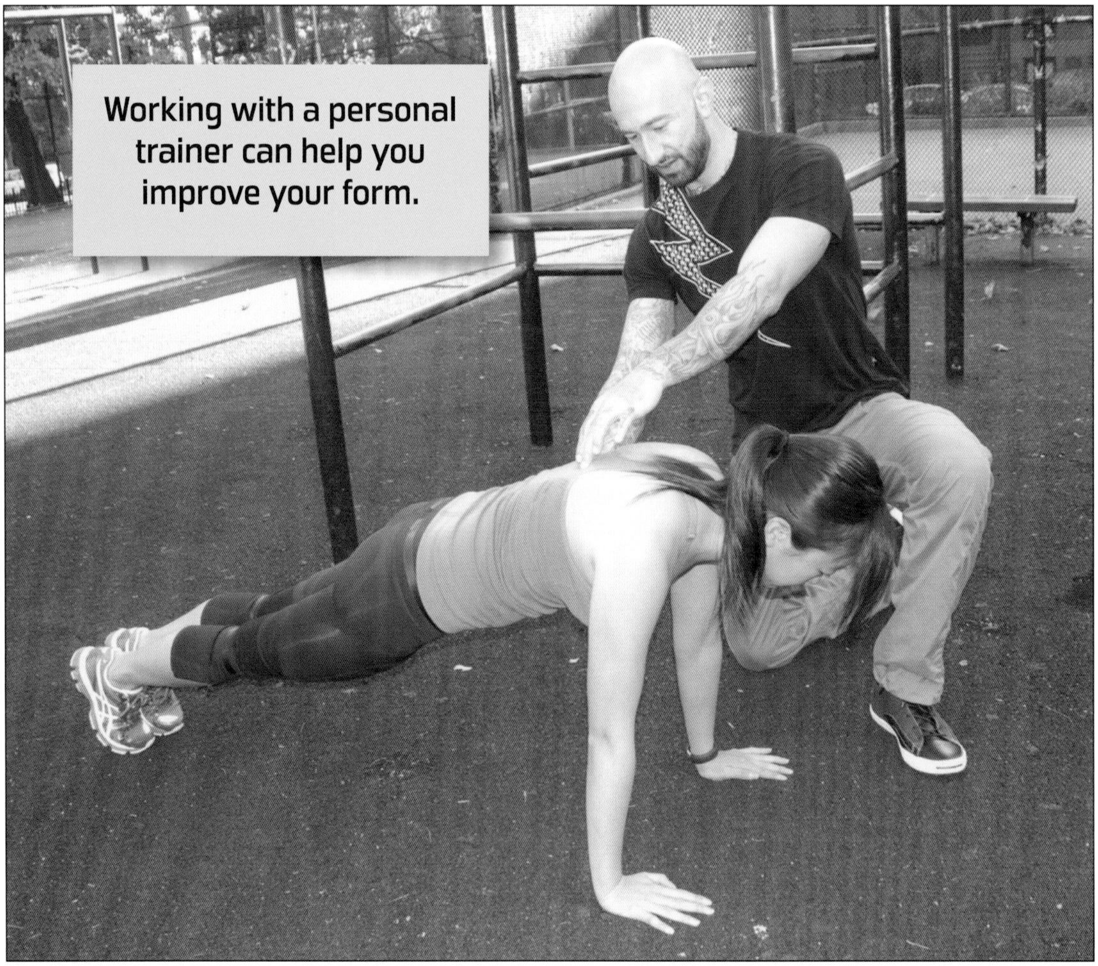

Working with a personal trainer can help you improve your form.

Healthy spinal alignment means that the bones in your spine (vertebrae) line up and fit properly with each one having as much contact as possible with the ones adjacent to it. Proper spinal alignment forms a slight inward curve in the lower back (the lumbar spine), a slight outward curve at the upper back (thoracic spine) and again curves slightly inward at the neck (cervical spine). The term "neutral spine" refers to the position of your spine when it is in proper alignment. Though your spine will be a bit curved, you should be able to draw a straight line down the side of your body passing through the center of your head, shoulders, hips, knees and ankles. This is the ideal position for your spine whether you are standing or doing a push-up.

So how do you stand up straight? For some people it will be as easy as simply bringing your attention to it. I sometimes catch myself slouching too, but once I notice, it's not hard to fix. However, if you're having a hard time figuring out how to stand up straight, here's something to try. Stand with your feet next to each other and start pressing your heels into the floor. Now squeeze your butt and think about gently gripping the ground with your toes. Without looking up, imagine you are reaching the crown of your head to the ceiling. Focus on lengthening your spine while taking a deep breath into your belly. Slowly exhale while tightening your abs and lifting your chest. Repeat as necessary.

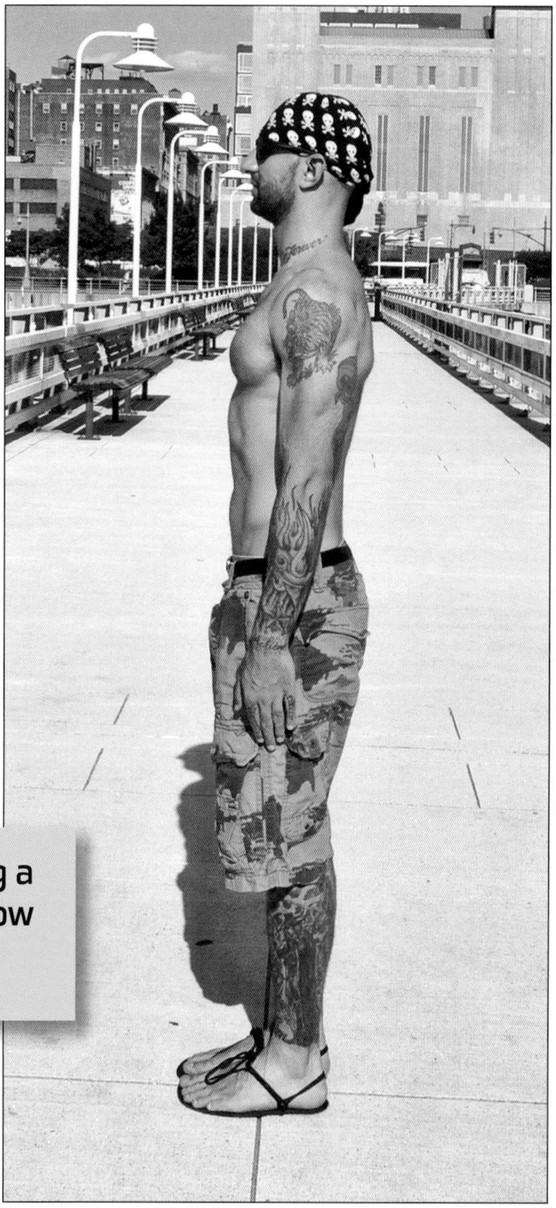

The initial step towards doing a proper push-up is learning how to stand up straight.

The Plank

Once you've got the hang of proper spinal alignment from standing, the next step is to learn to do it in a push-up position. Often known as the plank position, I recommend practicing this isometric hold on both your palms as well as your elbows. (Isometrics are exercises that require you to hold a fixed position, rather than moving through a range of motion.)

People who lack shoulder and arm strength will find it harder to hold the plank on their hands, while those who lack core strength will likely find the elbow plank to be more challenging. As the angle of the body gets closer to being parallel with the ground, it becomes harder for the trunk muscles to stabilize and maintain form, though having the elbows bent takes some stress off the shoulders and arms.

Remember, the same alignment guidelines apply to the plank as to standing. The key difference is that when you are horizontal, you have to use your muscles a lot more to maintain that neutral spine position. You'll need to squeeze your legs and glutes, suck in your stomach, and gently bring your shoulder blades down and back. Don't scrunch your shoulders or raise your hips in the air. Think about making your spine long, like you are being stretched out from top to bottom. Keep your shoulders directly over your hands (or elbows in the case of the elbow plank).

Pushing The Limits!

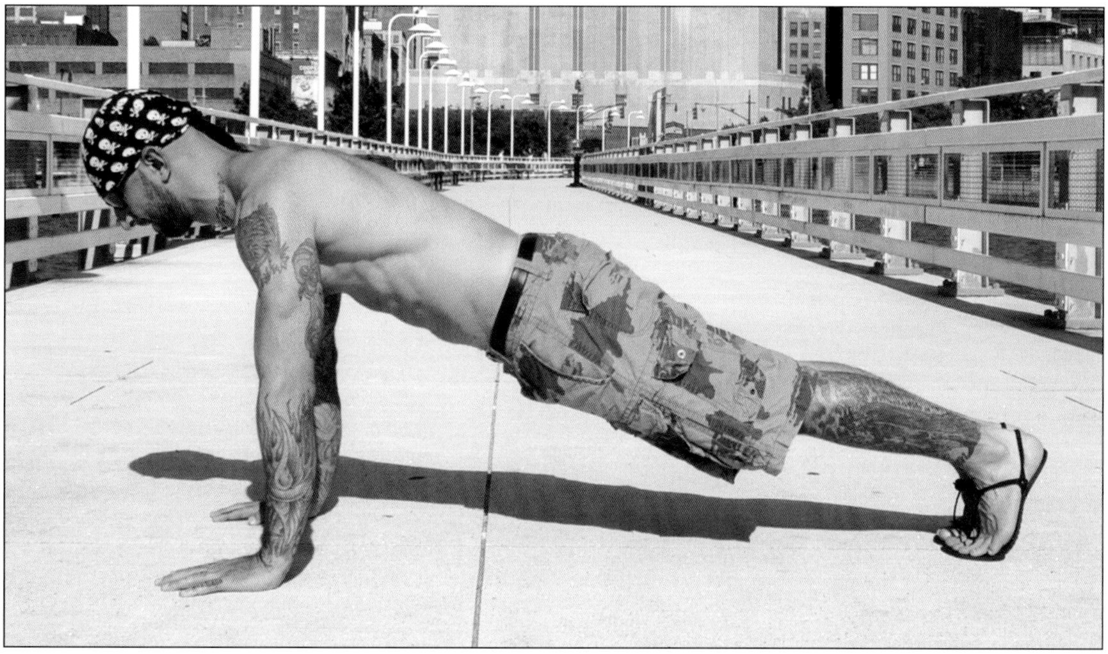

Beginners should be able to hold the plank position for at least a couple of seconds, but if you aren't able to yet, practice planking from your knees instead of your toes. Once you can do a standard plank, you should work up to holding the pose for longer amounts of time. One minute is a good target for a beginner to aim for, while intermediate level trainees should aim for two. With enough practice, plank holds simply become a test of will, as a strong body is capable of holding the pose for extended periods of time. The world record, held by George Hood, is over an hour and twenty minutes!

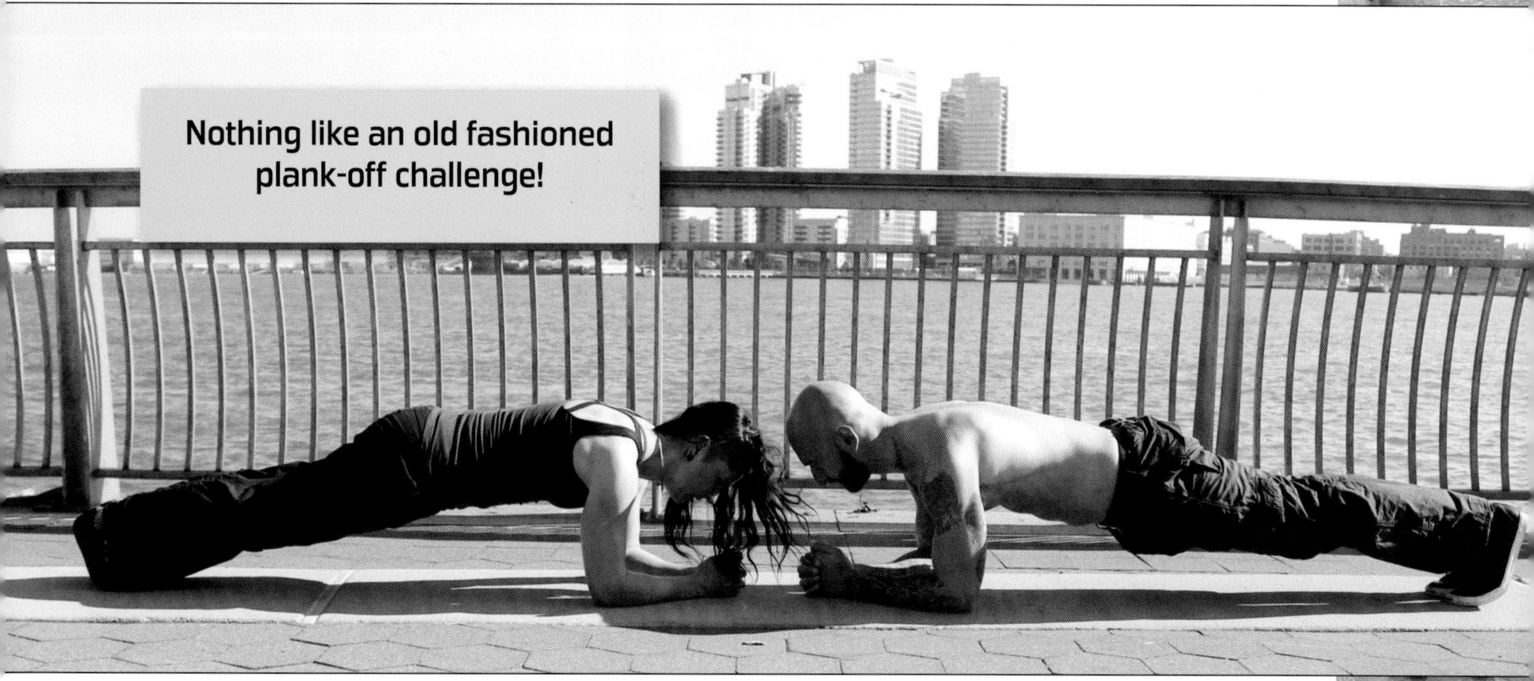

Nothing like an old fashioned plank-off challenge!

Wall Push-up

If you are new to push-ups, it's good to start off with wall push-ups. (I know I said the only equipment we needed was a floor, but I swear I'm not going to get much fancier than adding a wall into the mix.) A wall push-up just means you are working on holding that neutral spine position while you lean into a wall and press your body back to an upright position. This can be a great way to practice the movement pattern without having to worry about using much strength. For a deconditioned individual, however, this can become a challenging exercise after enough reps.

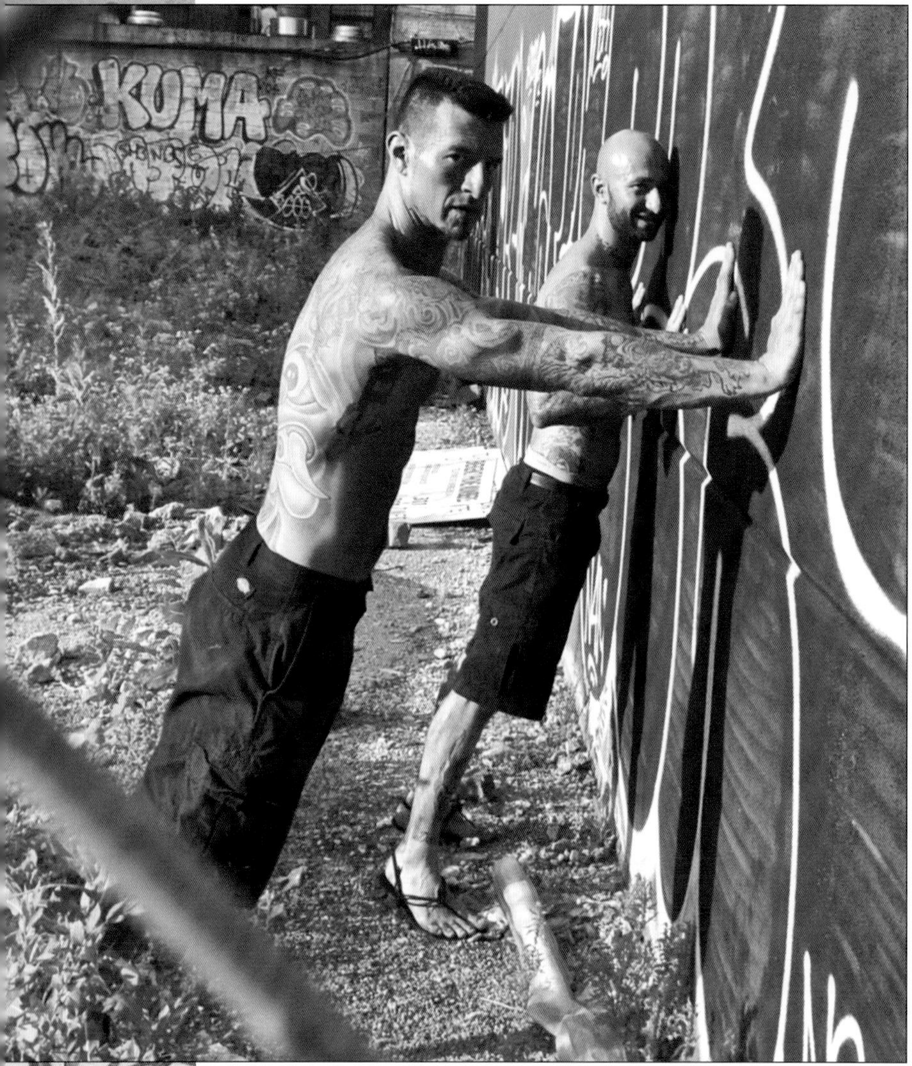

Wall push-ups can also be a good starting point for people with wrist or shoulder ailments. Even if your arms and chest are strong enough to do full push-ups, you may be better off starting with wall push-ups if you've had joint trouble of any kind. I urge you to get your wrists up to speed with wall push-ups if they are holding you back from doing full push-ups.

Everyone knows strength training is great for your muscles, but a lot of people don't realize that working out also does a lot for your bones, tendons and other connective tissue. It's true though; strength training makes the entire body strong. It's obvious when you really think about it — your connective tissue needs to be strong to support those muscles! Sometimes people are so concerned with aesthetic goals that they overlook the changes that can't visibly be seen.

If you have bad shoulders, wrists or elbows, in time your joints can be restored with lower intensity exercises. Once that is taken care of, you can safely move on. The body can only be as strong as its weakest link, and connective tissue tends to be slower to adapt than muscle. Stick with the basics for as long as possible. Don't let your ego sway you towards attempting to move on before your body is ready.

Since the intensity is fairly low, feel free to go for high repetitions with wall push-ups. A novice or even an injured person should still be able to start with at least 10 reps, quickly working to 20 and eventually 50 reps in each set.

Knee Push-up

The knee push-up is a more challenging variation for beginners on the path toward full push-ups. Knee push-ups involve bending your knees and resting them on the floor instead of your toes. By shortening the length of your body, the leverage changes, making the exercise less difficult. Again, this is a great way to practice proper spinal alignment during a push-up without requiring the full strength needed for a push-up on your toes.

Though sometimes known as a "girl push-up," the knee push-up is appropriate for a beginner of either gender. There is no shame in starting from scratch and practicing knee push-ups before moving on to full push-ups, even for a man. In fact, I find it quite respectable when a beginner can keep a humble mindset.

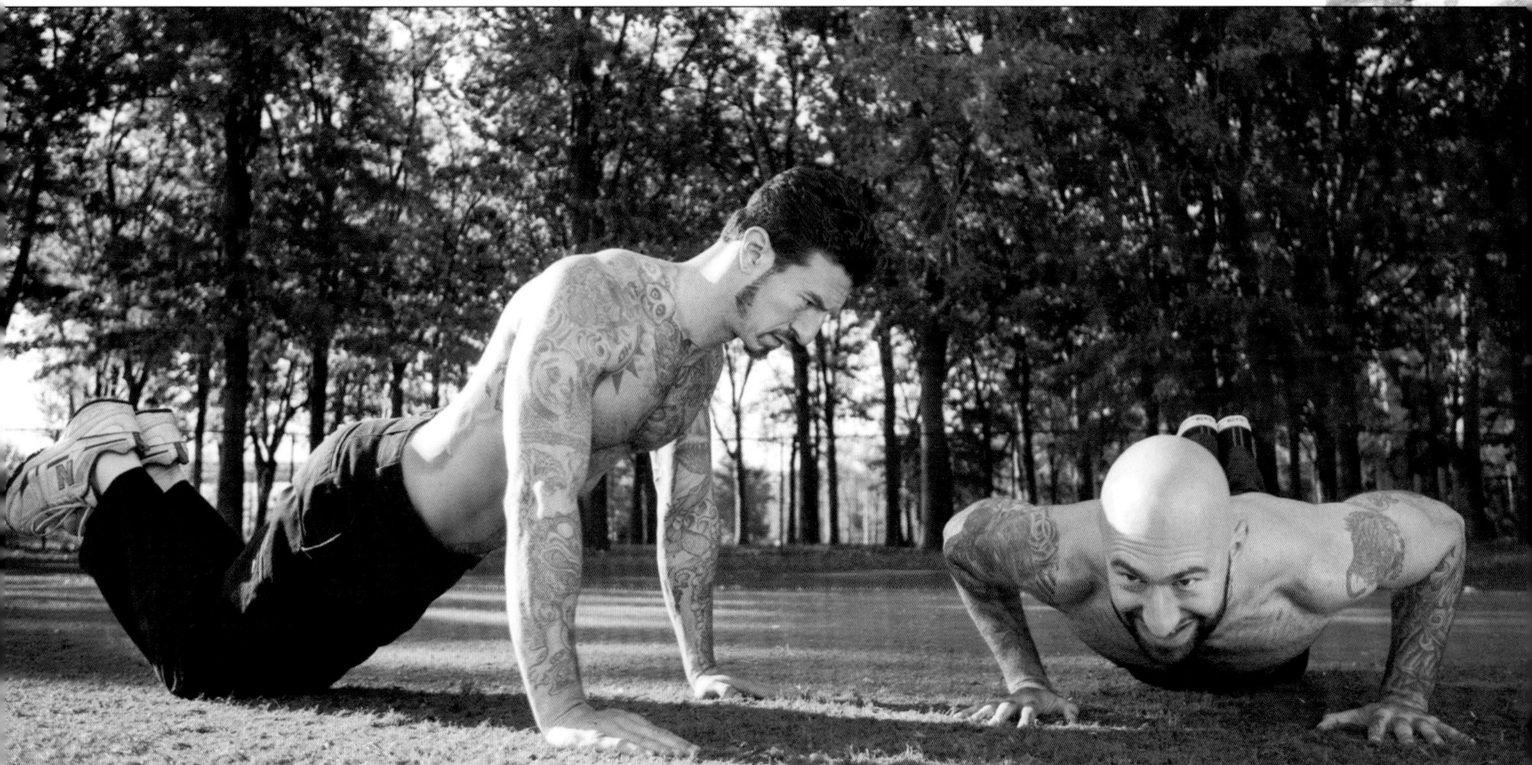

Incline Push-up

If wall push-ups and knee push-ups have gotten too easy for you, but full push-ups are still out of reach, incline push-ups can be a nice intermediate step. In fact, they can be several intermediate steps.

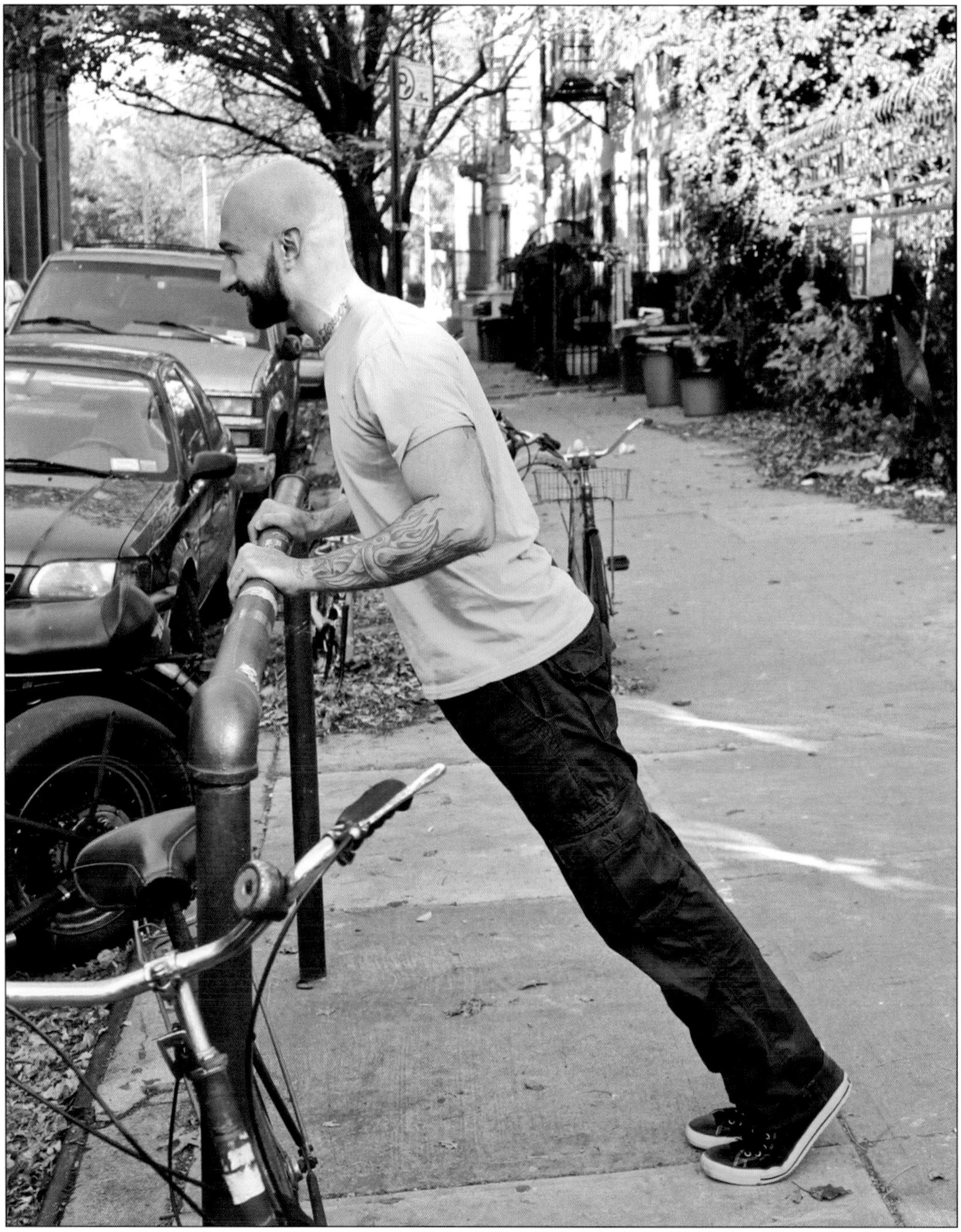

Pushing The Limits!

The higher your incline, the easier the push-up will be, the lower the incline, the harder it becomes. A high incline eventually becomes a wall push-up and a low incline eventually becomes a regular push-up, but there are many little levels in between. You can experiment with various household objects or things you may come across outdoors to find ways to incrementally lower yourself toward the floor.

Keep gradually working toward a lower incline.

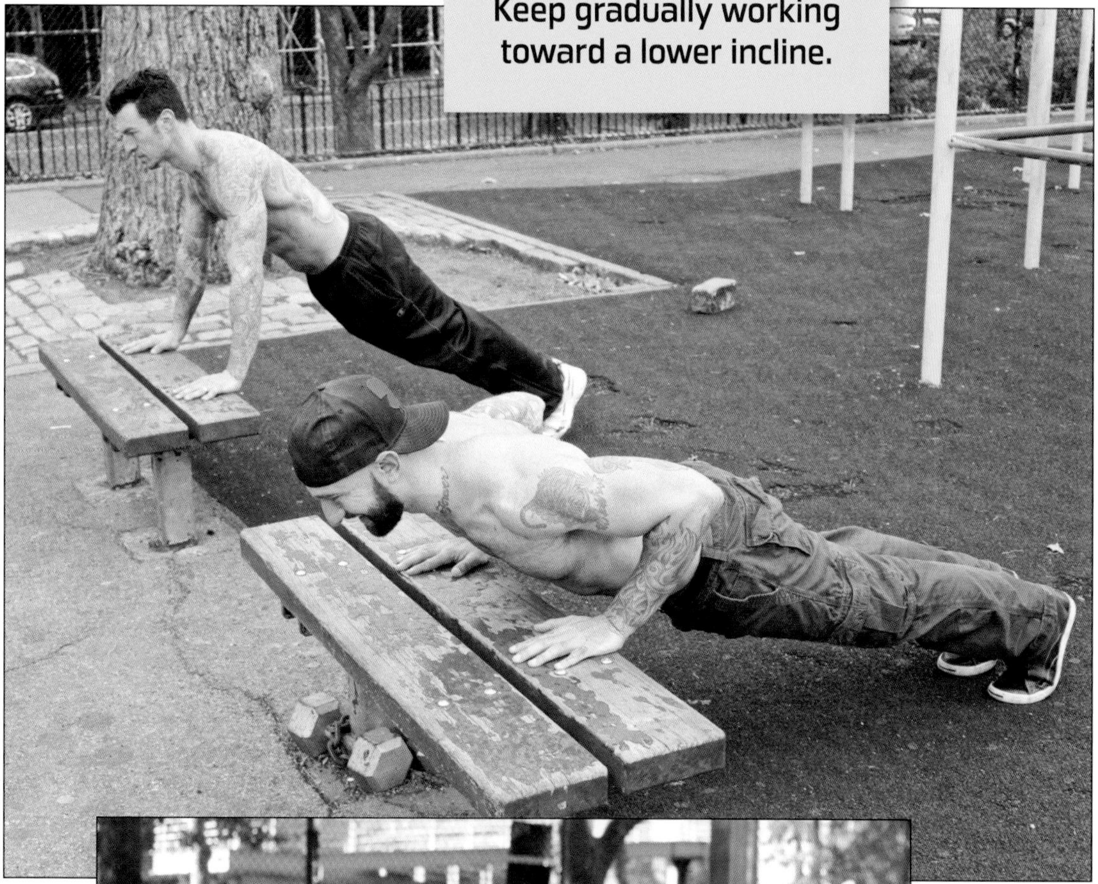

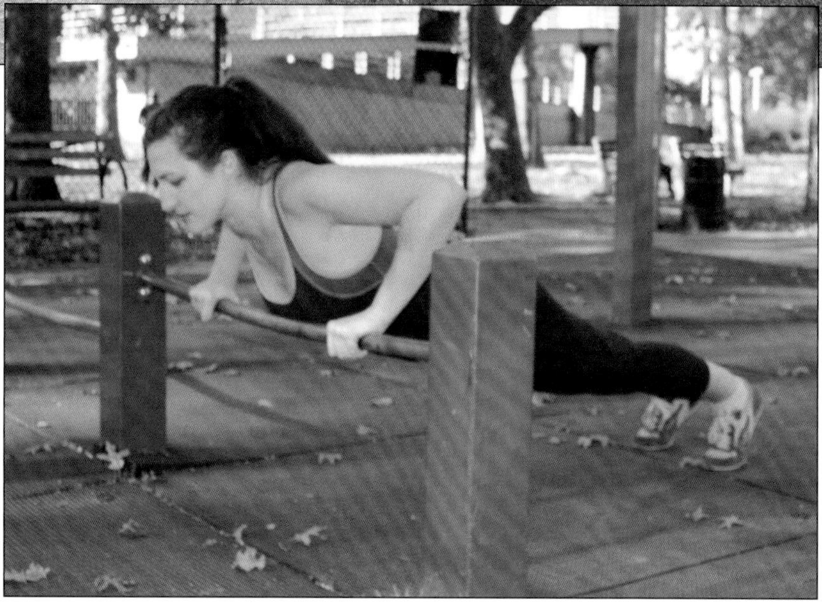

Full Push-up

Once you've gotten the feel for maintaining proper body alignment while performing wall push-ups, knee push-ups and/or incline push-ups (and you can comfortably do lots of reps of those easier variations) you'll be ready for full push-ups.

When doing push-ups, I recommend placing your hands just wider than your shoulders (your thumbs should wind up right beneath your armpits). Keep your elbows fairly close to your body and point them back; do not flare them out to the sides. Lower until your chest is just above the floor, pause for a split second and then press yourself back up.

Many beginners have trouble going low enough on their push-ups. Sometimes this is also the case for people who've practiced for years. Your arms should bend past 90 degrees as measured along the *outside* of your elbow for the rep to count; the lower the better. You may find it helpful to place a tennis ball, brick or other object on the ground under your chest in order to have a reference point for how low to go. You could even try to touch your chest to the floor if you want to extend the range of motion. The ability to do clean chest-to-floor push-ups with proper alignment demonstrates excellent strength and mobility in the upper-body. You might not be here yet, but it should be an eventual milestone.

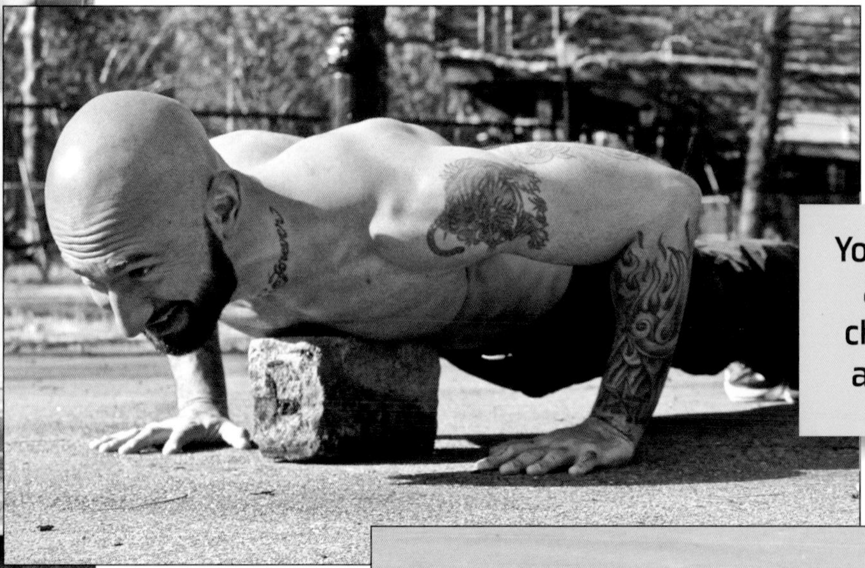

You may choose to place an object under your chest to make sure you are going low enough.

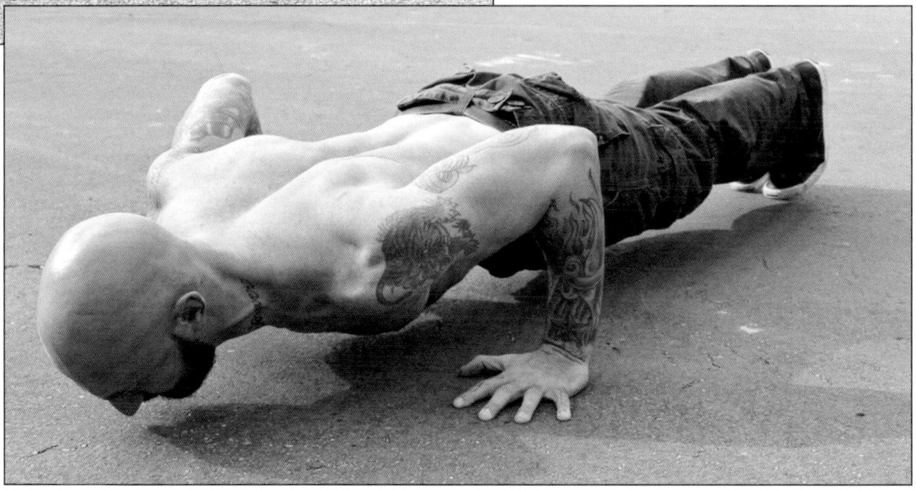

Lock It Out

It is essential to do push-ups with a full range of motion. Just as I want you to make sure that you get all the way down, I also want you to make sure that you get all the way up. I've heard many coaches advise against fully locking out your joints when performing strength training. While this may be true if you are lifting heavy external weights, it is most certainly not the case when dealing with bodyweight exercises like push-ups. In fact, our skeletons are actually designed to support our bodies as much as possible when our joints are locked. (This same concept is why spinal alignment is important.) Yogis, gymnasts and other hand-balancers often support their entire bodyweight on locked out elbows for extended amounts of time with great results.

If you don't get in the habit of performing your push-ups with a full range of motion, you will not get the most out of them. You could even wind up reducing your active range of motion in the process. I've met lots of guys who practiced limited range of motion in their strength training and wound up losing the ability to fully extend their arms altogether. If you don't use it, you'll lose it!

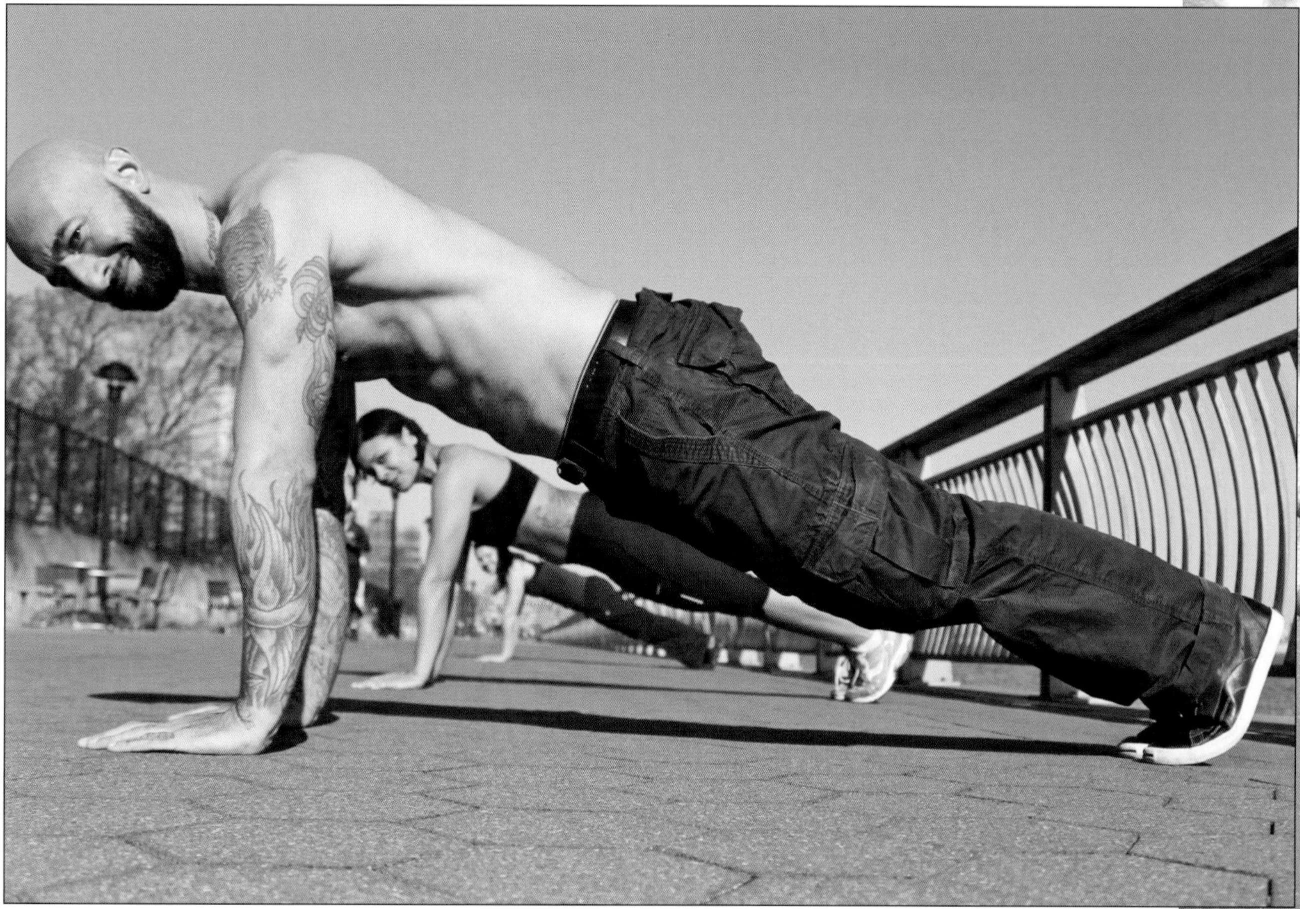

Push Yourself

The push-up is one exercise that you can constantly continue to refine. I've probably done more reps of push-ups in my life than any other single exercise and I still find myself discovering nuances that I hadn't previously noticed. It can be surprisingly challenging to keep yourself completely controlled when performing push-ups. The human body is never perfectly symmetrical, yet I like to use that ideal as a reference point for form. Aim for perfection and you might achieve greatness.

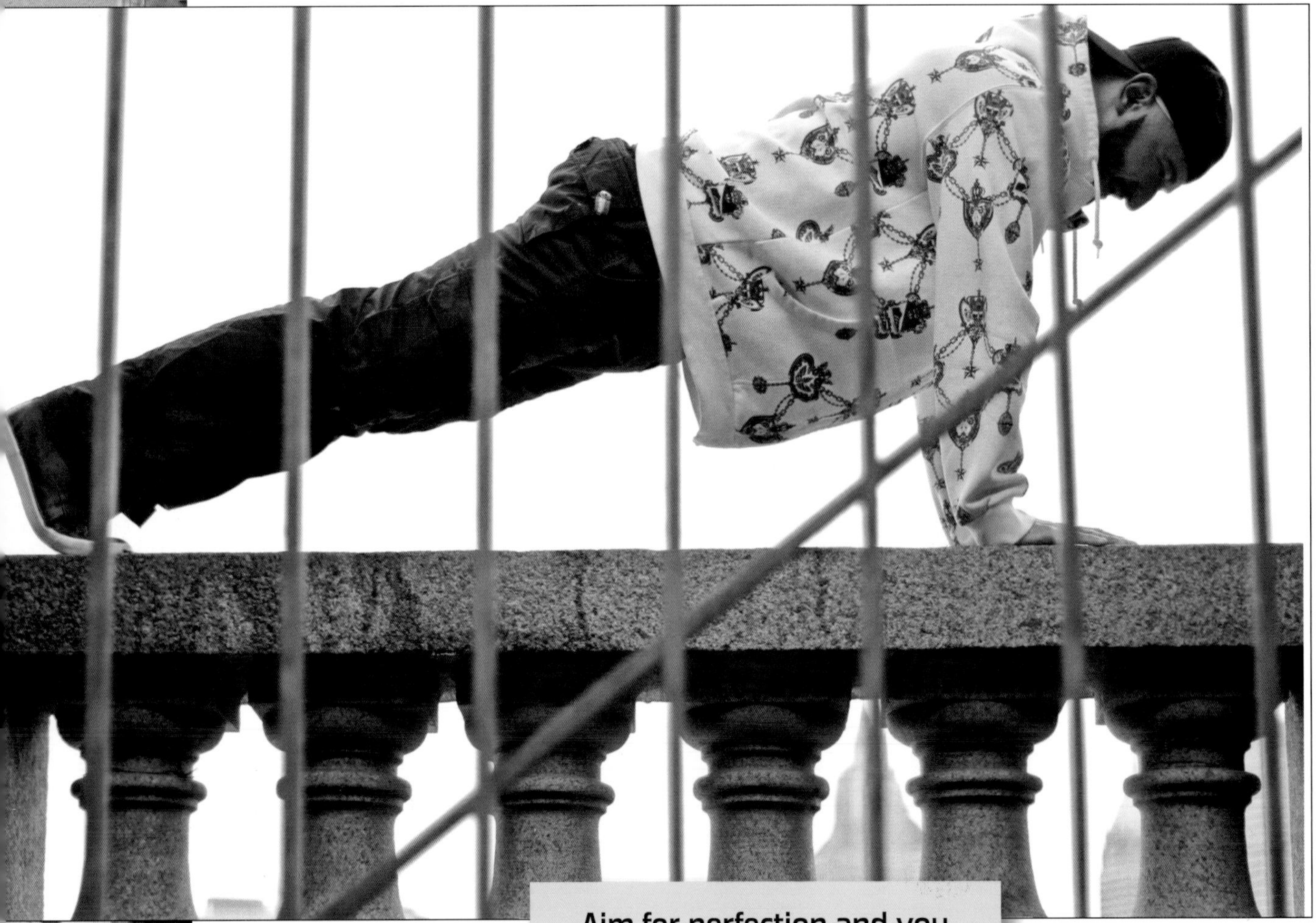

Aim for perfection and you might achieve greatness.

Get into a push-up position in front of a mirror and make sure your thumbs are directly under your shoulders. Your hips, legs and feet should be in a straight line so you can see your toes directly in between your hands. Now try performing a couple of slow reps while watching yourself. Once you do a few of these, stop craning your neck and go back to your neutral spine position. Visualize your entire body staying straight as you move up and down. Don't let your hips go up in the air or shift from side to side. Keep your whole body tight. The push-up is not just an upper-body exercise!

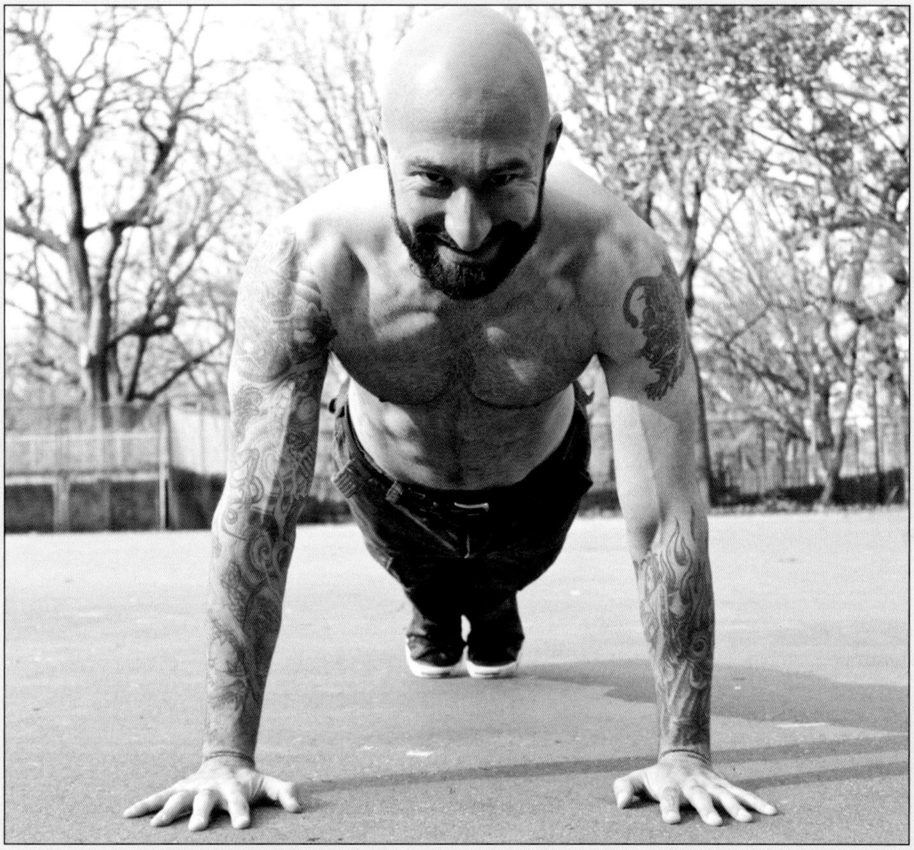

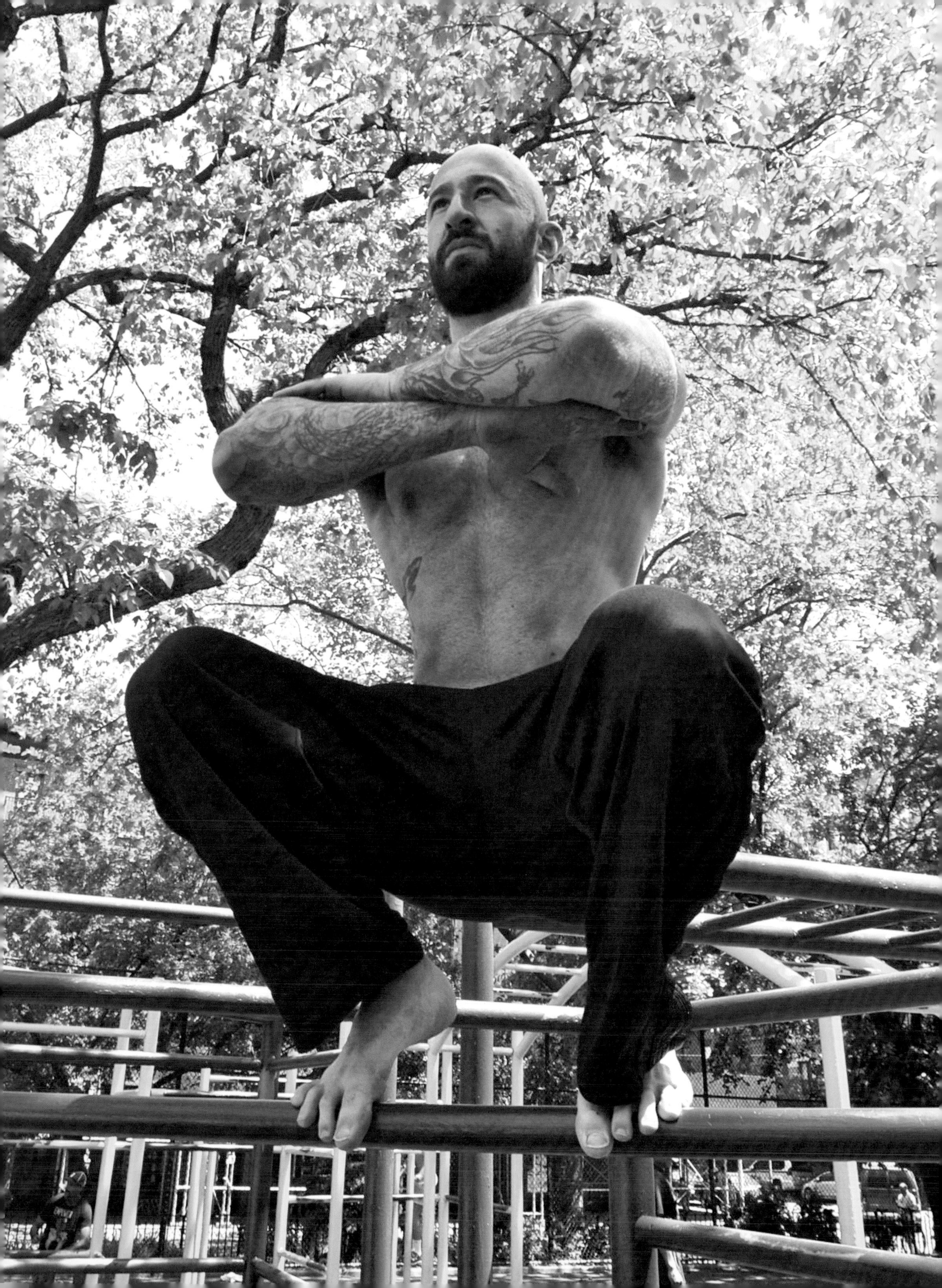

Chapter Two:

Knowing Squat

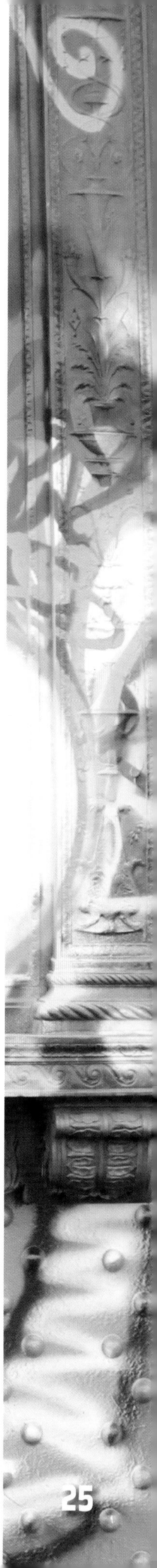

The squat is the king of all lower body exercises. In fact, I could have left the words "lower body" out of the previous sentence and it would still reflect my opinion of squats. Without squatting, it's virtually impossible to build a functionally strong body. Squats work every muscle in your legs as well as your abs and lower back. Since your legs are such large muscles, they require lots of blood and oxygen to perform squats. This makes squatting a great way to give your heart and lungs a workout too.

Though squatting is typically something that children will do instinctively, most adults have spent so much of their lives relaxing in chairs (and being lazy in general) that they have lost the movement pattern entirely. The good news is, the body can usually relearn it fairly fast (though some people will require more remedial work than others).

There are lots of methods of learning how to perform a squat, but I like to keep things as simple as possible. As far as I am concerned, there are really only three things you need to think about when squatting in order to perform the movement correctly: keep your heels down, stick your butt out and keep your chest upright. If you can do these three things while performing a full range of motion, there is little else you could do wrong.

Though squatting involves bending from both your hips and your knees, when learning to squat, it helps to think about bending your hips before your knees. Only once your hips have started moving back should you involve your knees. This can take some practice if you are new to squats. I mentioned keeping your chest up, but bear in mind that this doesn't mean you cannot lean forward. In fact, you have to lean forward in order to squat or you'll fall on your butt. The trick is to lean forward from your waist, not through your spine.

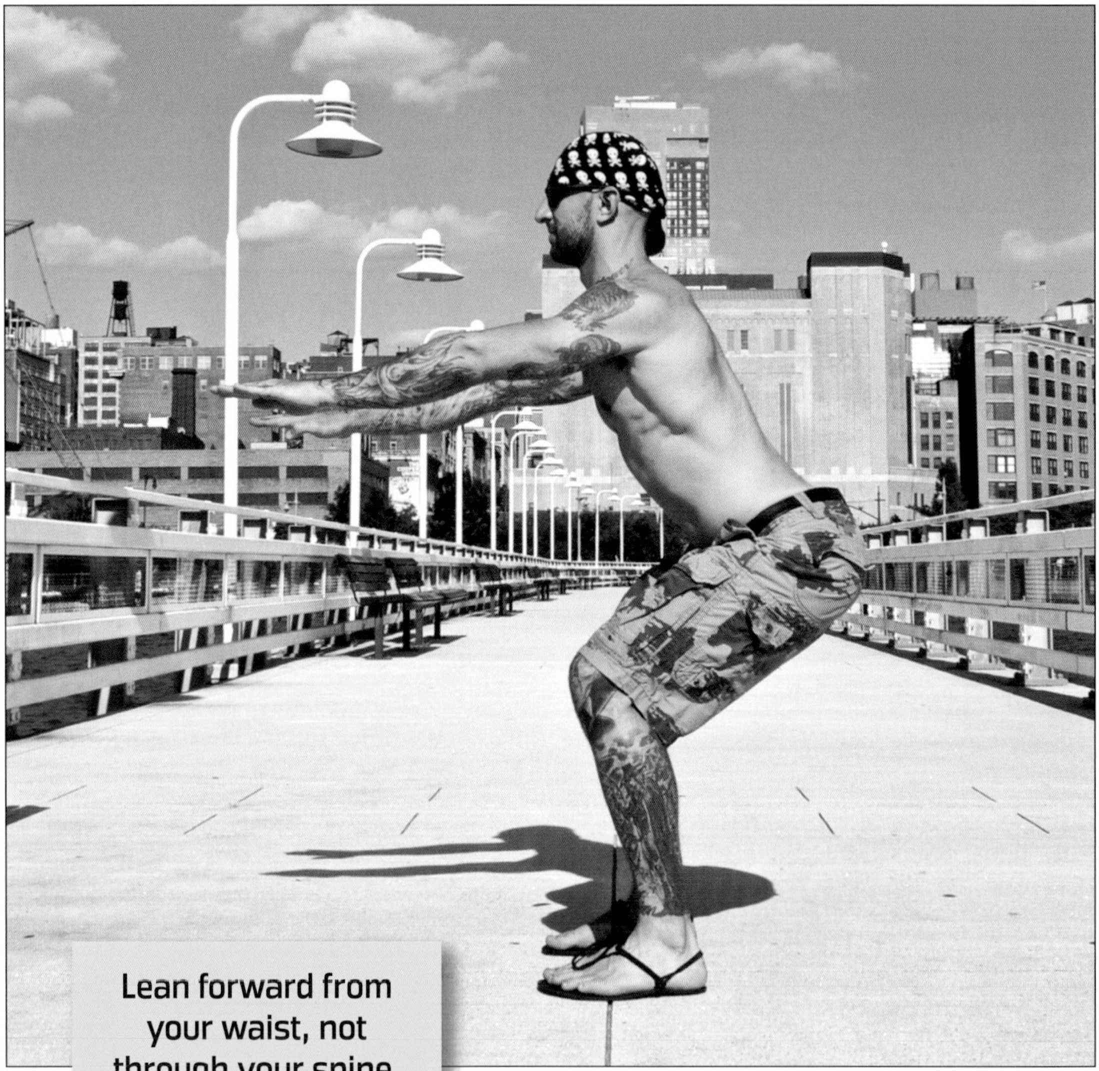

Lean forward from your waist, not through your spine.

As your hips go behind you, your torso should pitch forward to counterbalance the weight of your hips moving back. Your ankles should also bend, allowing your knees to move forward slightly, though your heels must stay on the ground. It can be helpful to reach your arms out in front of you to assist with this.

Pushing The Limits!

Remember the vertical line I mentioned before that should be running from your ear to your heel when standing upright? When you are at the bottom of a squat you should still maintain a straight line from your ear to your heel, only your hips will have moved back and your knees will wind up a bit in front. You should still be able to draw a straight line passing through your head, shoulders and heels at the bottom of a squat.

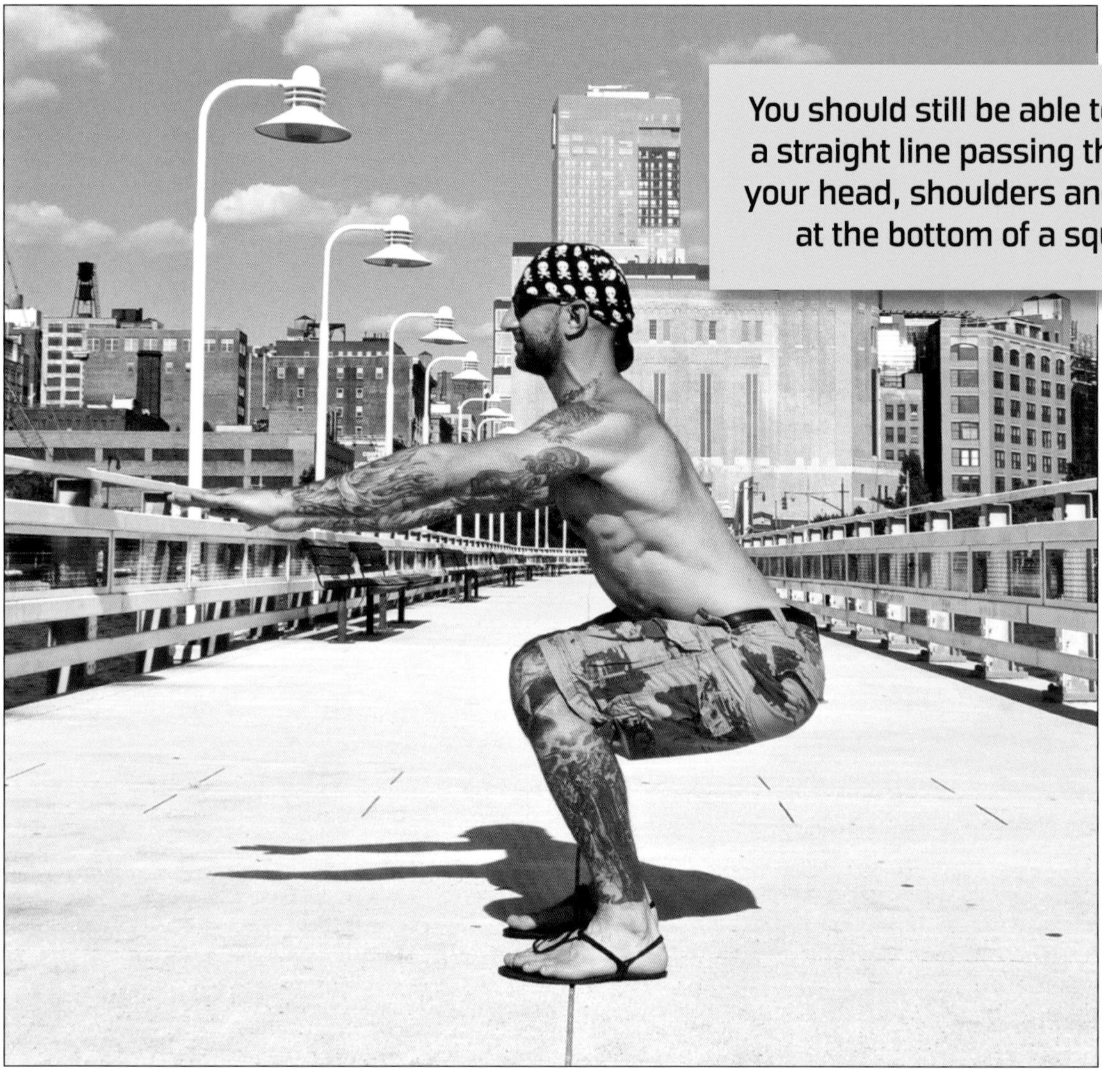

You should still be able to draw a straight line passing through your head, shoulders and heels at the bottom of a squat.

Just like learning to hold a push-up position, when you perform a squat, it takes a lot more effort to maintain your spinal alignment than it does when you're just standing there. As you move your hips out, you will have to contract your lower back and your abs in order to keep from losing the curve of your lumbar spine. You'll also need to engage the muscles of your upper back to keep your thoracic spine in alignment and prevent your shoulders from shrugging upwards. It helps to think about pulling down and back through your shoulder blades to maintain this posture.

Everybody Get Low

A lot of coaches still perpetuate the myth that deep squatting is inherently dangerous for the knee joint — this is total malarkey! In an ideal world, everyone would be able to squat so deep that their hamstrings and calves would be totally flush against one another at the bottom with their spine in a natural position the whole time. In fact, in many countries, this is the only way that people can go to the bathroom!

Unfortunately, in America most people are lucky to get half that far without losing form. The answer to the question "how deep should one squat" then becomes a question of "how deep *can* one squat?"

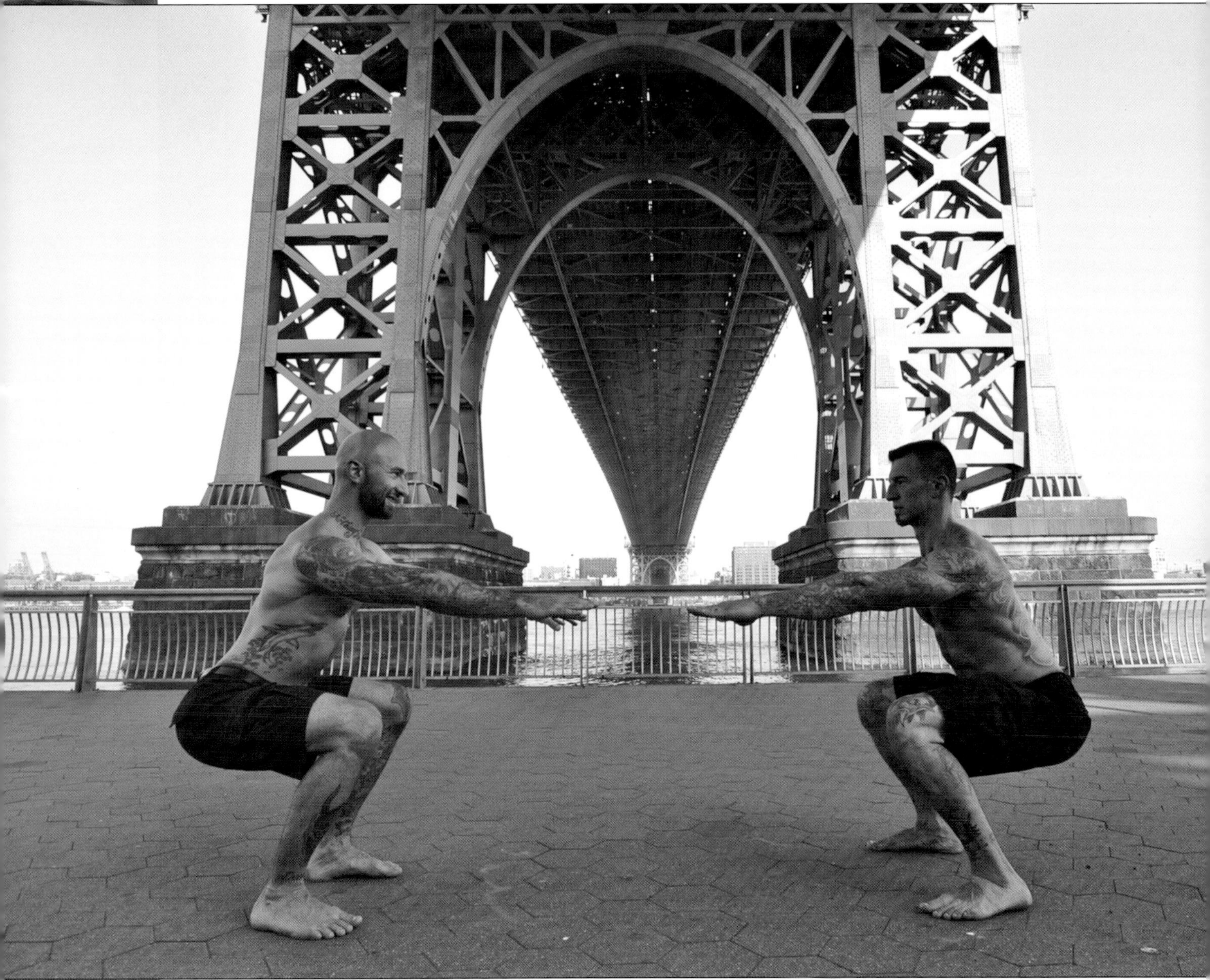

For some people this will simply mean that they can only squat until the bottom of their thigh is level with the ground, which is barely half of the ideal range of motion. However, if that's all they can do, then it's all they should do. Since I prefer to live in reality and not some hypothetical world of textbooks and formulas, the ideal range of motion for that person is until the bottom of the thigh is parallel to the ground.

When people in the fitness industry talk about squatting to parallel, however, this is not what they are talking about. True parallel depth means that the *top of the thigh* is parallel to the ground, which is lower than many people can go right away. The great thing about squatting, however, is that it becomes an active stretch that can improve your range of motion, allowing you to eventually work towards deepening your squat. When performing bodyweight squats, always go as low as you can — in time that range of motion should start to increase.

When performing bodyweight squats, always go as low as you can – in time that range of motion should start to increase.

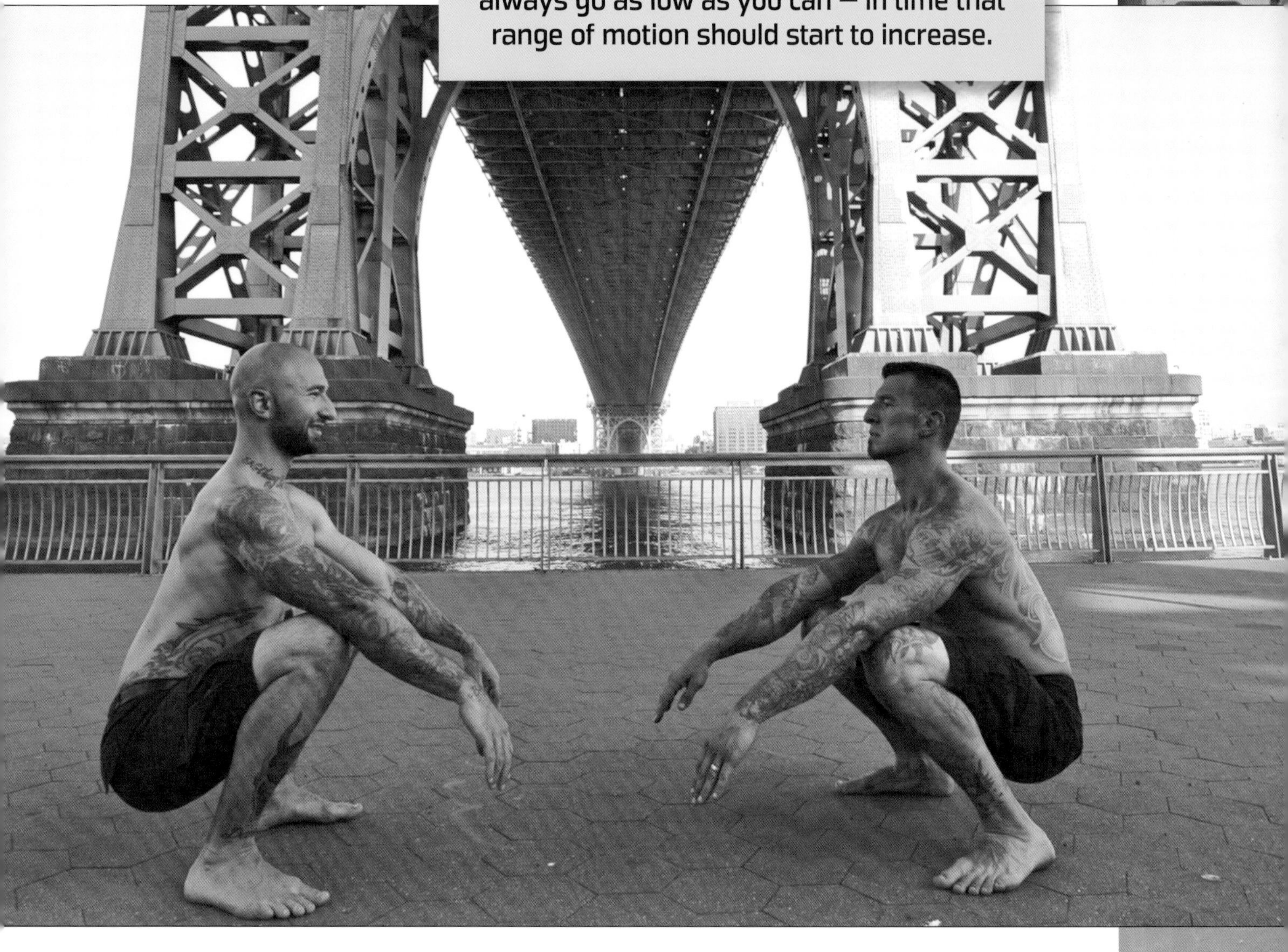

Spinal Jeopardy

Though there is more leeway for the spinal alignment in a bodyweight squat than one performed with a barbell on your back, you'll get the most out of each rep by keeping mindful of your spine. Your back is obviously designed to bend and flex, but standing and moving with a neutral spine is generally a good habit to develop in your strength training practice.

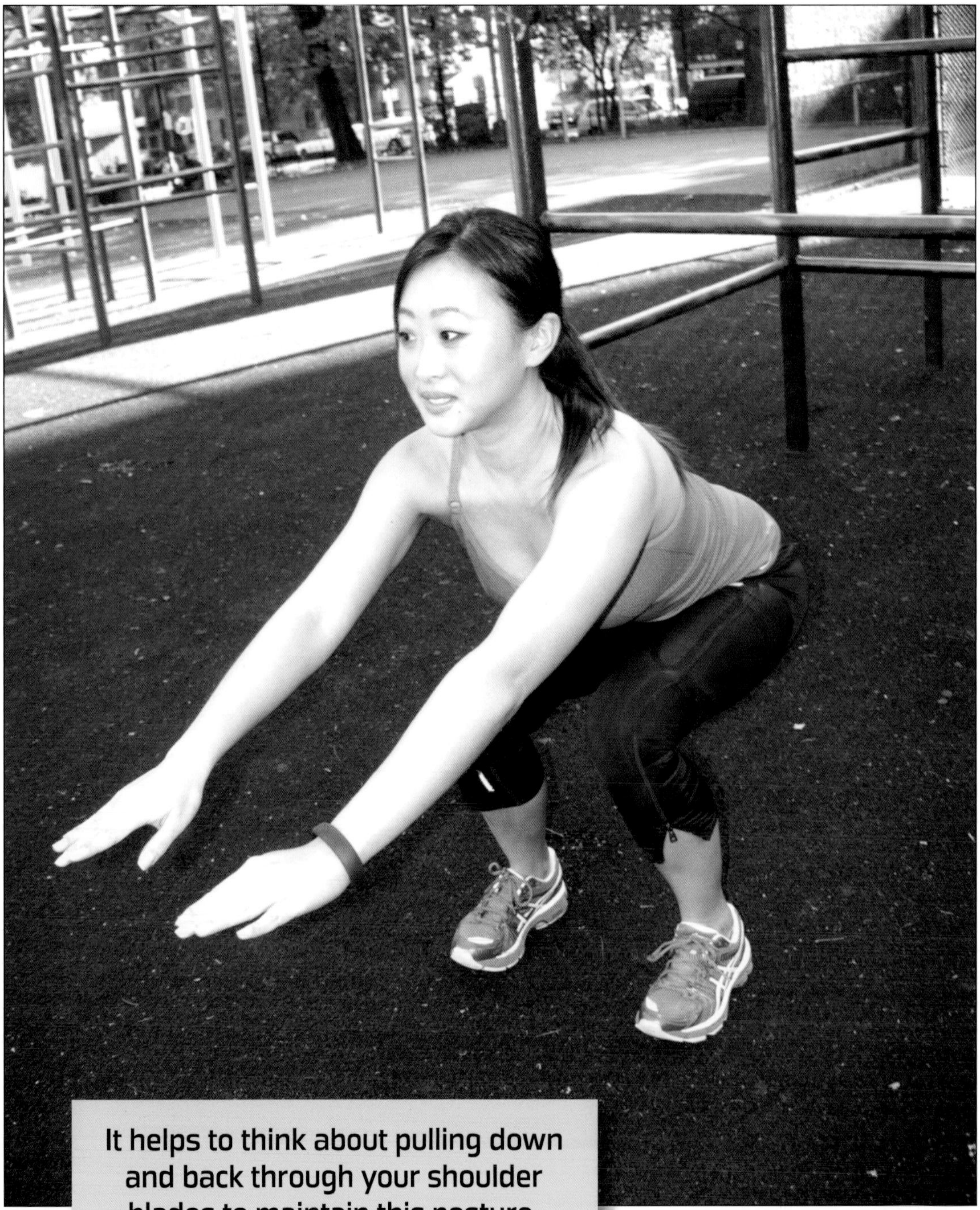

It helps to think about pulling down and back through your shoulder blades to maintain this posture.

Foot Position

A standard squat is typically performed with the feet about hip distance apart. However, varying the distance between your feet can change the subtleties of muscle recruitment. Some people will find that a slightly wider stance feels more natural and allows them to get deeper without losing spinal position. If this is the case for you, feel free to begin with a wide stance. Turning your toes out slightly can also facilitate opening your hips, which can help improve the range of motion, too. On the other hand, squatting with your feet parallel and close together can be quite challenging and effective (more on close-stance squats in Chapter Five).

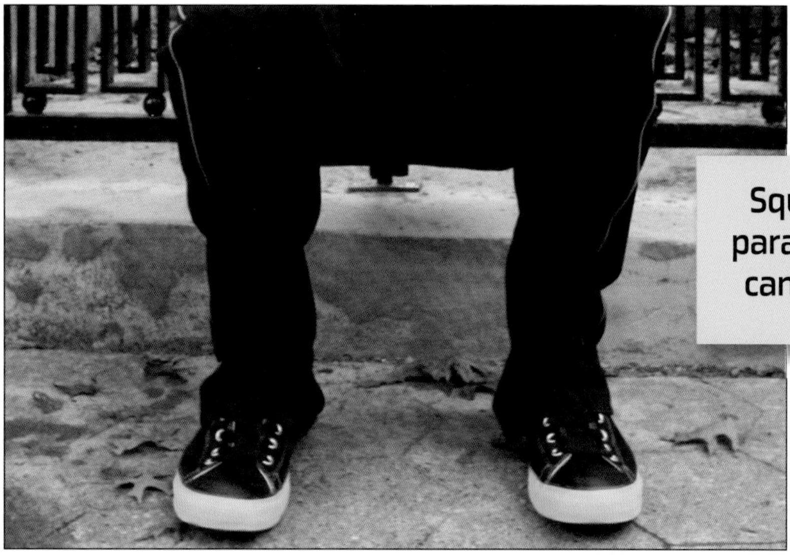

Squatting with your feet parallel and close together can be quite challenging.

Try a slightly wider stance with your toes pointed out if you are having trouble squatting with your feet parallel.

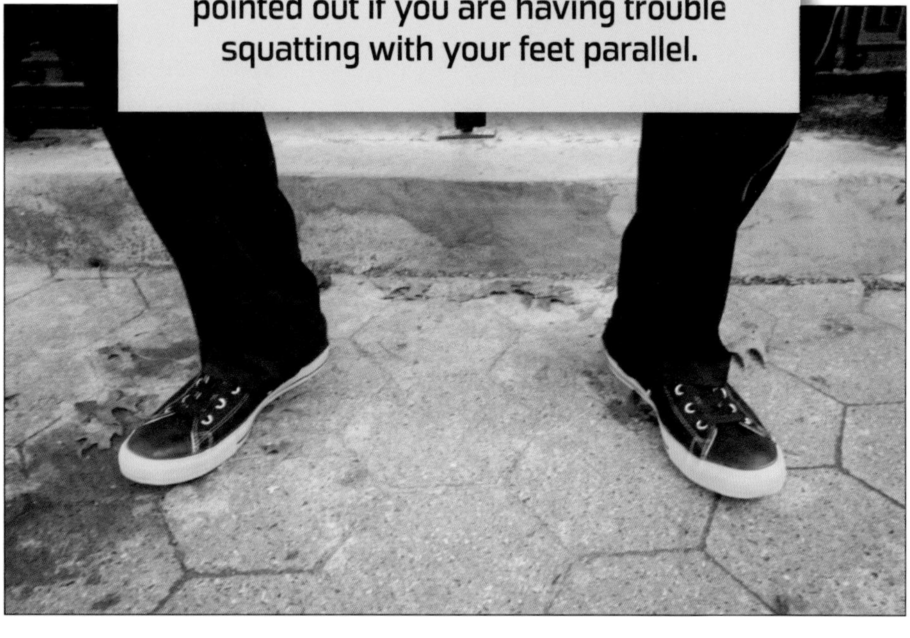

Bench Squat

If you feel like you are going to fall on your butt when you try to squat, it can help to use a bench (or other object) to assist (there I go with the equipment again!). You want to use an object that is sturdy and low. Start with something that will leave you with the top of your thigh just about parallel to the floor when you're seated.

To perform a bench squat, simply stand in front of the object and sit back onto it. If you can't maintain your balance during the descent, just plop down on the bench, stand back up and try it again. With practice you'll get better at controlling yourself on the way down. Eventually you can move to a lower object. In time, you'll be squatting ass-to-ankles without needing to fall back on anything.

Even once you are comfortable with free-standing squats, however, you can still use bench squats in your routine. Coming to a full stop and resting on an object at the bottom of the rep can offer its own challenge. Initiating the upward movement from a full stop requires a unique type of strength and stability.

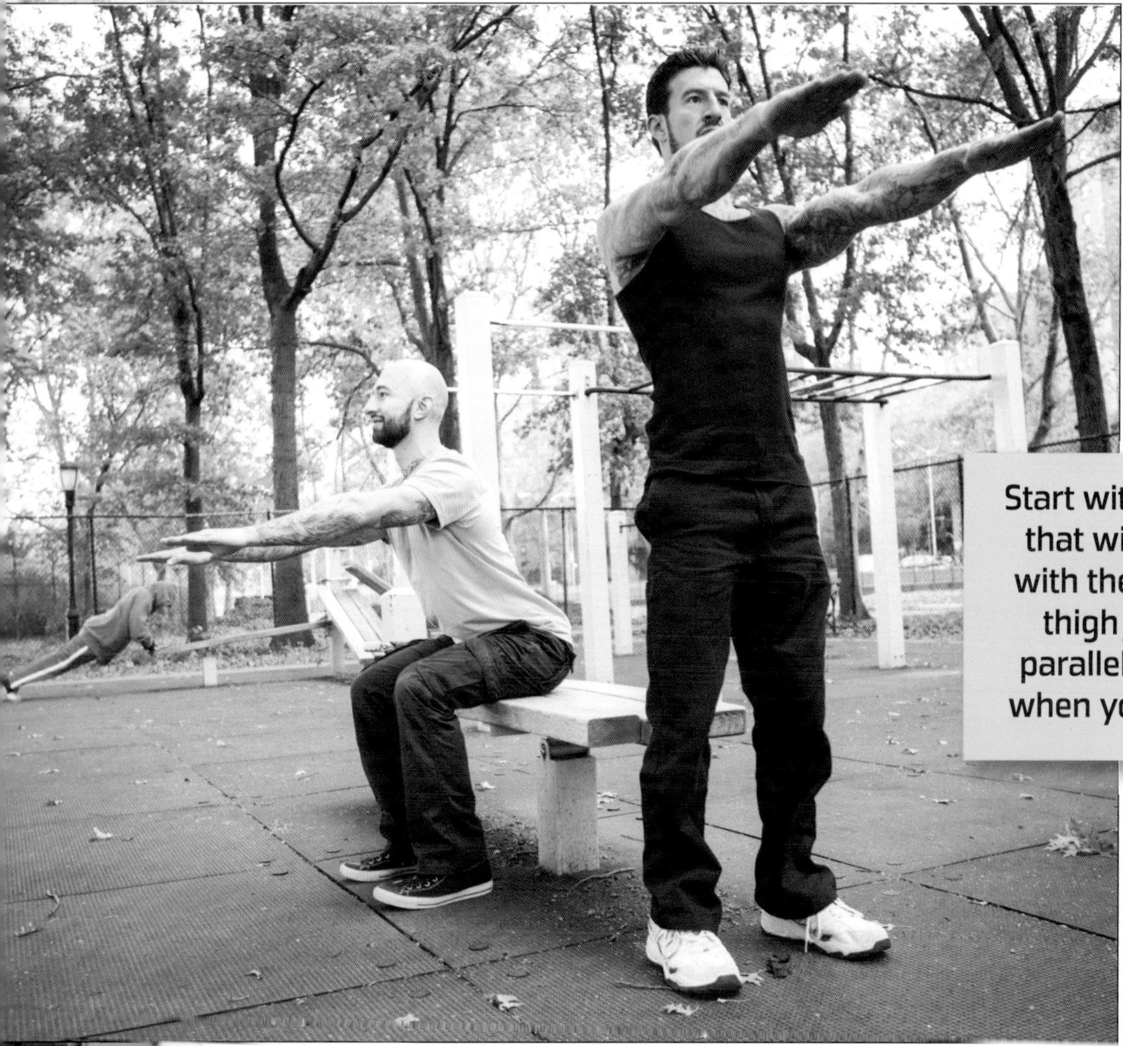

Start with something that will leave you with the top of your thigh just about parallel to the floor when you're seated.

Sumo Squat

Named for an entirely different wrestling style than the one I loved as a kid, the sumo squat is an exaggerated wide-stance squat with the toes turned almost all the way out to place additional emphasis on the muscles of the hips and inner thighs. Similar to a ballet style plie, sumo squats can potentially be easier for beginners. If you're having a hard time maintaining your balance and/or posture when squatting, the sumo squat might be a good way to ease in. Regardless, it is a worthwhile exercise to have in your arsenal if you want to give extra attention to your inner thighs.

Though you should be aware of your leg alignment during any type of squat, when practicing sumo squats, give extra attention that your knees are tracking in line with your toes and not bowing in towards the middle.

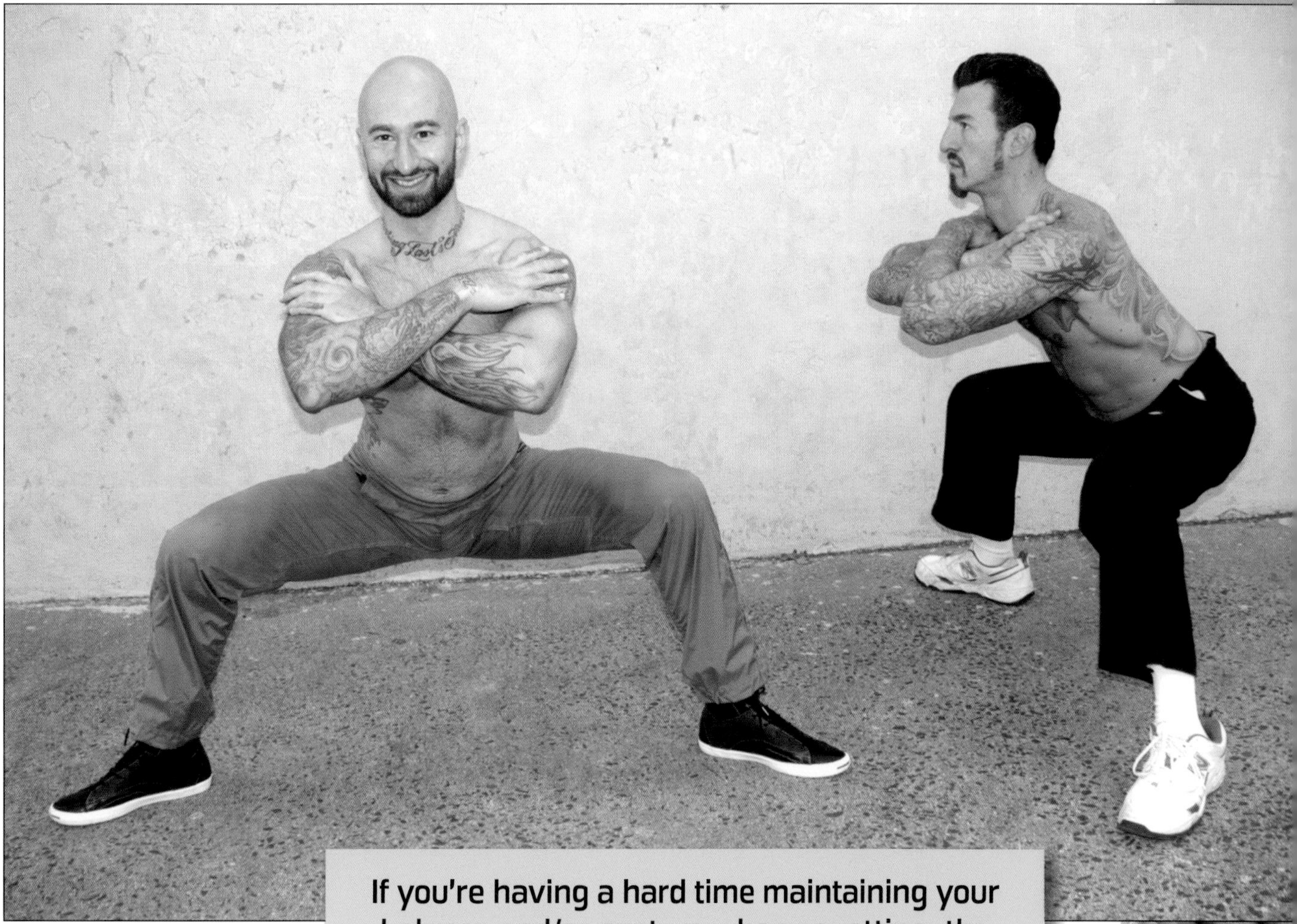

If you're having a hard time maintaining your balance and/or posture when squatting, the sumo squat might be a good way to ease in.

Split Squat

The split squat is a wonderful variation on the squat that changes the balance as well as changing the angles at which you are working your muscles. Instead of standing with your feet next to each other under your hips, a split squat involves standing in a split stance with one foot in front of your body and one foot behind. The front foot should be totally flat on the ground while your back foot stays up on the toes. I find it best to keep the arms relaxed at your sides during a split squat, though some people will find placing their hands on their hips to be helpful; either way is fine by me.

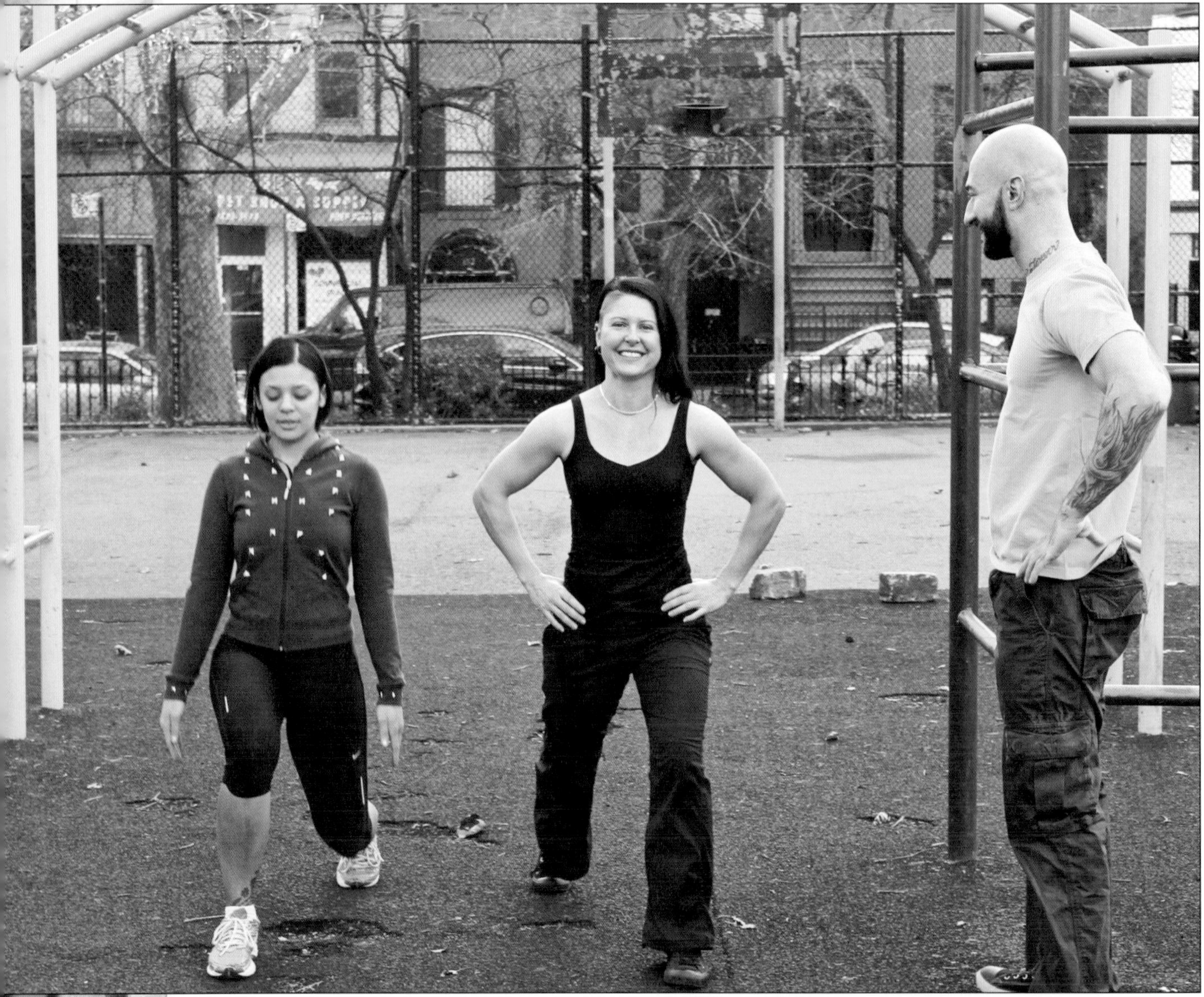

From here the objective is to keep your torso upright while you lower yourself down until both knees are bent to approximately 90 degrees, then return to the starting position. Think about initiating the movement by bending the knee of the leg that is in back, otherwise you might wind up with too much flexion in the front knee and not enough in the other. Your center of gravity should be about halfway between the two legs.

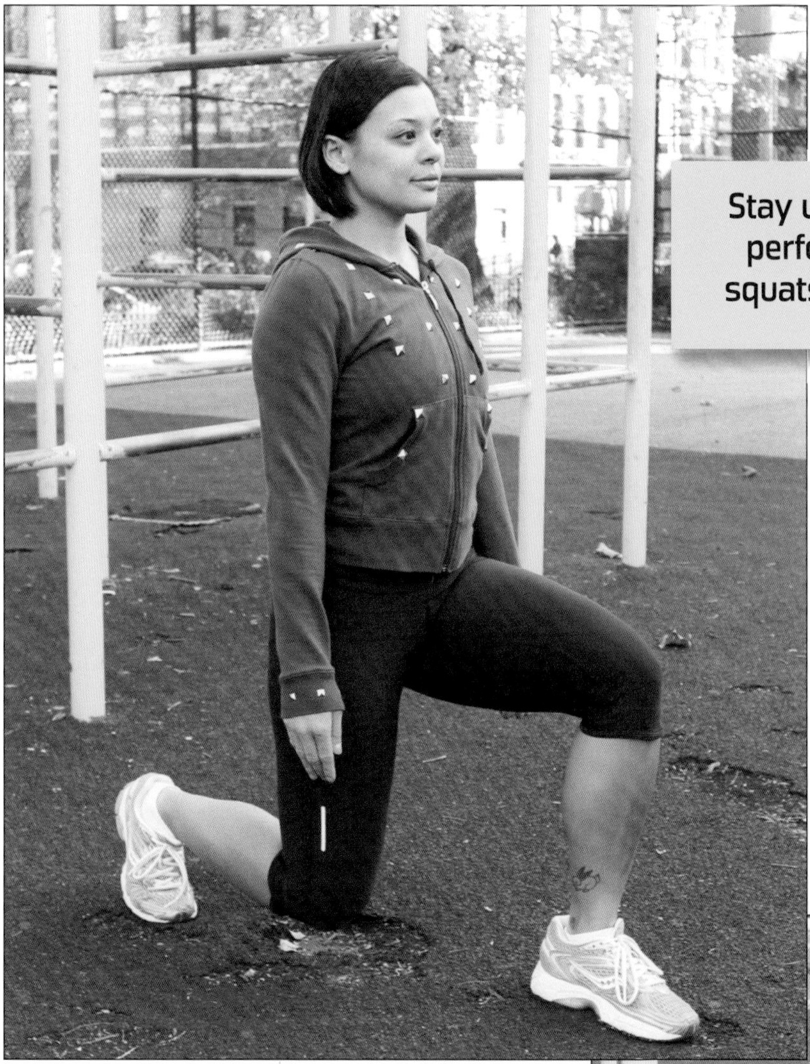

Stay upright when performing split squats and lunges.

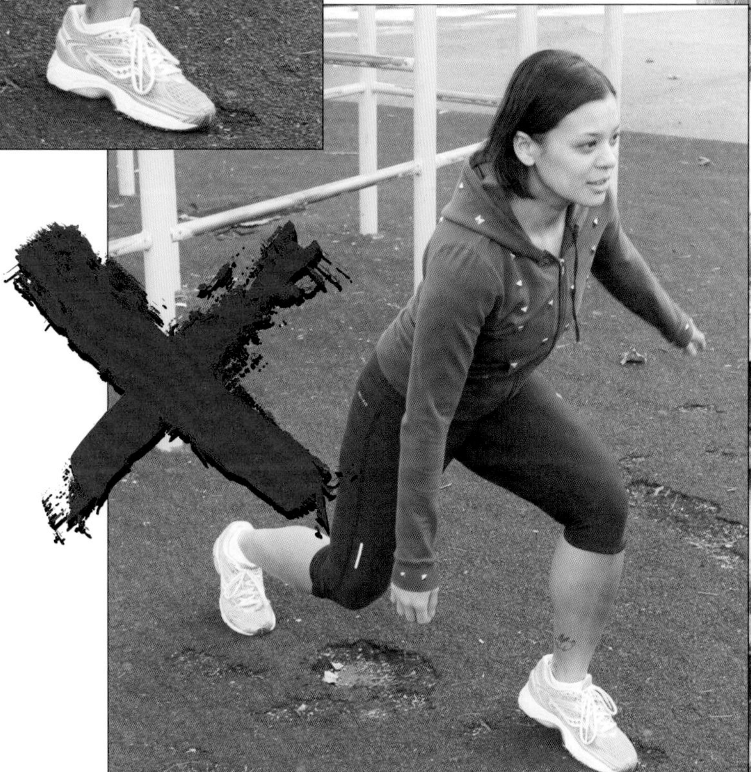

Walking Lunge

Once you get the hang of split squats, you can get moving with lunges — literally! The walking lunge is one of my favorite exercises (I sometimes call them "*fun*-ges"). A walking lunge involves stepping forward into each rep, rather than maintaining the split stance. When performing a walking lunge, it is still essential to maintain your posture and avoid letting the heel of your front foot come off the ground. Think about breaking the walking lunge down into three distinct phases. First forward, then down, and then up and together in one motion. This will help you avoid losing form.

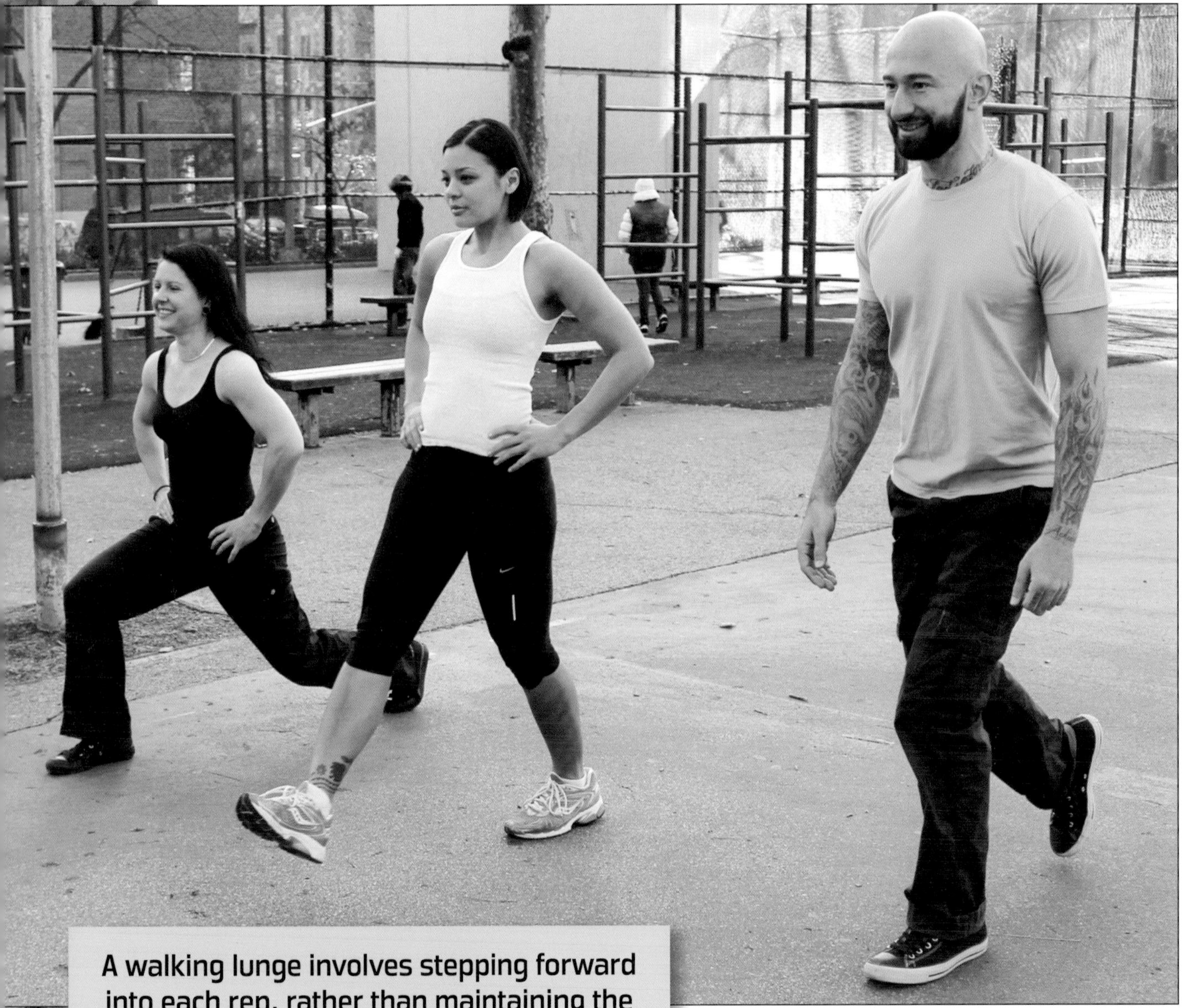

A walking lunge involves stepping forward into each rep, rather than maintaining the split stance.

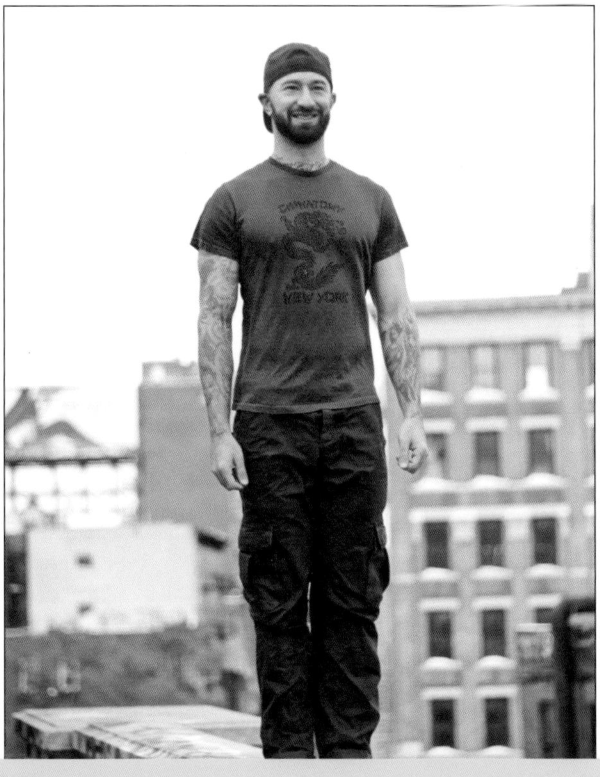

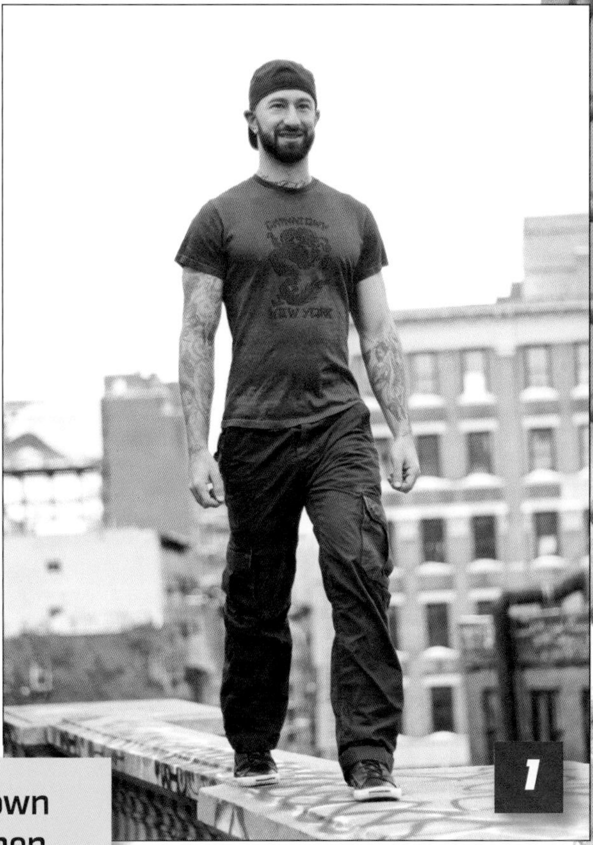

Think about breaking the walking lunge down into three distinct phases. First forward, then down, and then up and together in one motion. This will help you avoid losing form.

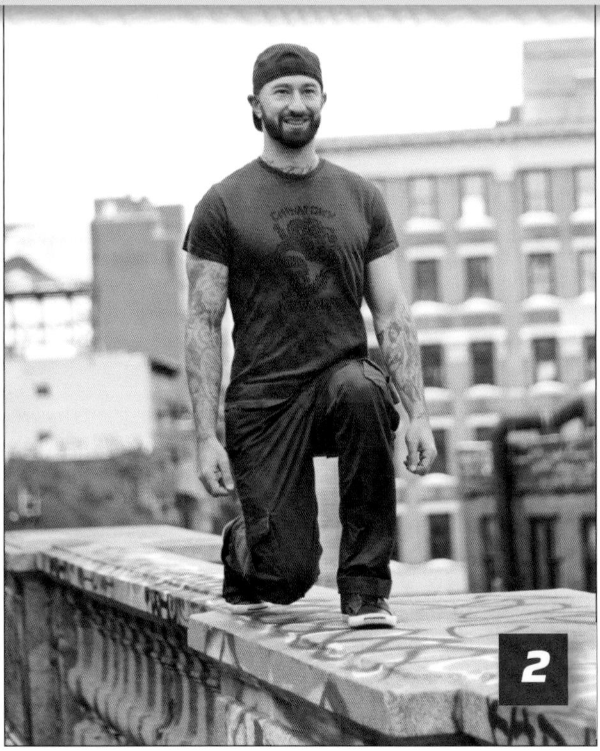

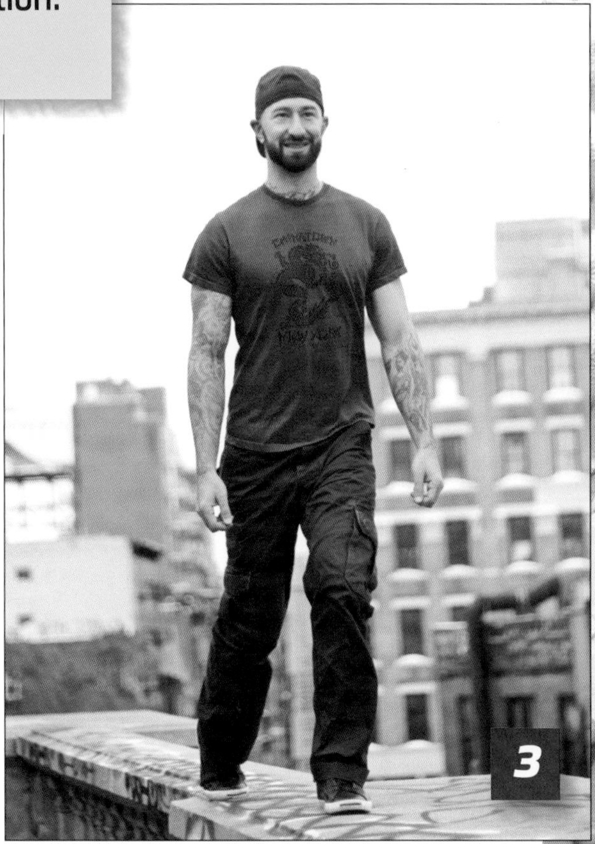

Back Lunge

Another common variation on the split squat involves stepping back into the split stance from a standing position. Compared to the walking lunge, back lunges tend to have less impact on your joints, as people naturally land harder when stepping forward than when stepping back, plus you don't need much space to do them. When coming up from a back lunge, just step right back to where you started so you can begin the next rep. Like all the lunge variations, back lunges can be performed by alternating legs or repeating each leg for a set number of reps before switching sides.

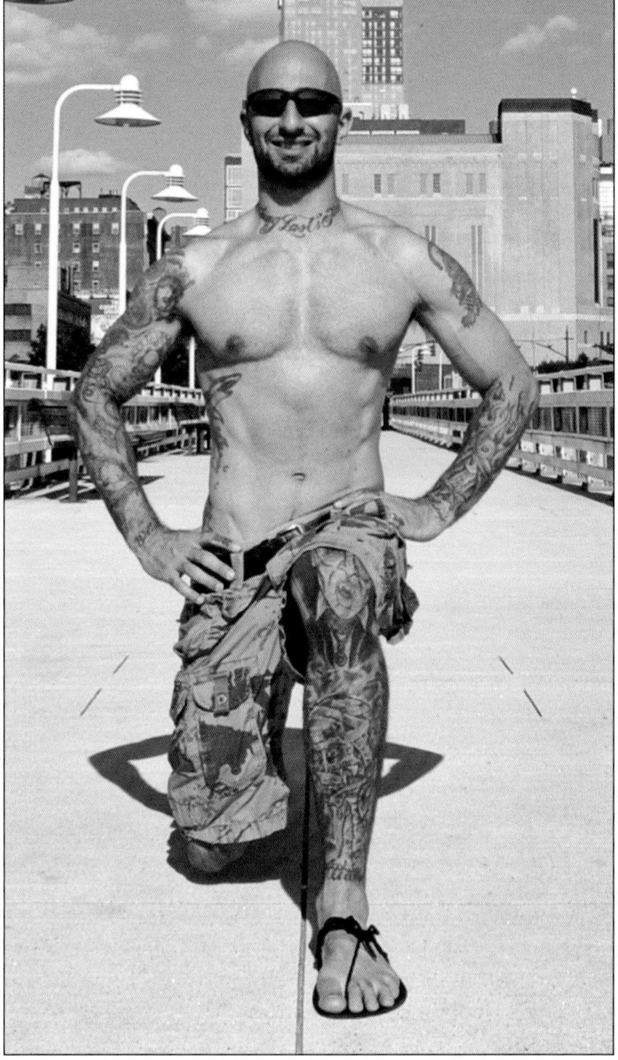

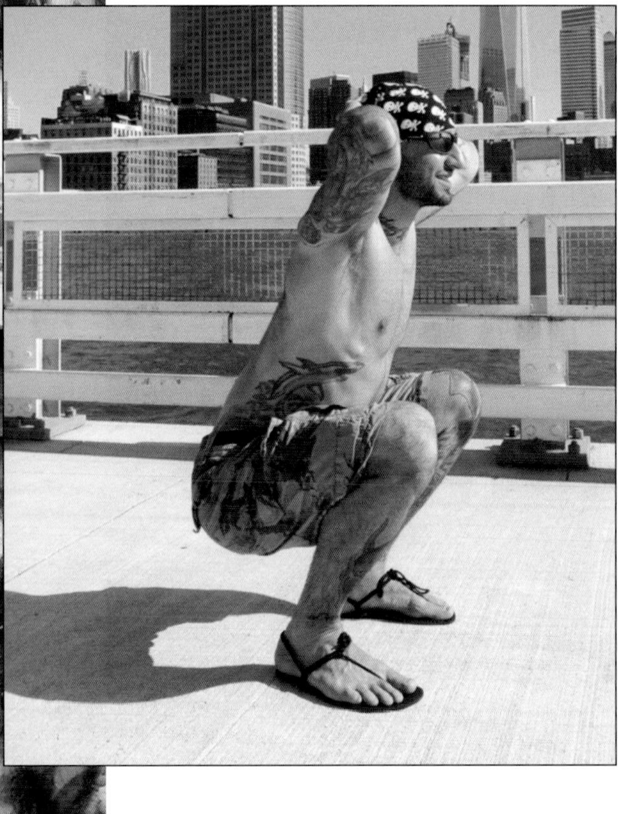

Prisoner Squat

When learning to squat, I typically instruct my clients to reach their arms out in front in order to counterbalance the weight of their hips going back. Once you can do that without much trouble, a great way to progress the exercise is to change the leverage by placing your hands behind your head. This can also turn the squat into a stretch for the upper body. Think about actively retracting your shoulder blades and keeping your chest up in order to avoid caving inward.

Wall Sit

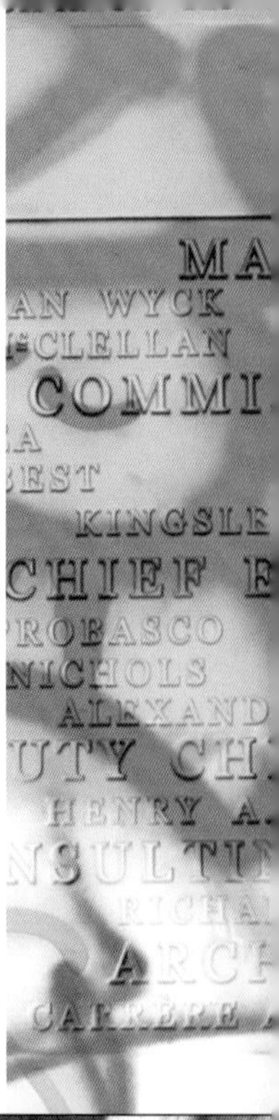

Also known as the "Chinese chair," this exercise will challenge you mentally as much as physically. Stand with your back against a wall, then walk your legs out and squat down until the top of your thigh is parallel to the ground. Lean against the wall and stay upright, but don't use your arms to press on your thighs for assistance — keep them at your sides or cross them in front of your chest. It's almost like you are sitting in a chair with no bottom.

Like the plank, the wall sit is an isometric hold, so stay in position for as long as possible. Take deep breaths and try to relax your mind. Beginners should be able to manage 30 seconds, eventually building to several minutes. Like holding the plank position, it simply becomes a question of will after a certain point.

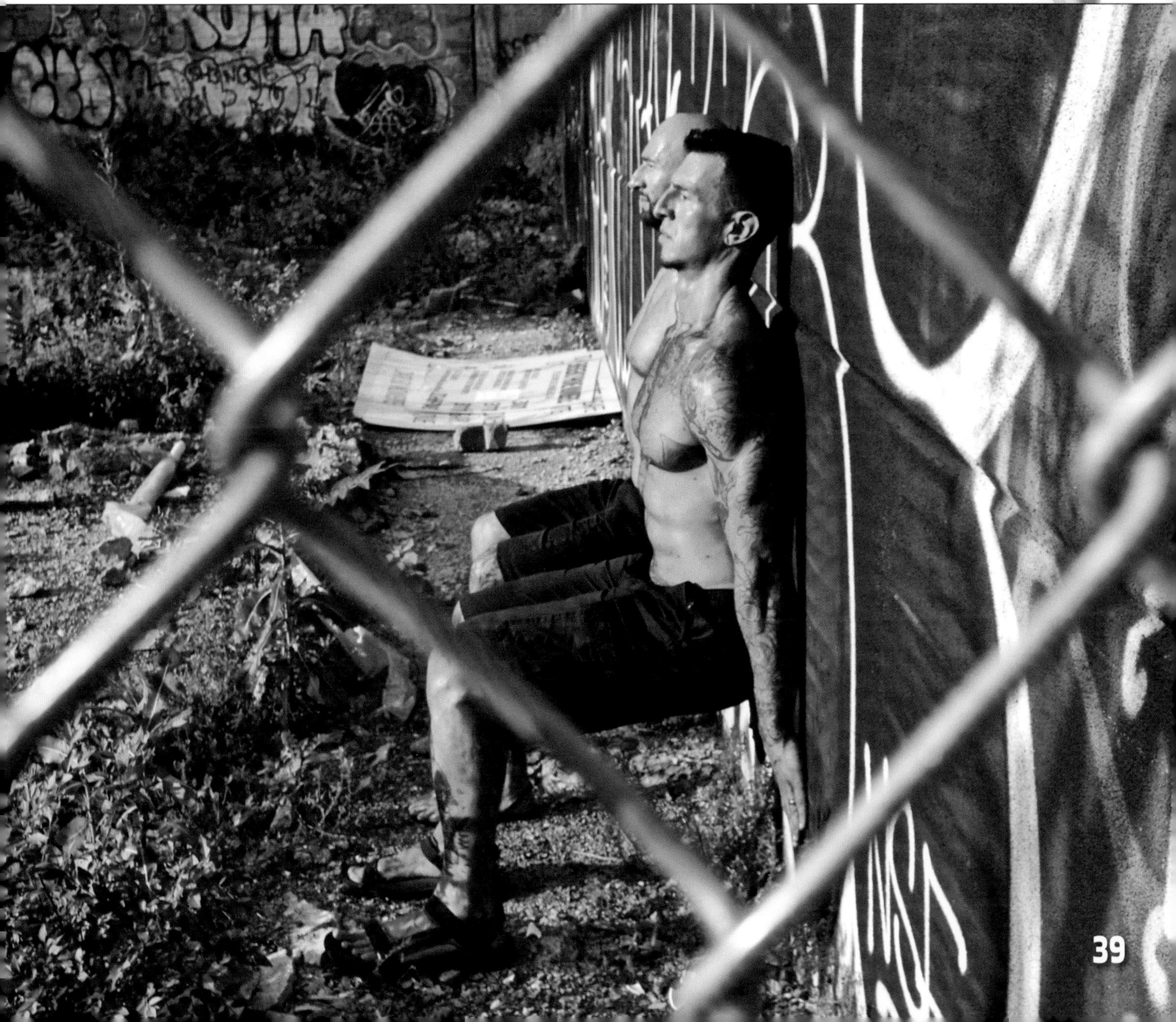

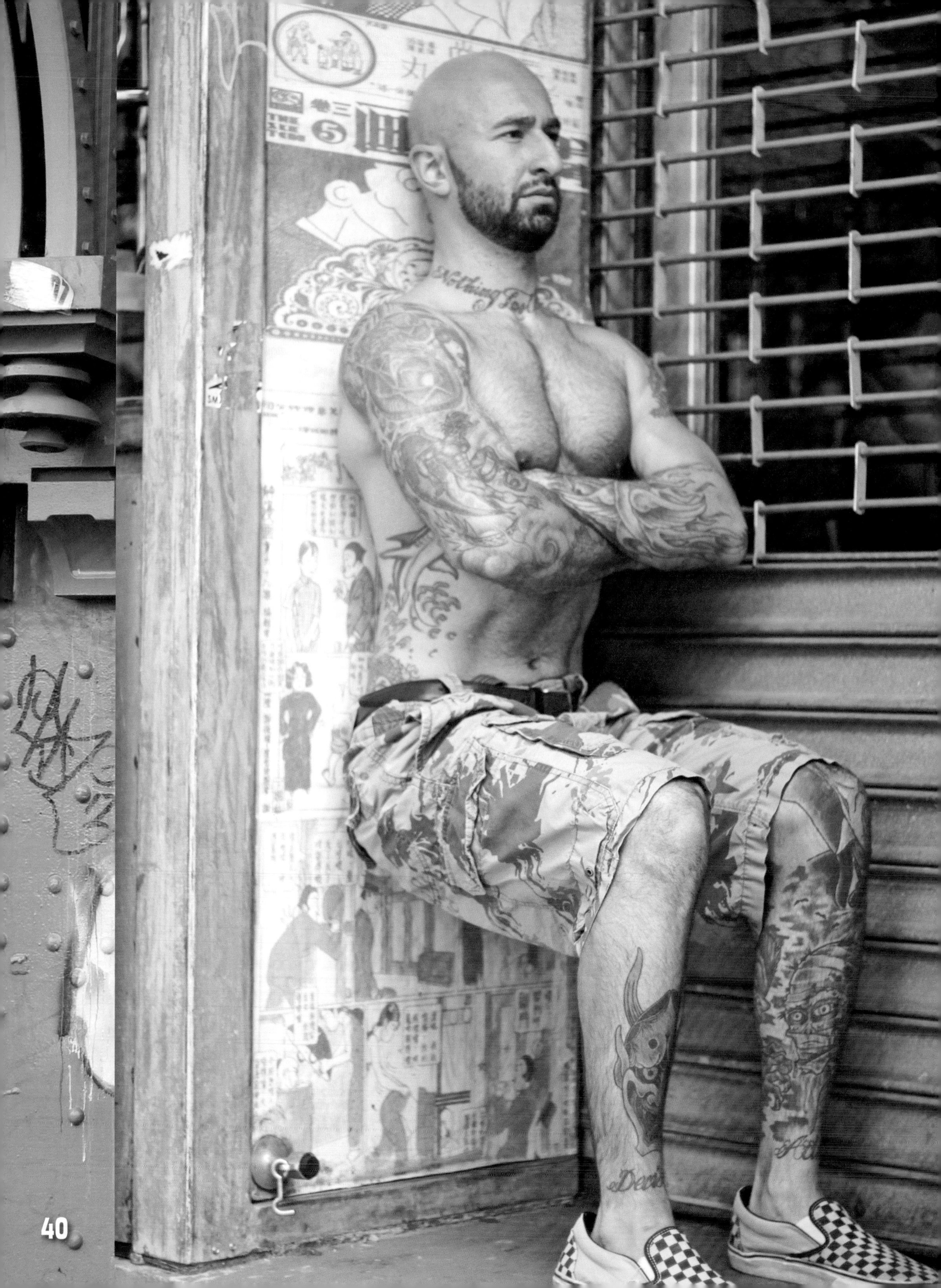

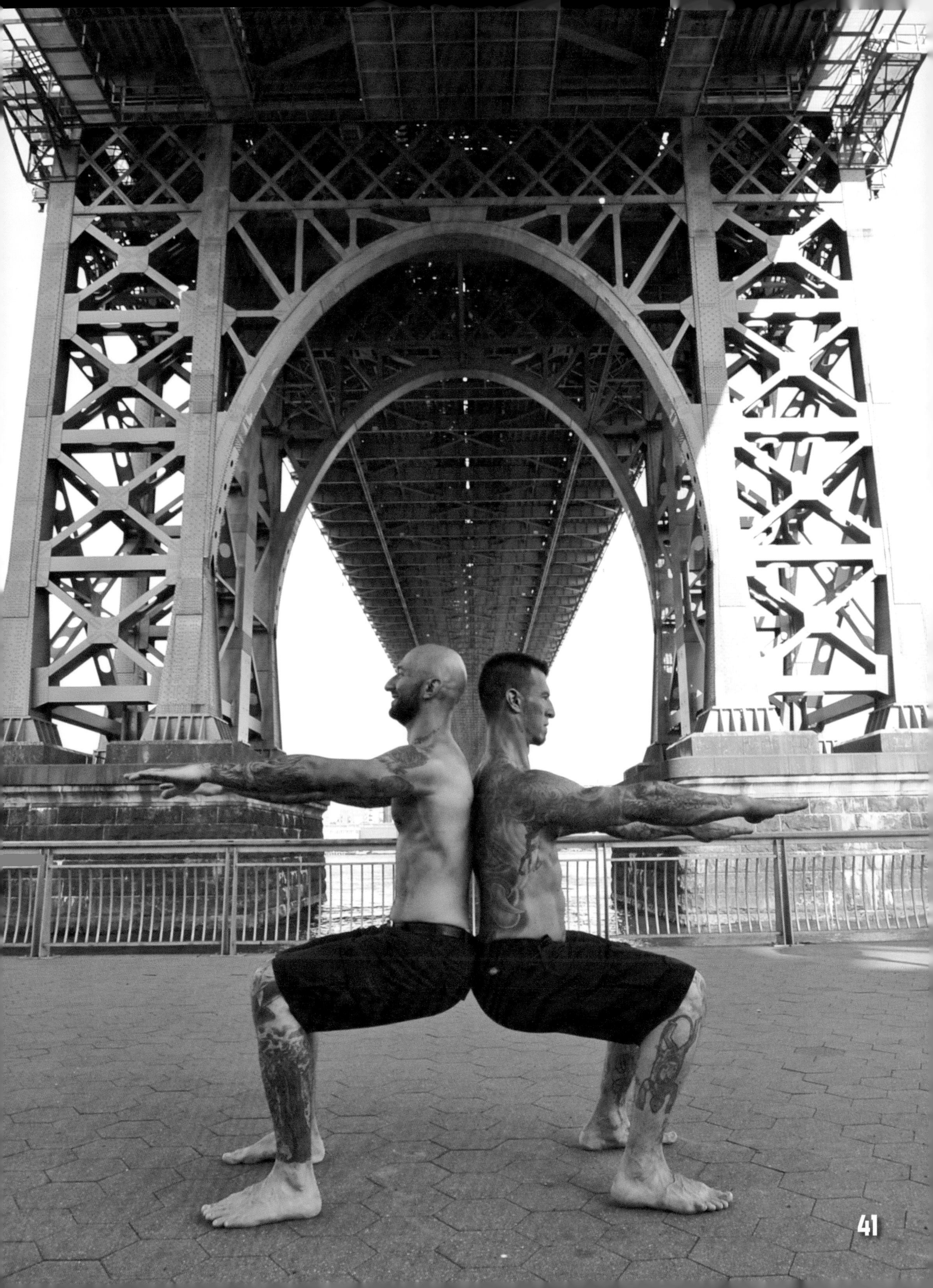

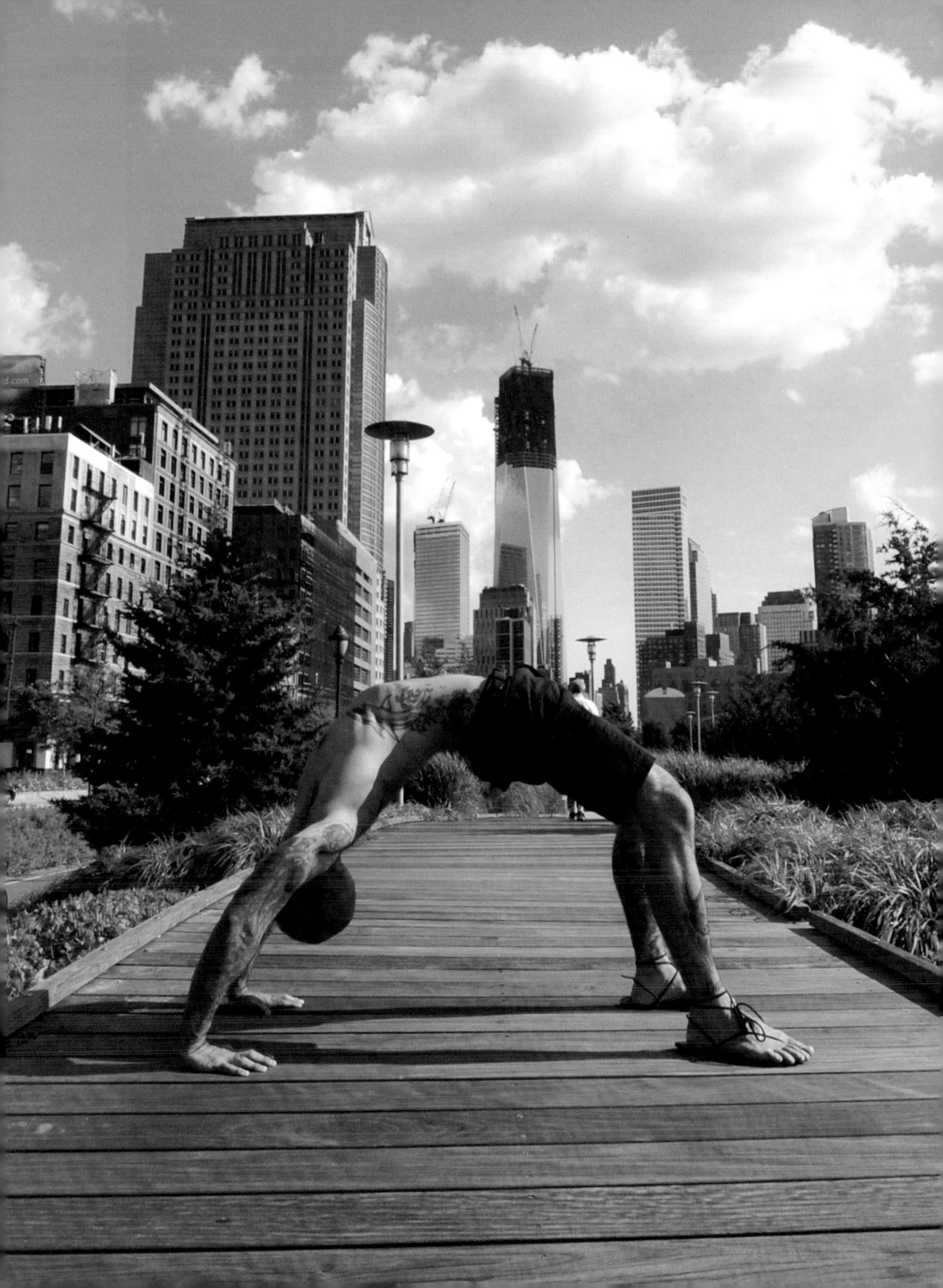

Chapter Three:

Bridging The Gap

Back bridging is probably the most underused exercise in modern fitness, though it is vital to practice bridging in order to counterbalance the time you spend sitting with your back bent forward (like right now, probably). Bridges are also a wonderful introduction to the world of inversions. Though headstands and handstands generally come to mind before bridges, any posture that involves your heart being higher than your head is an inversion. Back bridges can prepare you nicely for full inversions where your legs are in the air, as they give you the feeling of being upside-down. But unlike most full inversions, they're also great for strengthening the muscles of your back, glutes, hamstrings and calves.

A full back bridge involves holding your body face-up on your hands and feet with your spine fully extended and your hips way up in the air. You want to make sure that the arc of your spine is relatively even throughout, and not too heavily arched in the lumbar region. If your upper back is stiff, which is quite common, you'll need to be especially mindful of this. I like to perform bridges as isometric holds, gradually trying to ease deeper into the position with each breath.

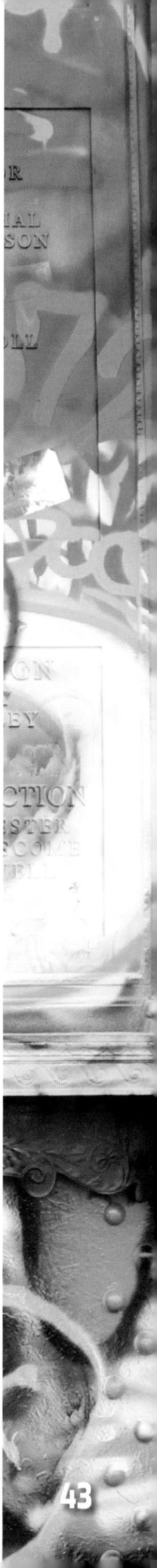

Pushing The Limits!

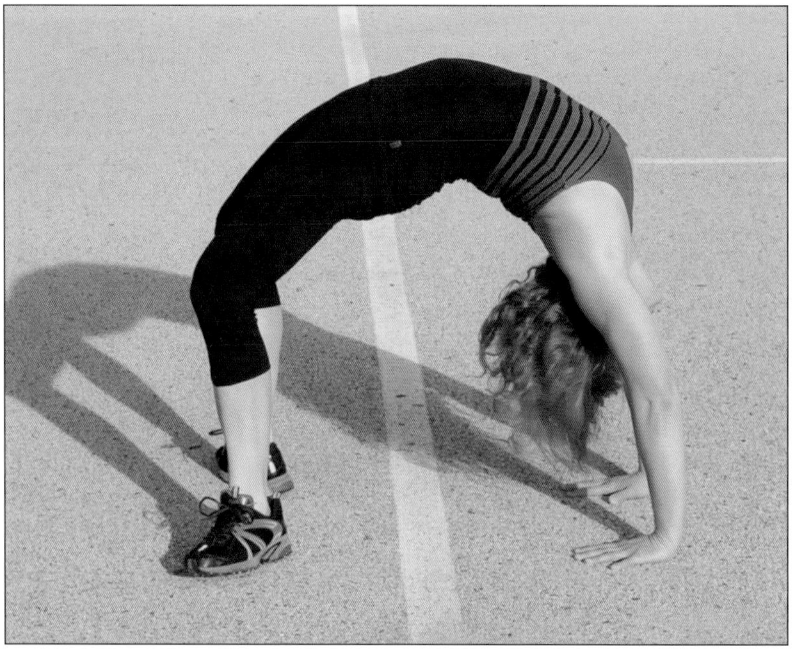

While some people will struggle with the flexibility needed to perform a full bridge, others will be able to find the hold without much trouble. The better your flexibility, the closer you'll be able to get your hands and feet. This is also a simple way to add intensity to the exercise.

The better your flexibility, the closer you'll be able to get your hands and feet.

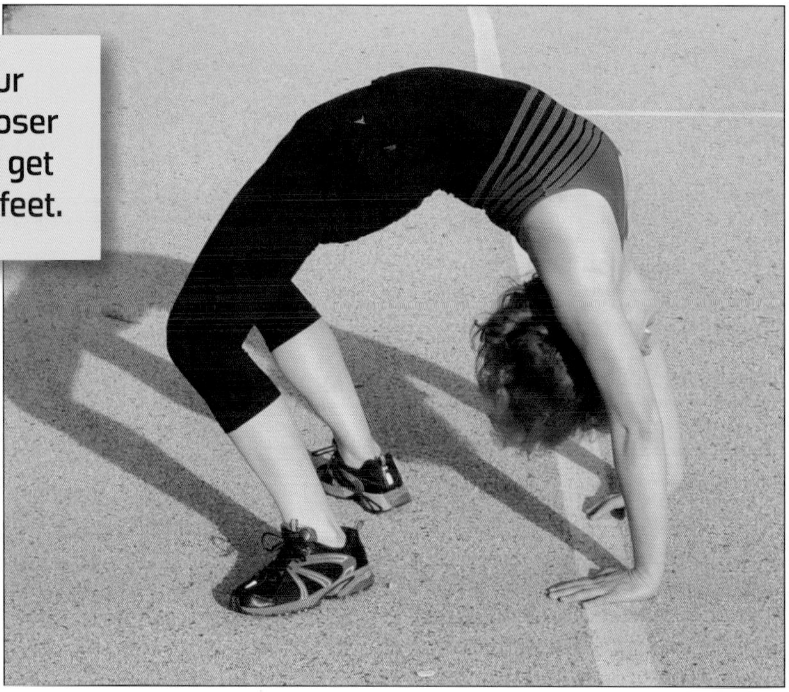

Beginner's Bridge

Before we worry about adding intensity though, let's focus on how a beginner can safely progress. If you're new to the world of back-bridging, your best bet is to start off with a partial bridge. Lie on your back with your knees bent, feet flat and arms by your sides. Roll up onto your shoulders, puff out your chest and try to get your hips as high up as you can. It also helps to wiggle your shoulder blades together and grab your hands in a palm-to-palm grip for more leverage to make your arch higher.

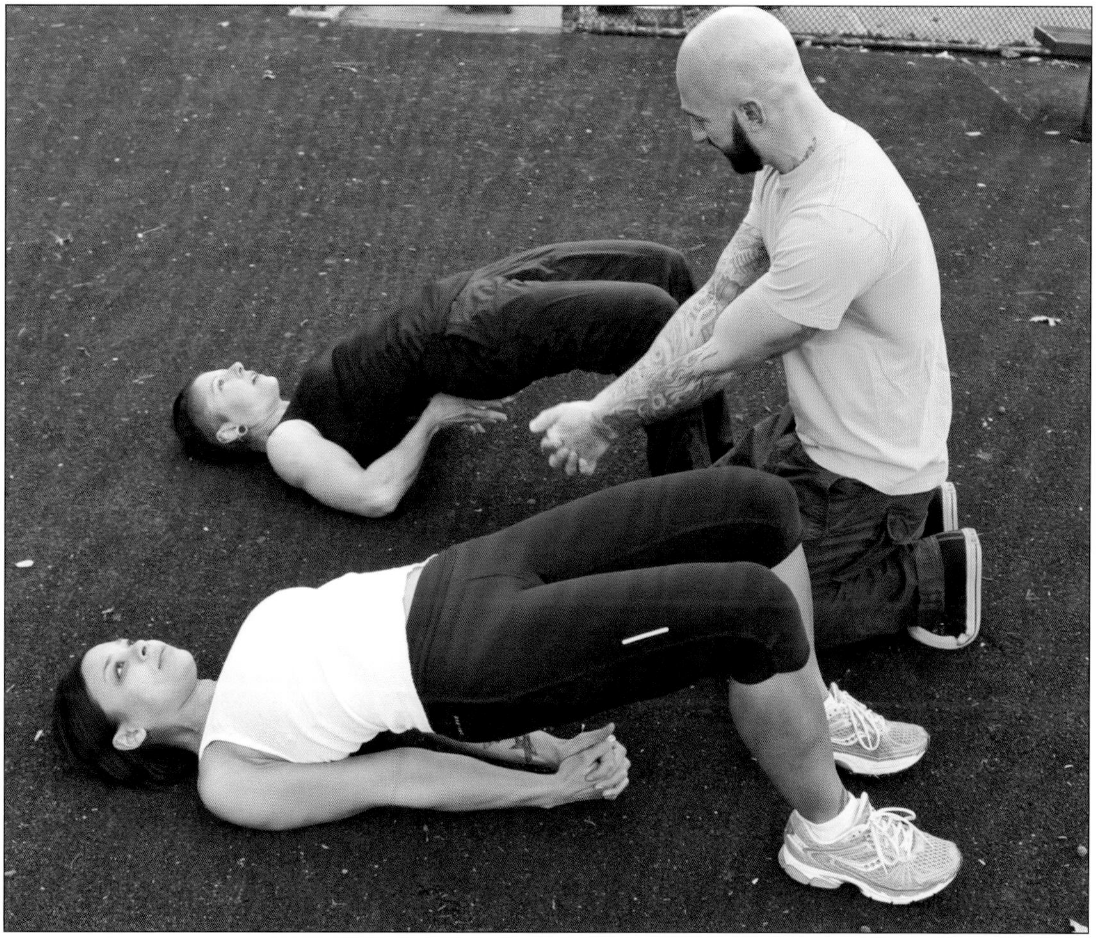

Straight Bridge

Once you get the hang of the partial bridge, you should start working on a straight bridge. This time you're going to sit with your legs directly in front of you, almost like you were going to perform a seated toe touch, except your hands will be on the ground just behind your hips. From here, lift yourself up and straighten out your body by contracting your hamstrings, glutes and other posterior musculature. Drop your head back, press your chest out and try to look behind you. You'll wind up looking like an upside-down plank. The straight bridge will give you a deep stretch in your chest and shoulders. Even once you move on to the full bridge, it's still a great exercise to keep in your routine for a long time to come.

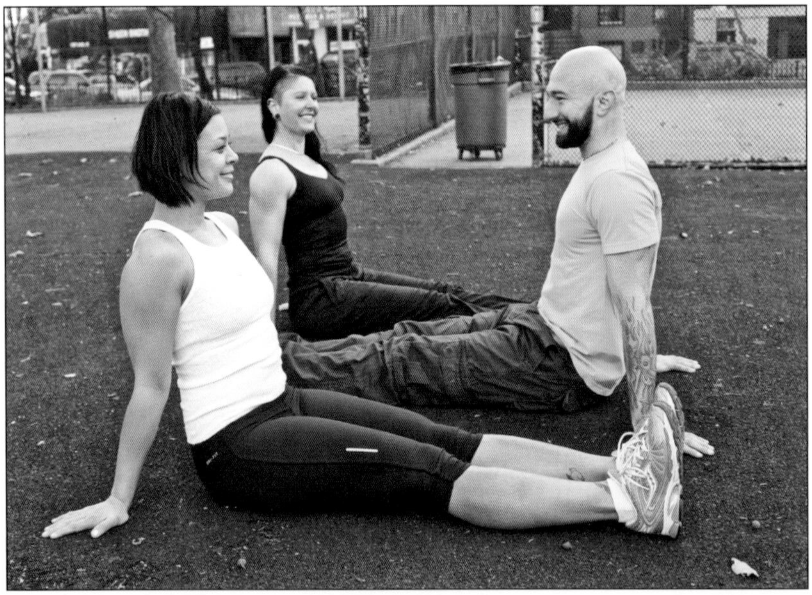

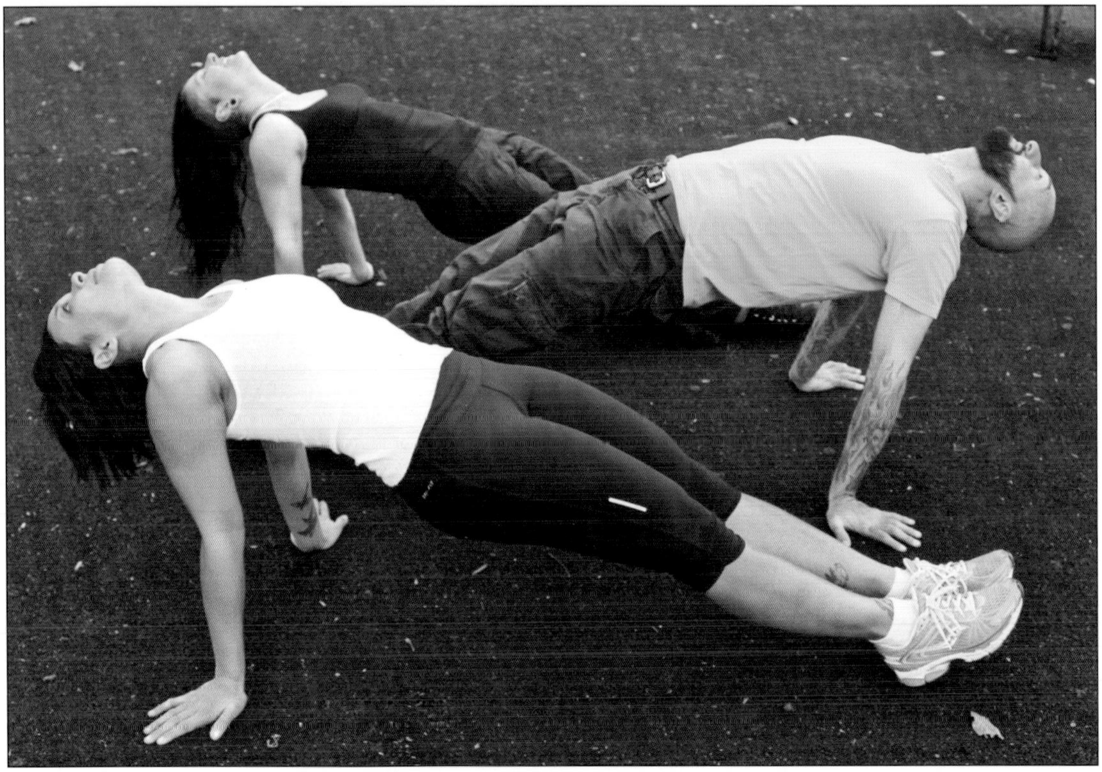

Table Top

As an alternative, you may try bending your knees to ninety degrees during a straight bridge, which will bring you to the table top position. The change in shoulder position leads to an even deeper opening of the chest, while having your knees bent allows for better leverage with the hamstrings and can facilitate deeper glute activation.

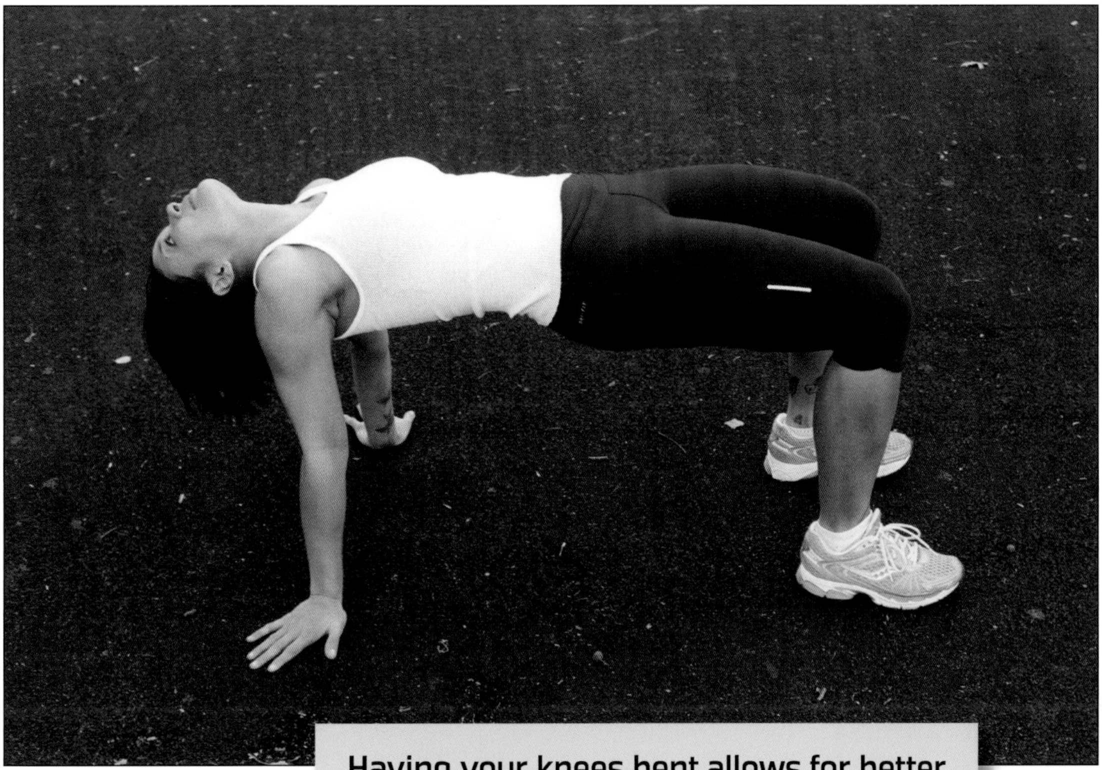

Having your knees bent allows for better leverage with the hamstrings and can facilitate deeper glute activation.

Neck Bridge

This variation starts off in the same position as the partial back bridge except your palms are placed shoulder width apart on either side of your head with your wrists bent back behind you. From here, press yourself off your back and roll onto the top of your head. You might want to place a towel or other soft object between your head and the ground when starting out.

Though a good deal of your weight will be supported by your skull, this exercise can do a lot to strengthen your neck muscles. Remember to push your chest forward and arch your spine as much as possible while contracting your glutes, hamstrings and lower back. Once you get comfortable with the hand-assisted neck bridge, work toward taking your hands away for an added challenge.

Though a good deal of your weight will be supported by your skull, this exercise can do a lot to strengthen your neck muscles.

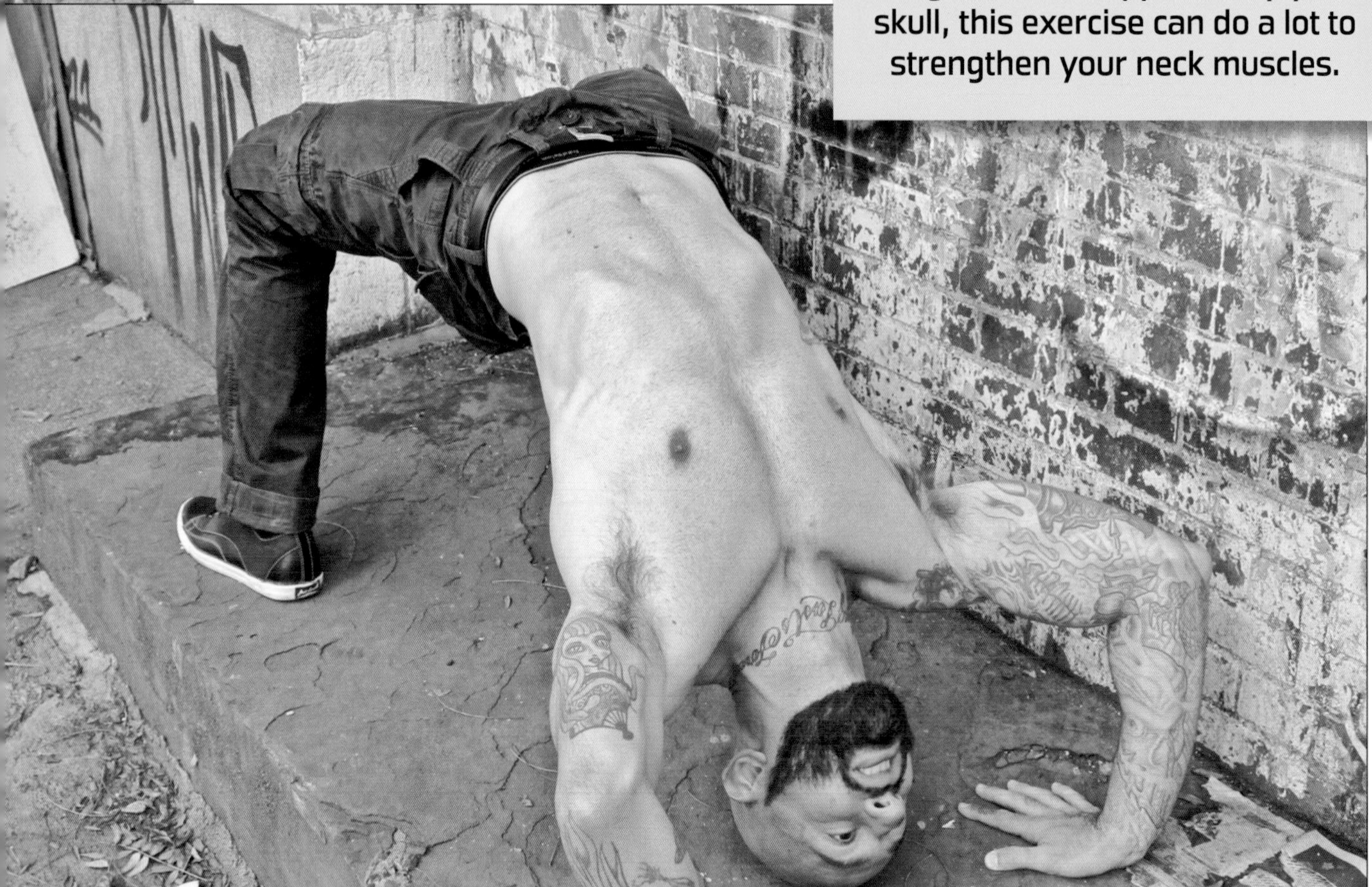

Full Bridge

When you are ready to try a full back bridge, I recommend beginning in the neck bridge position with your palms flat on the floor a few inches from your ears. Press your hands into the ground, drive your heels down and push your chest forward. That last part is particularly important for those of us with tight shoulders, as pushing forward with the chest will encourage a deeper stretch through the thoracic region. Think about trying to make your neck and spine lengthen as they bend back. It may help to look in between your hands to further facilitate opening your upper back and chest, though once you're fully in position, you can relax your head and let it hang naturally.

It will likely take some practice, but your intention should be to get the arc of your body virtually symmetrical on either side of your hips. Think about actively lifting your hips up as high up as you can to achieve that aesthetic. You may also find that gently shifting your weight from side to side can gradually open your upper back and help with fully extending your elbows. Be careful when doing bridges on potentially slippery surfaces, however. It can be helpful to practice on grass or rubber so that your hands and feet don't slide.

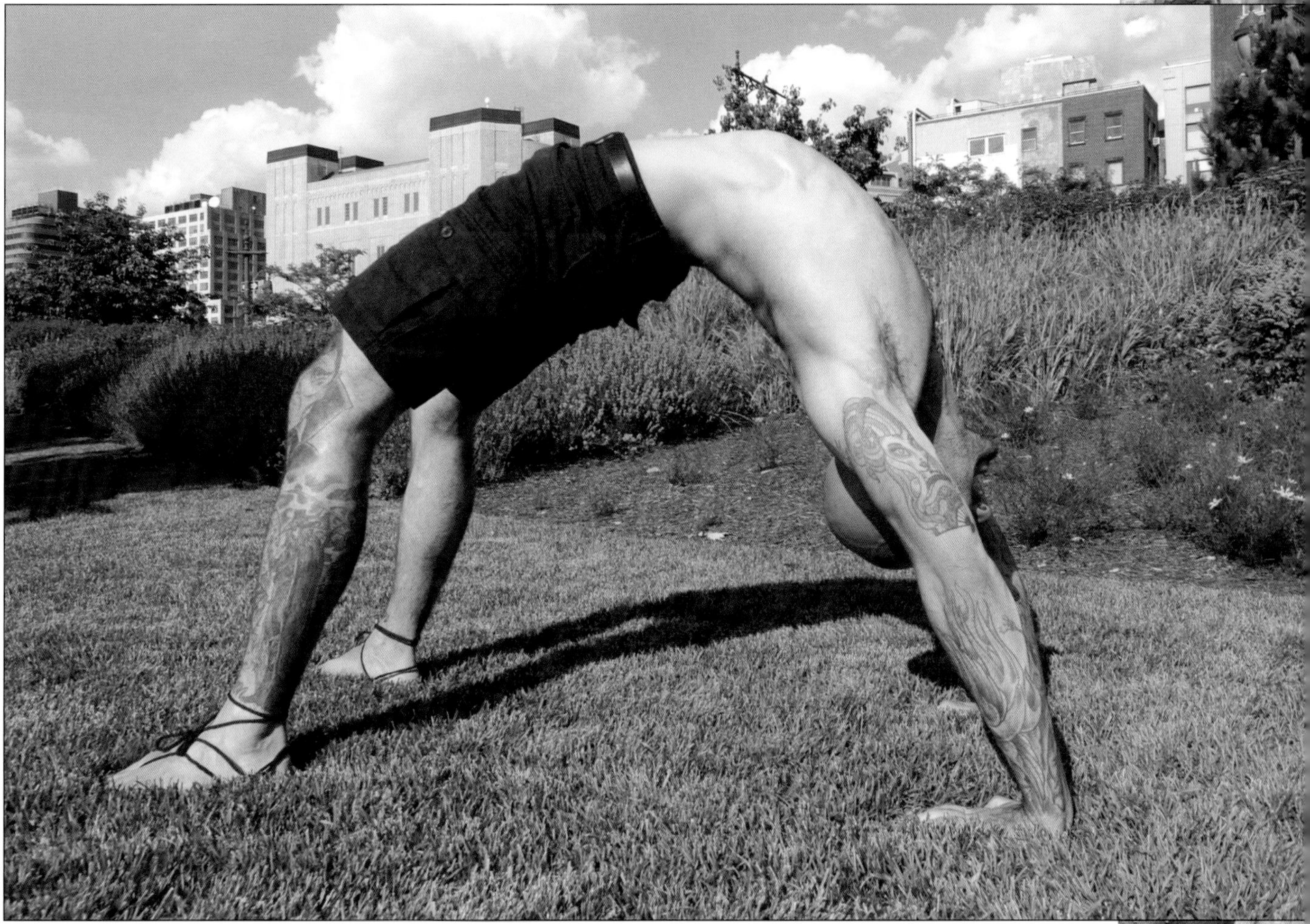

Heels Or Toes?

One of the most common questions I get about bridging is whether it is best to keep your heels flat or come up on the tips of your toes. Most of the time, it's ideal to keep your heels down when bridging, but there are exceptions to every rule. If you find yourself having a hard time fully locking out your arms in the bridge, you can try shifting your weight off your heels to allow some leeway for your chest to press forward. You should be able to add a bit more extension through your arms this way. Once you've achieved that, lower your heels back down while maintaining the additional stretch in your upper body. Feel free to repeat the process a few times during an extended hold.

Keep in mind that while going up on your toes will give you better leverage to open up your thoracic region, coming off your heels reduces the strength benefits for your legs and spine. Additionally, when you place your heels back down after deepening the stretch, you'll need to be especially mindful of engaging your glutes and lower back extensors or the added pressure on your spine may be too much. There aren't always simple right and wrong answers to everything. Different approaches have their pros and cons. Play around with various techniques and experiment for yourself.

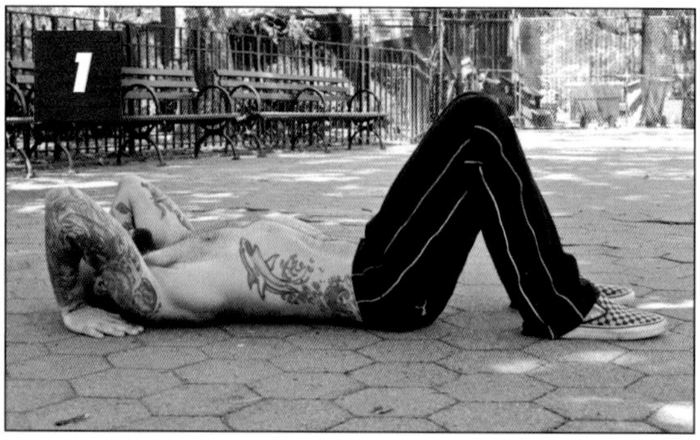

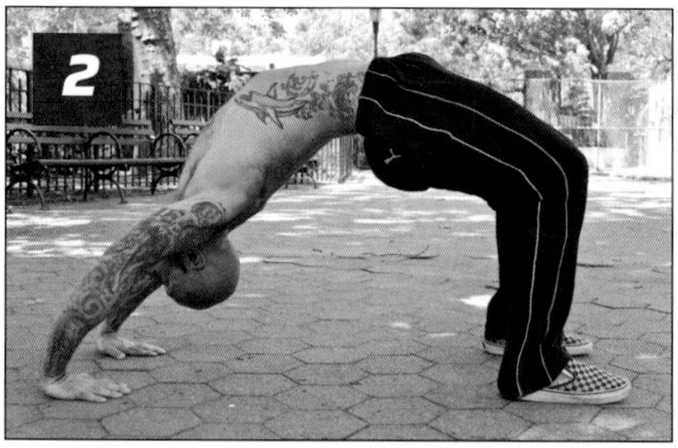

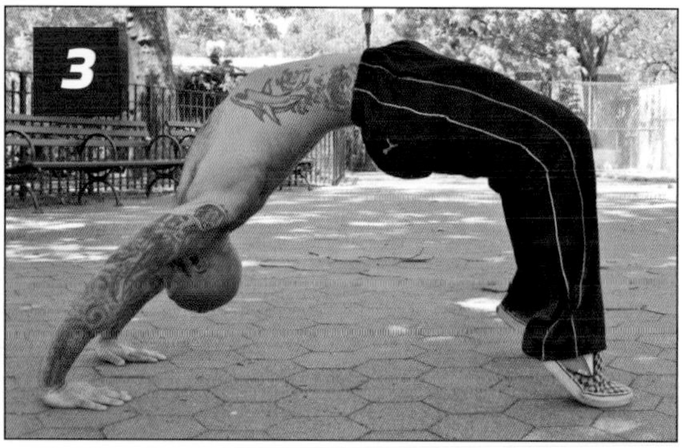

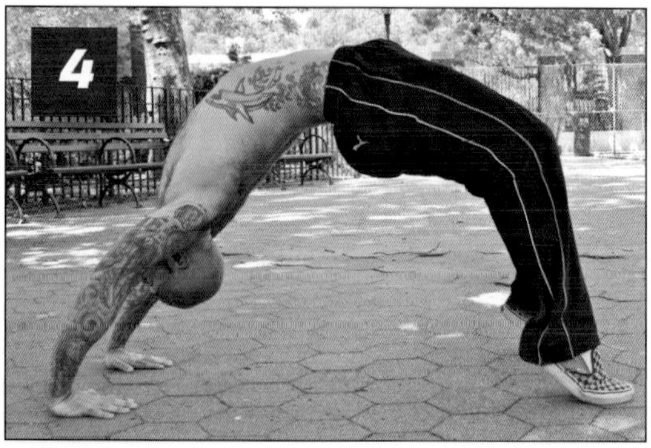

If you're having a hard time fully extending your bridge, try shifting your weight off your heels to allow some leeway for your chest to press forward.

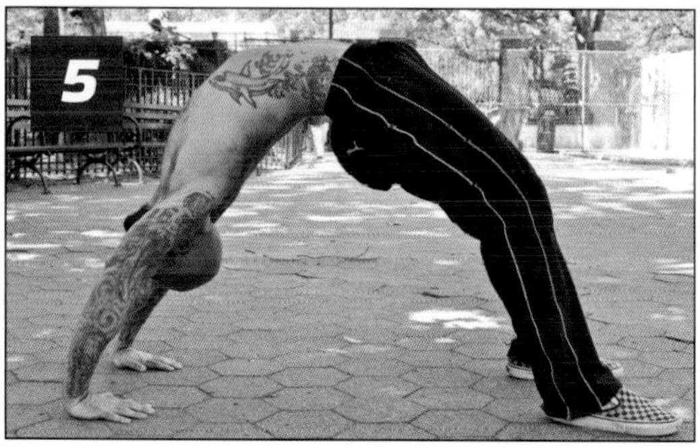

If you're having a hard time bending your wrists all the way back or you feel like your hands are going to slip out from under you, try practicing your bridge right up against a wall. Allowing your hands to rely on the wall for leverage can be a good way to ease yourself into full bridges.

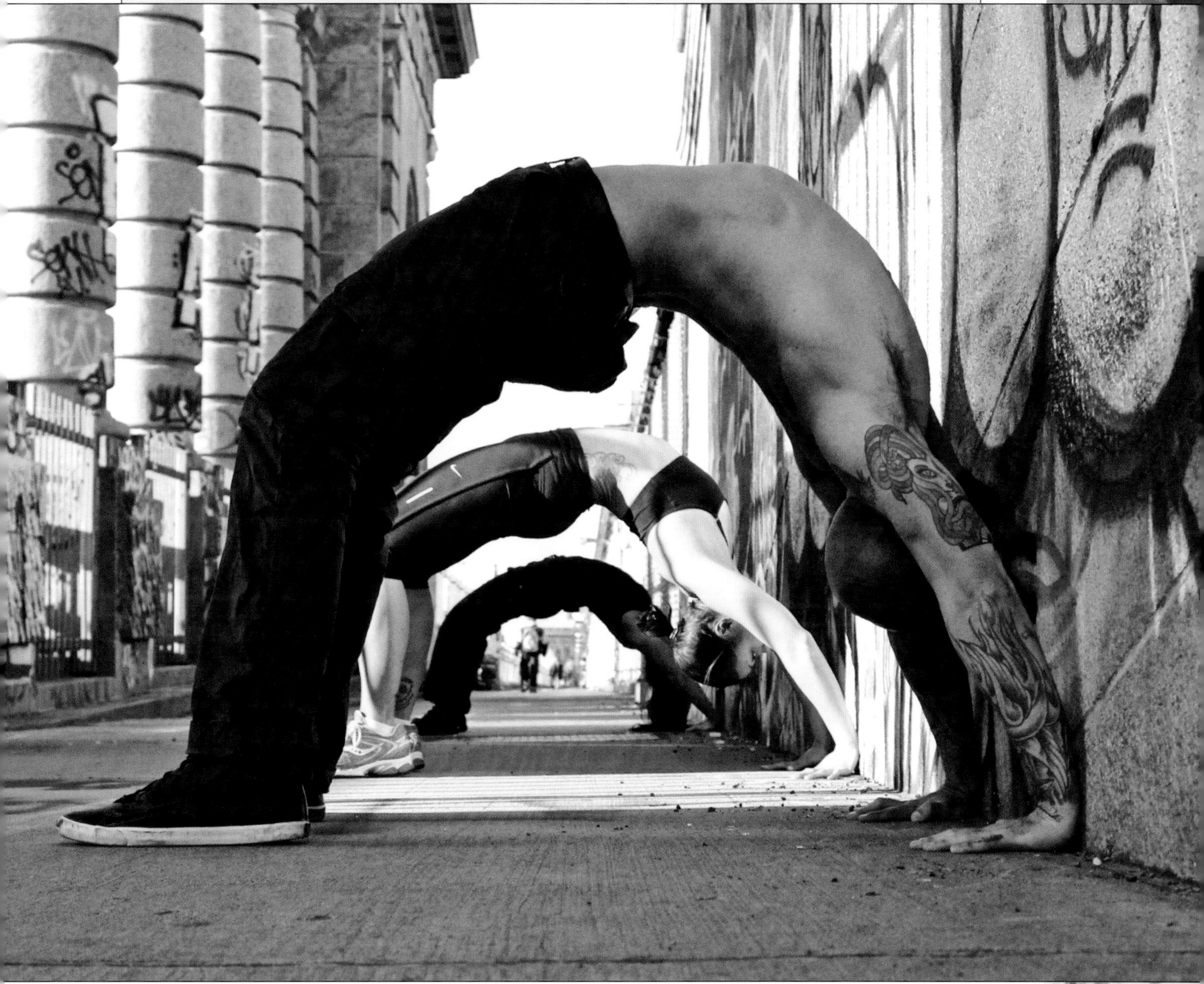

Wall Crawl

Once you can do a full bridge, you can try walking yourself in and out of position by using a wall, pole or other sturdy, vertical object. Stand a few feet away with your back to the object, place your hands on your hips, and bend backward as far as you can. Once you can see the object behind you, reach your arms out and press your hands against it for support. Slowly walk yourself down into a bridge position, then crawl your way back to the top. Make sure to squeeze your glutes tight and stretch your arms away from your body as much as possible. On the way up, aim to pull yourself off the wall with your core and legs — don't do too much of the work with your arms.

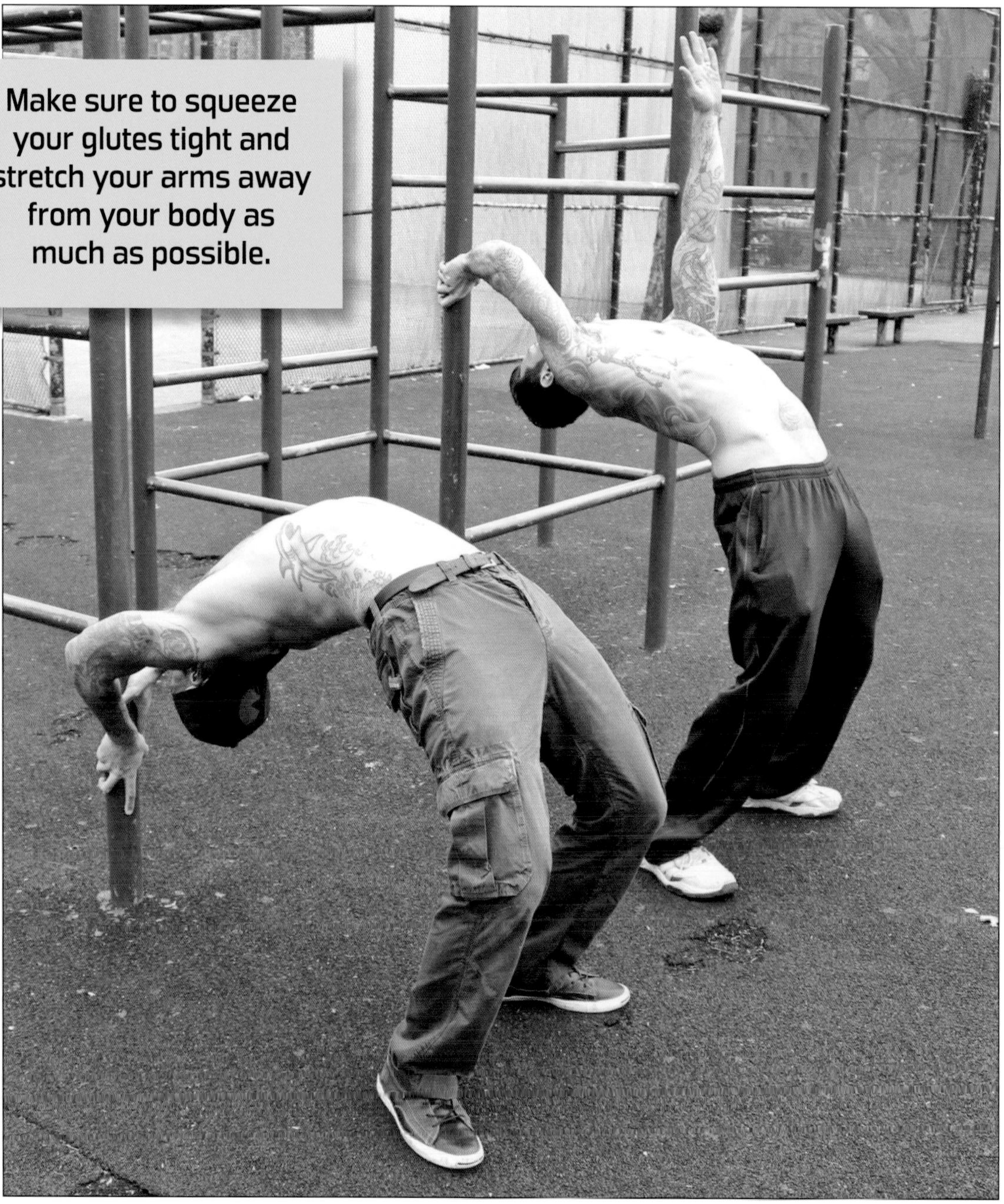

Make sure to squeeze your glutes tight and stretch your arms away from your body as much as possible.

Pushing The Limits!

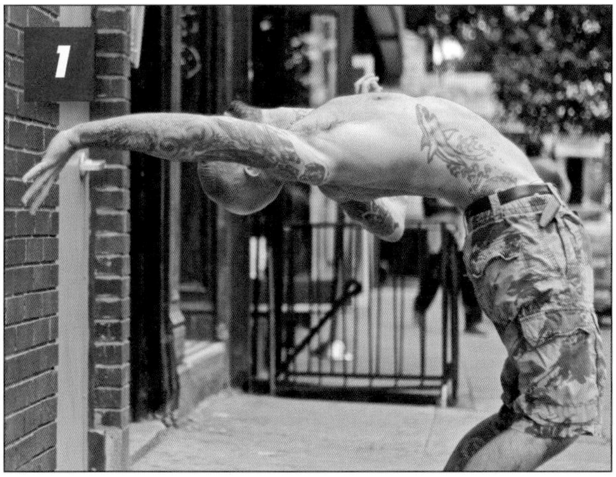

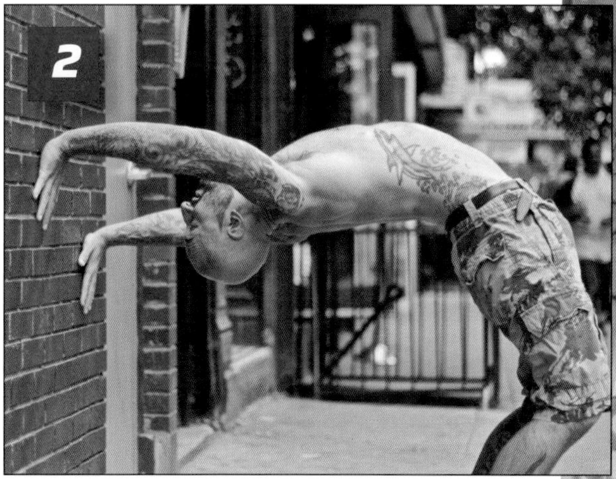

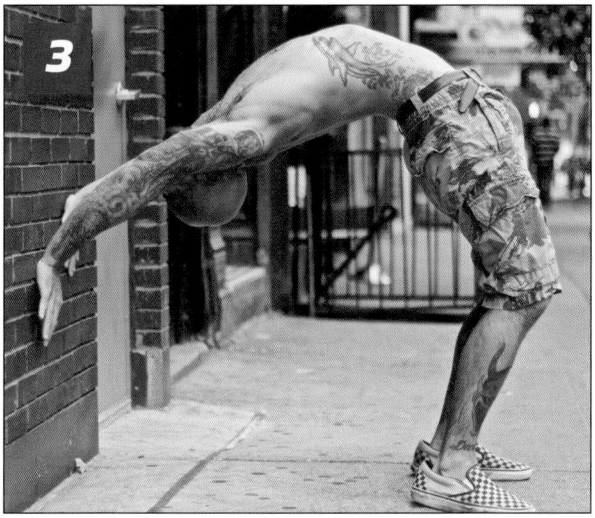

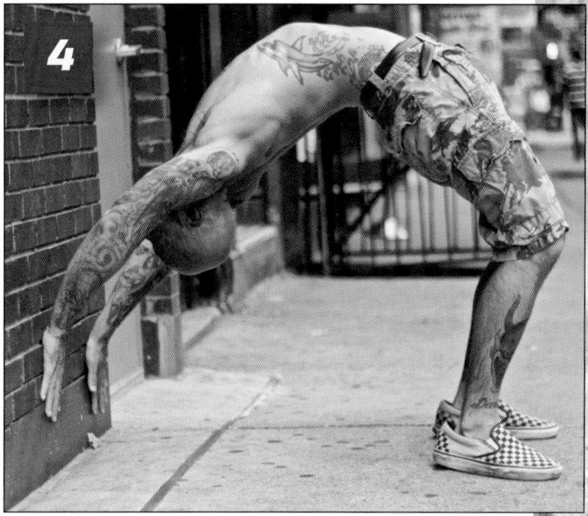

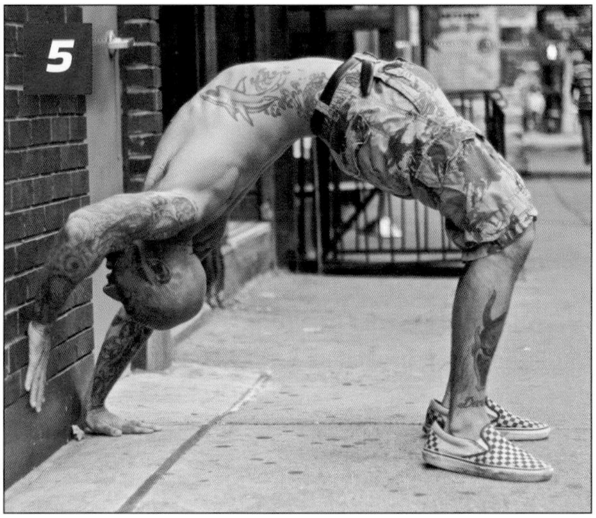

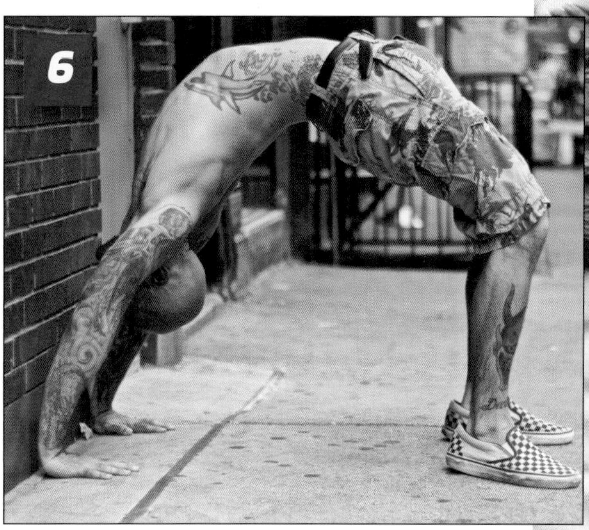

Drop Back

When you've done lots of wall crawling, you may eventually get comfortable enough that you aren't relying on the wall much anymore. When you've gotten to that point, you're ready to attempt to drop back into a full bridge from standing. When starting out, I suggest using a spotter and/or practicing on a soft surface. You'll want to think about pushing your knees and hips forward as you bend back toward the floor. Place your hands on your lower back, and look behind you, gradually going deeper with each breath. Keep trying to look farther and farther behind your back until you can almost see the floor. At this point, remove your hands from your back and reach for the ground.

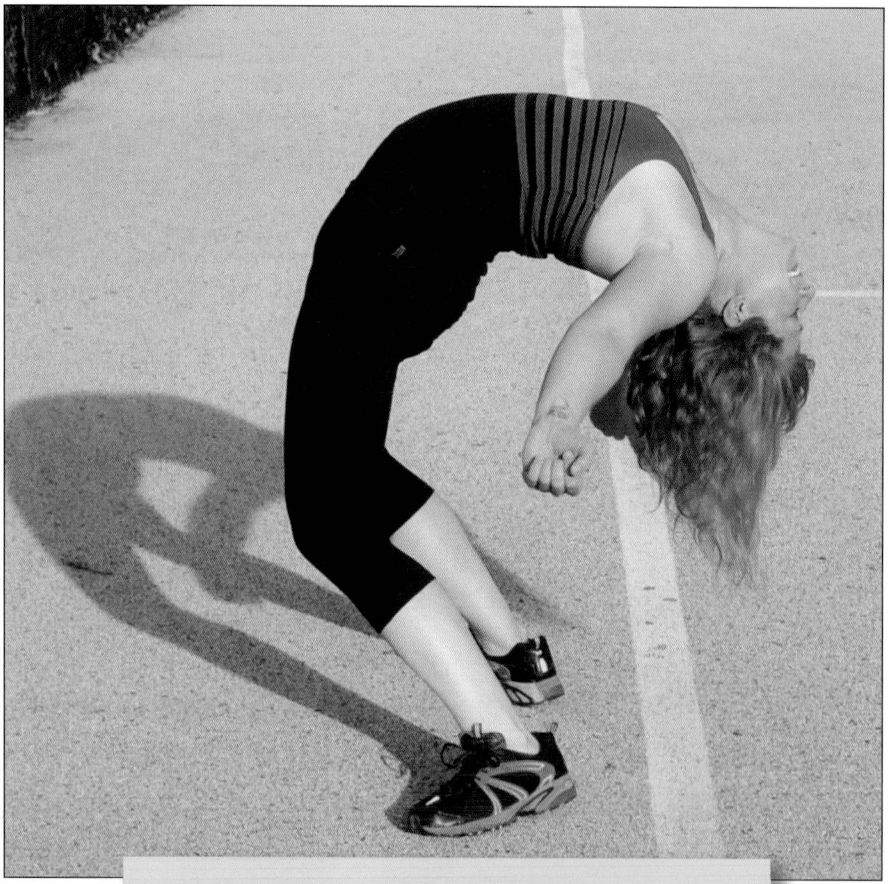

At this point, remove your hands from your back and reach for the ground.

Stand-to-Stand Bridge

Once you get the hang of the drop back, you can attempt to return to an upright position by reversing the movement. This is often referred to as a stand-to-stand bridge. From the full bridge position, think about pushing your knees forward as you contract your legs, lower back and glutes while pushing off the floor with your hands. This is another exercise where having a spotter to support you can be very helpful. A difficult move to execute cleanly, the stand-to-stand bridge is a wonderful display of strength, flexibility and total body control.

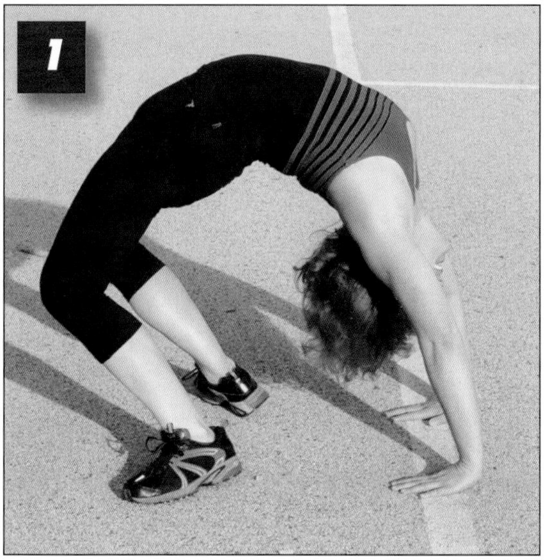

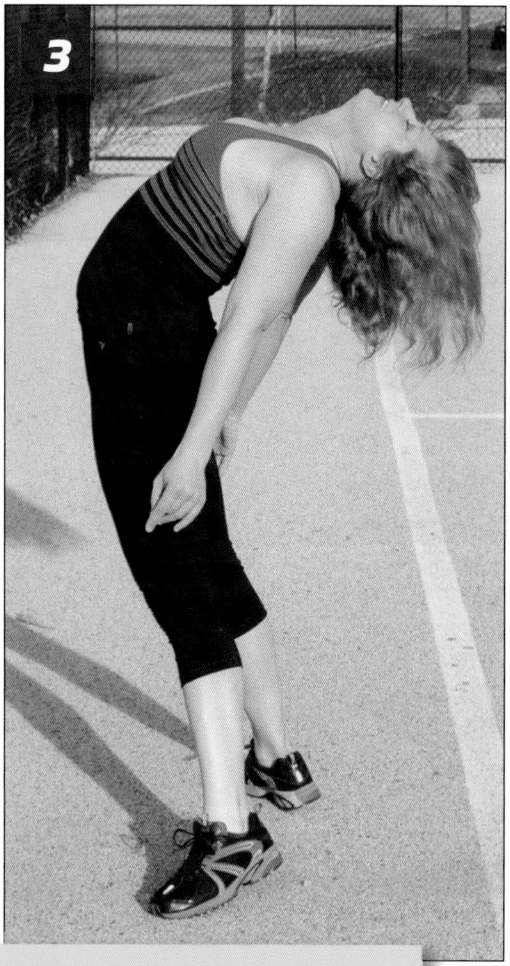

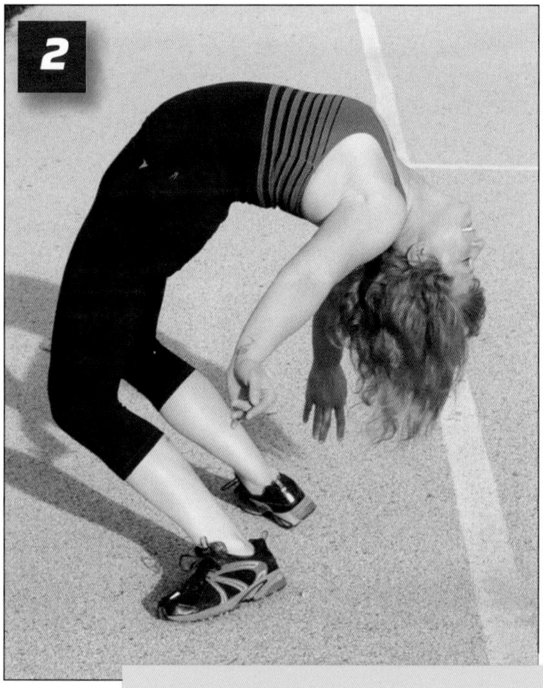

A difficult move to execute cleanly, the stand-to-stand bridge is a wonderful display of strength, flexibility and total body control.

Walkover

Unlike the stand-to-stand bridge, when you perform a walkover you return to an upright position from the bridge by continuing backward in the same direction after you drop back. This can be a very difficult move, especially for people who are tight through the upper back and shoulders.

If you want to learn a walkover, start by getting comfortable reaching one leg into the air while holding a bridge position. From here, you may eventually be able to kick with your other leg and get your hips over your shoulders to bring yourself back around to a standing position. Using a bench to elevate your feet can be a good way to practice toward a full walkover. Again, it can also help to have a spotter.

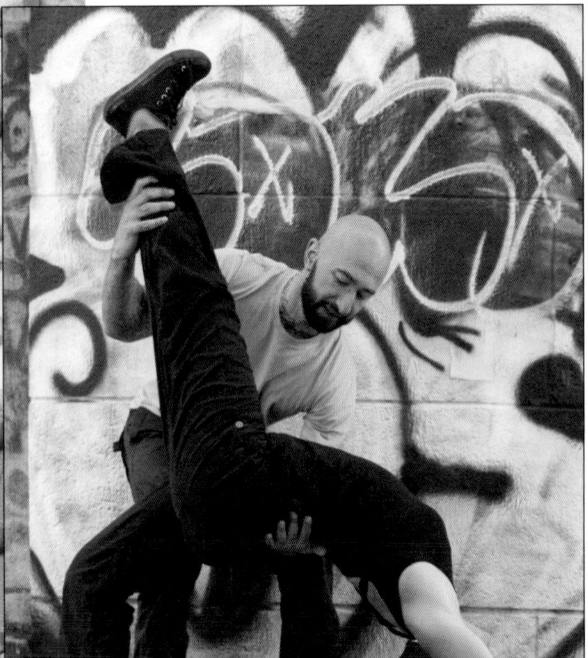

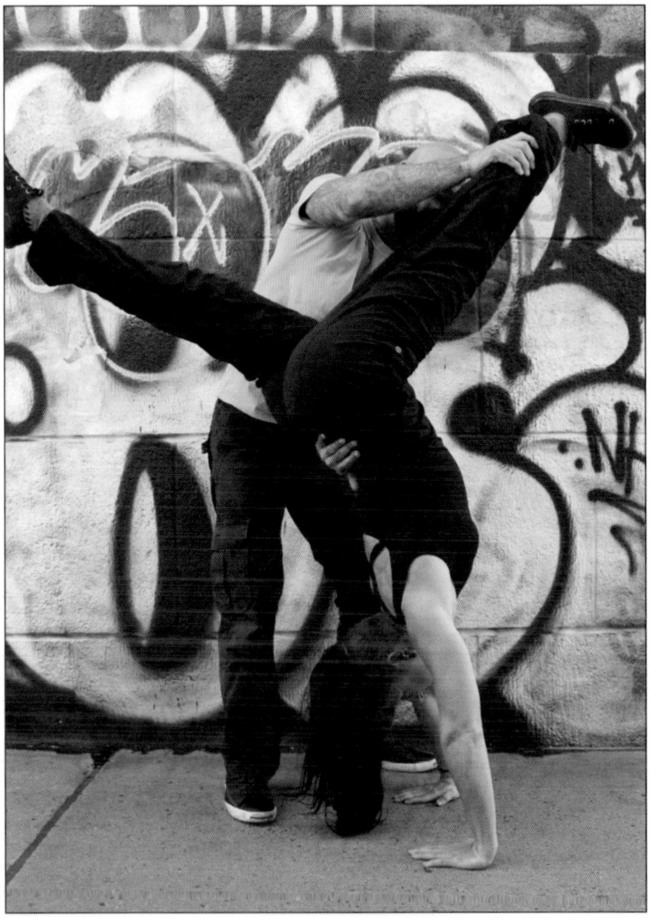

Single Leg Bridge

Once bridge holds have gotten less challenging for you, try holding a bridge on just one leg. It's a great way to build additional strength in your glutes and hamstrings as well as adding a stability challenge. The beginner bridge position becomes an intermediate exercise when held on one leg, the straight bridge becomes advanced and a full bridge becomes, well, a lot harder!

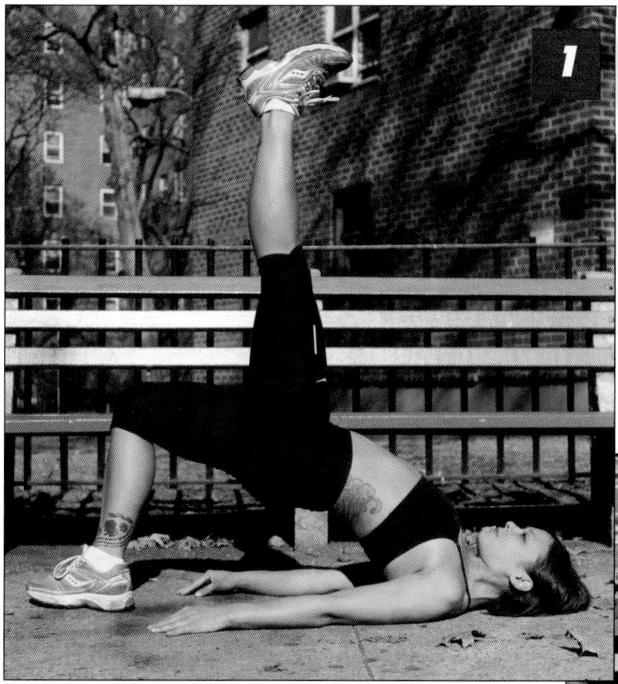

Even once you get comfortable with straight bridges and full bridges, single leg bridge work from the beginner position can be very valuable. Your best bet is to begin the whole progression again on one leg. Keep in mind that you'll need to bring your leg in toward the middle, halfway between the width of your arms, in order to maintain your balance.

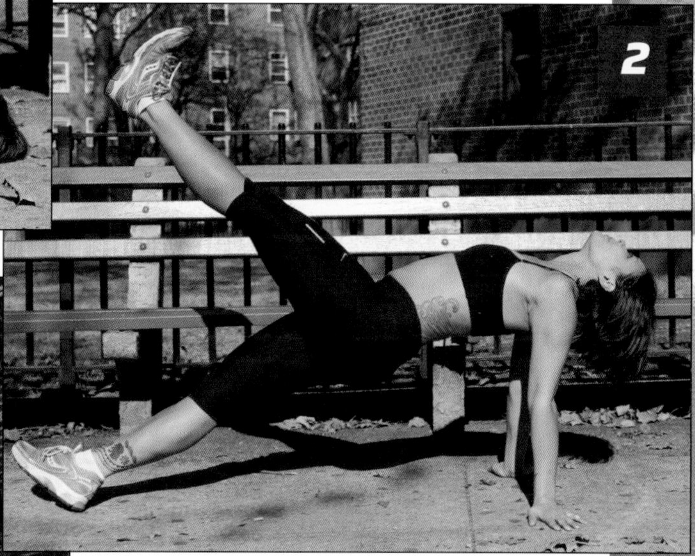

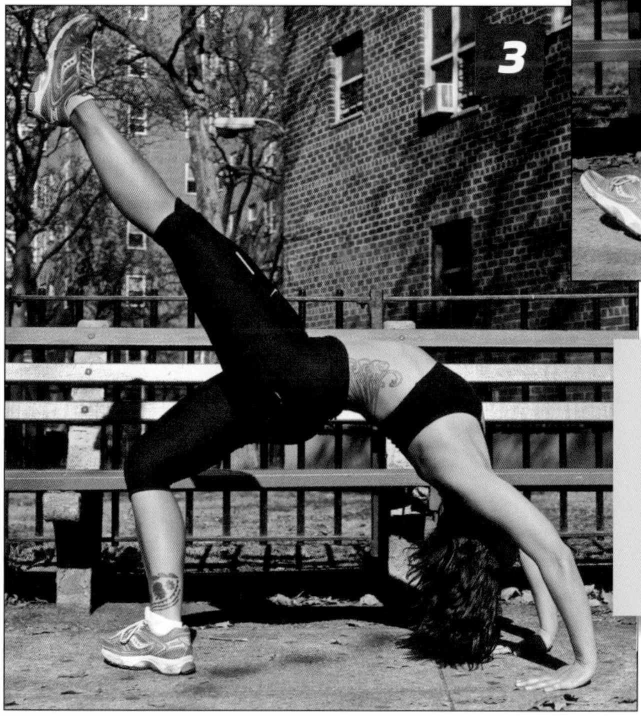

The beginner bridge position becomes an intermediate exercise when held on one leg, the straight bridge becomes advanced and a full bridge becomes a lot harder!

Feet Elevated Bridge

If you want to build monstrously strong shoulders while simultaneously increasing their range of motion, try holding a bridge with your feet elevated. Raising your feet changes the exercise in two ways: it takes some of the stress off your lower back by decreasing the degree to which it must bend, and in doing so it also puts more of the weight in your hands. This makes the feet elevated bridge more work for your shoulders, while the change in leverage also allows you to push your chest out farther to intensify the stretch in your thoracic spine. If the hardest part of holding a standard bridge is the range of motion in your upper body, this is a great variation to practice. I recommend using a bench that's about a foot and a half high. The higher up your feet are, the harder it gets to support your bodyweight. Eventually you're just in a handstand.

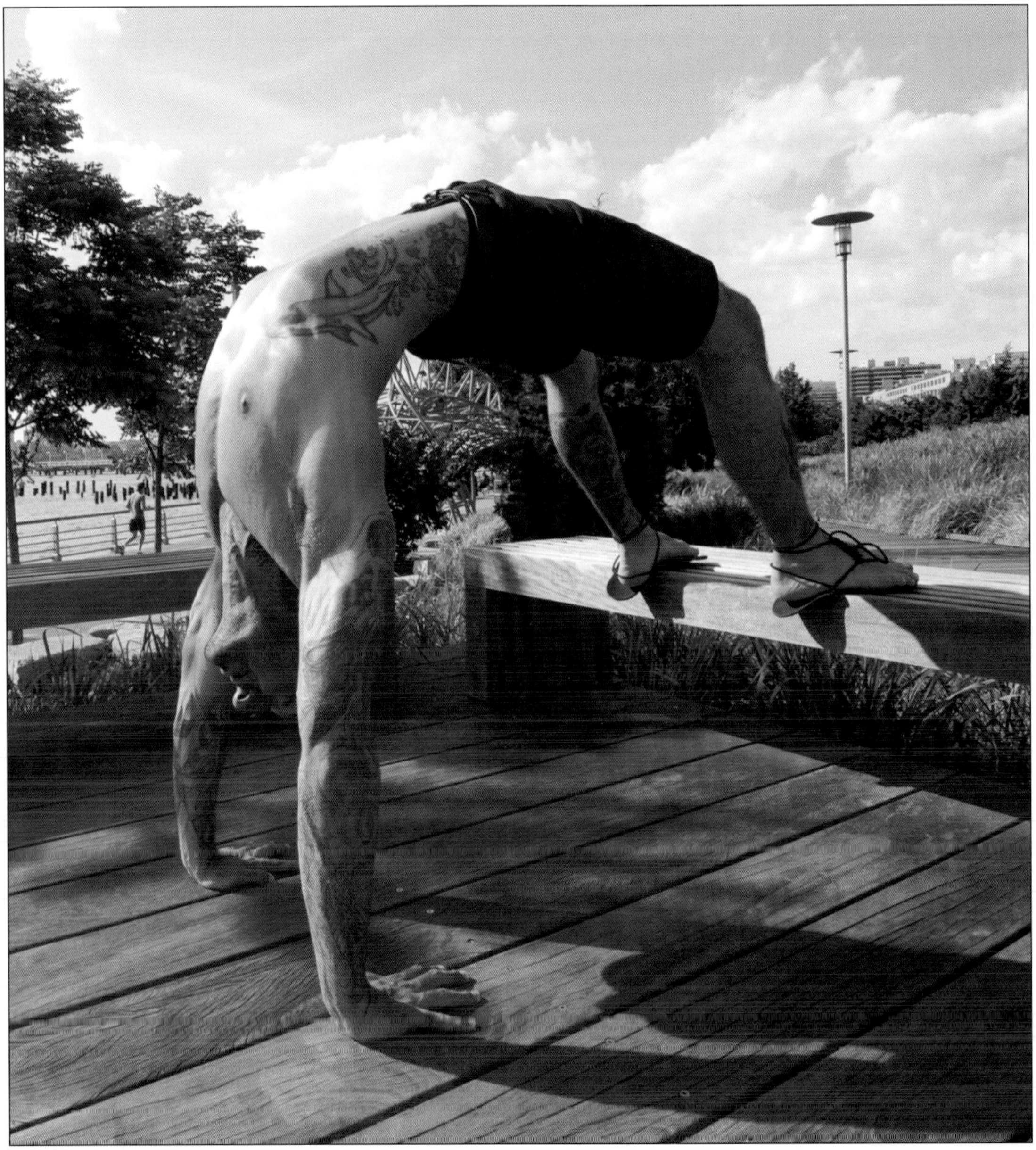

Bridge Push-up

Though I generally like to treat bridges as isometric holds, the exercise can be performed for reps. Going in and out of the bridge can be a nice way to add intensity for someone who feels like they can get into and hold the full bridge easily. If the full range of motion doesn't come easily for you, however, you're probably better off just holding the top position, as the peak contraction will likely be the most worthwhile part of the movement. With practice, your body can eventually loosen up and accept this position more comfortably for longer amounts of time. On the other hand, the bridge push-up is pretty much a combination of two of my favorite exercises, so I can't really be mad at it.

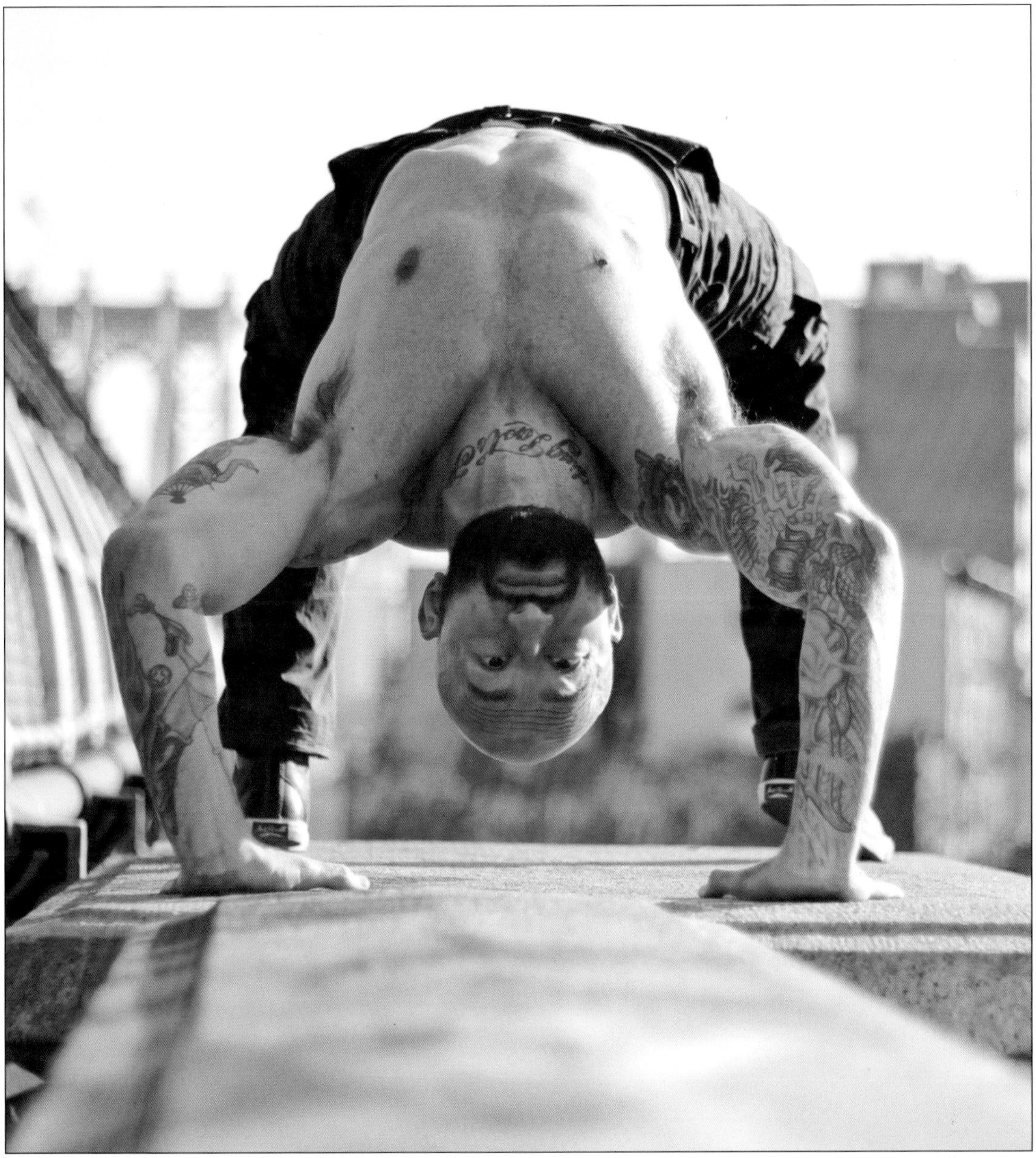

Single Arm Bridge

A bridge can also be performed on just one arm. Though this doesn't apply much from the beginner bridge position, an advanced practitioner who is looking for a challenge can attempt to lift one arm after getting into a full bridge. Aim to gradually move your weight onto that arm to prevent from falling. Once you get the hang of that, you might try pressing into the bridge using just one arm. This can be surprisingly difficult, so be patient.

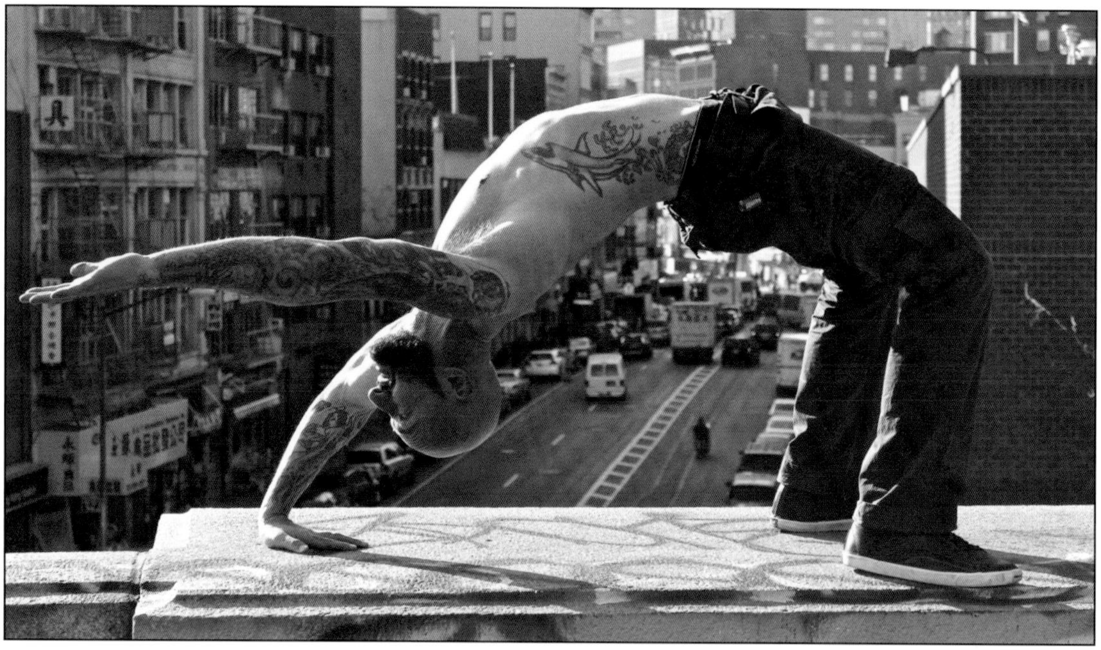

You can also do a straight bridge with one arm. I recommend starting with a wide stance for this variation, though with practice you may be able to perform the exercise with your feet together.

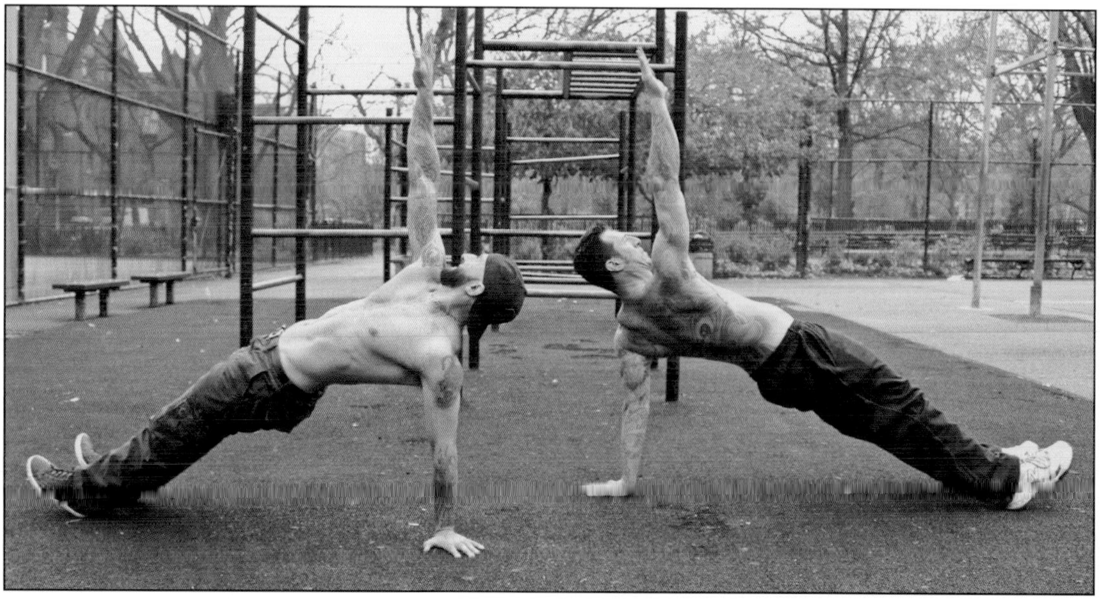

One Arm/One Leg Bridge

When you've been practicing single leg bridging and single arm bridging long enough, you may eventually be able to put the two together. The cross-stability required for this move is tremendous, and it also requires major posterior chain power. I recommend easing into the one arm/one leg bridge very gradually. Start by picking up one hand first and then try lifting your opposite foot. Make sure to think about bracing your entire body. If you can hold this variation for even a few seconds, you are off to a good start. In time, you can work towards lifting the hand and foot simultaneously and holding it for longer periods of time.

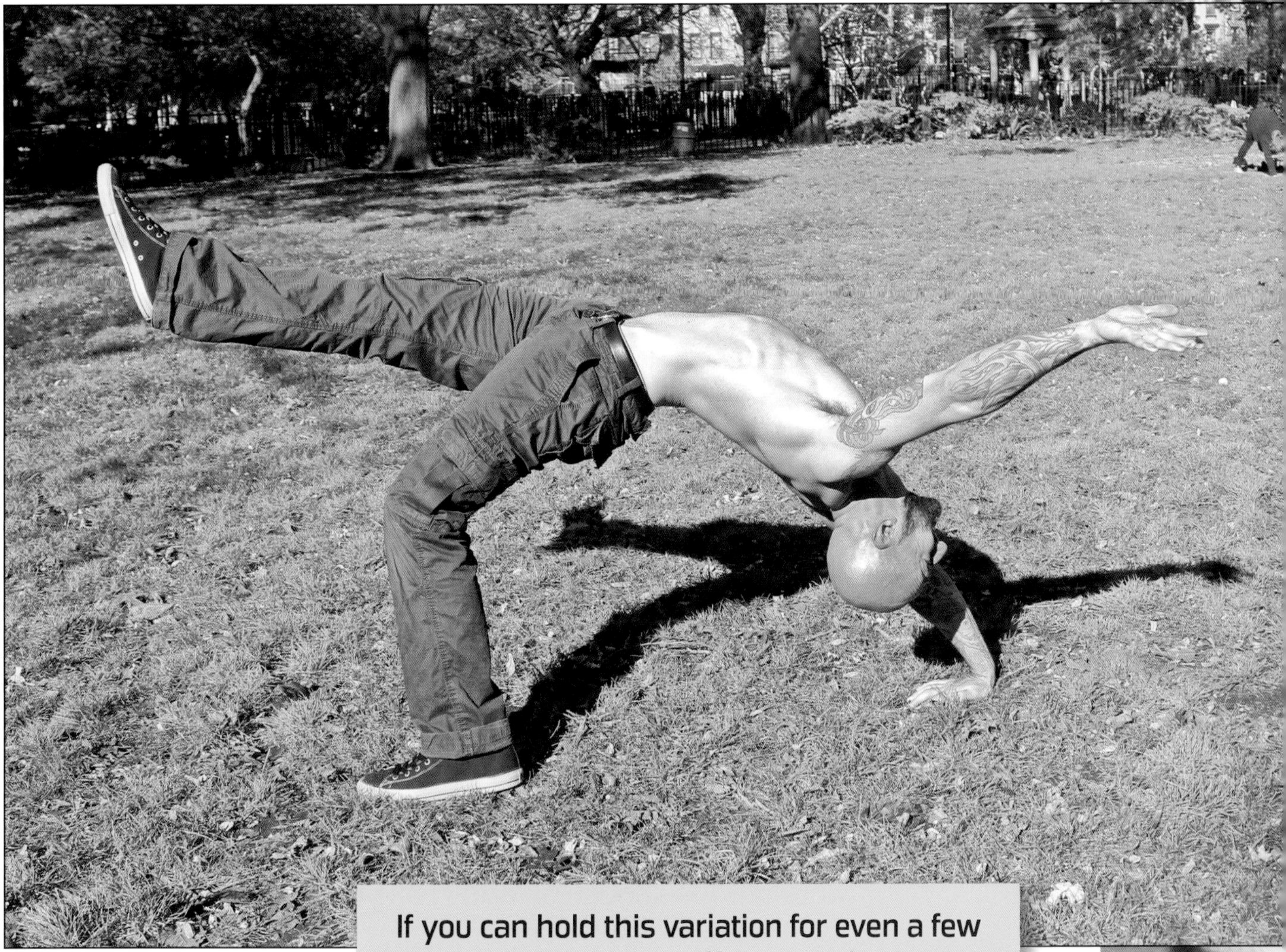

If you can hold this variation for even a few seconds, you are off to a good start.

Bridge Partners

Once you get familiar with the full bridge and its variants, you might experiment with using a training partner to provide additional resistance. Get into a full bridge, then have your partner gently press down on your hips. This will force you to contract your posterior chain harder in order to stay up. After 5-10 seconds of resistance, have your partner back off. You should instantly feel your bridge opening up and becoming stronger. In exercise science, this concept is known as proprioceptive neuromuscular facilitation. Basically, pushing against your partner's resistance causes your stretch inhibitors to relax once the resistance is removed, allowing you to ease deeper into the hold.

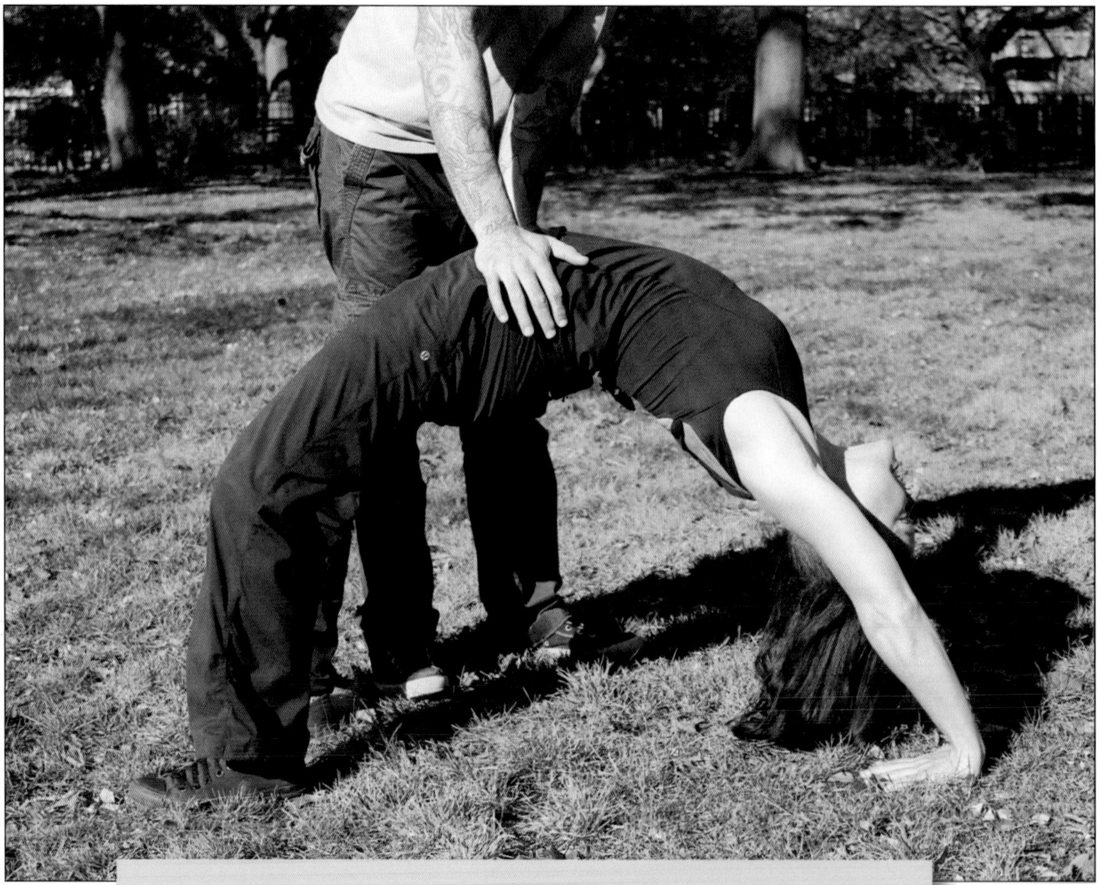

After 5-10 seconds of resistance, have your partner back off. You should instantly feel your bridge opening up and becoming stronger.

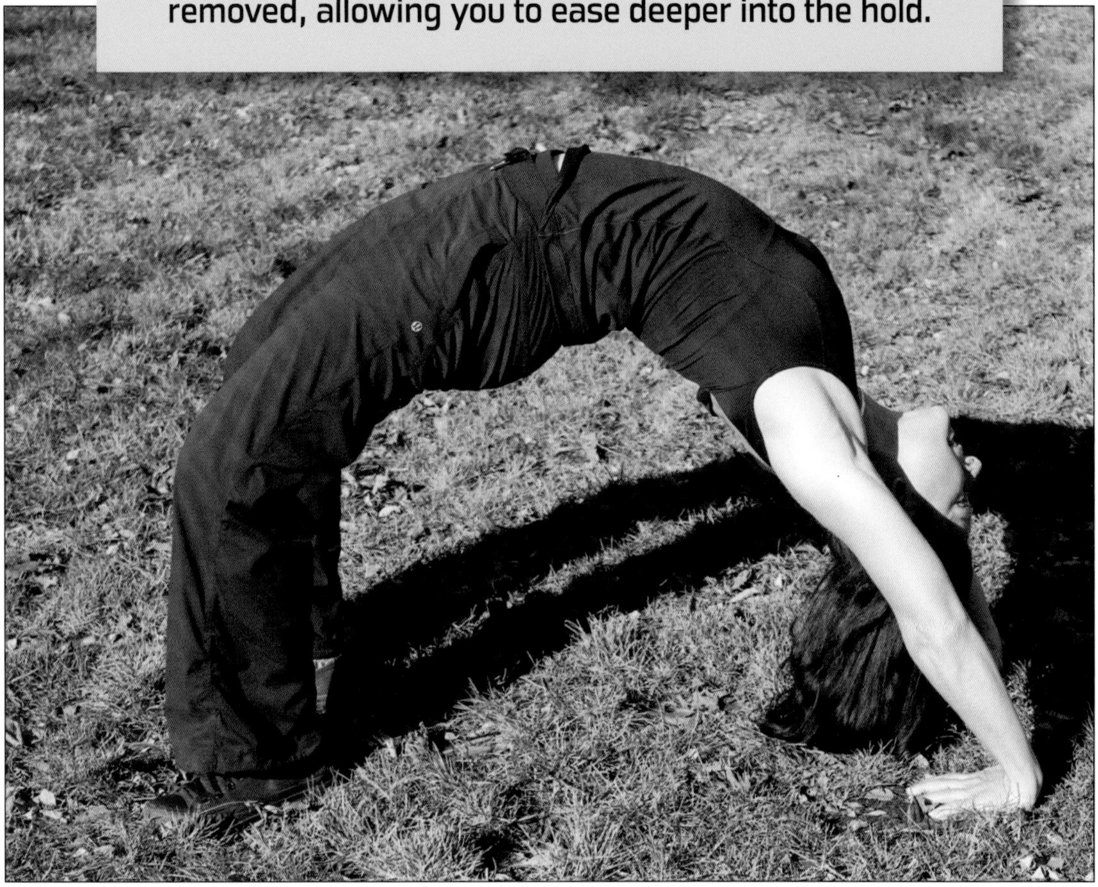

Pushing against your partner's resistance causes your stretch inhibitors to relax once the resistance is removed, allowing you to ease deeper into the hold.

Additionally, contracting your bridge against resistance will cause your body to adapt in the same way that adding resistance to any exercise would — you'll get stronger. As that happens, you can have your partner gradually put more of their weight on you with each training session. Eventually you may even be able to support their entire body weight.

Remember to take your time with these progressions; back bridging can be fun but it's not a game! Many people will need to stick with the earlier progressions for several weeks or longer before attempting a full bridge. Trying too much, too soon can often lead to injury.

Things like partner bridges can make you super strong, but it takes practice and dedication to get there. Put in the work and the rest will take care of itself. With consistent training, ordinary people can do amazing things.

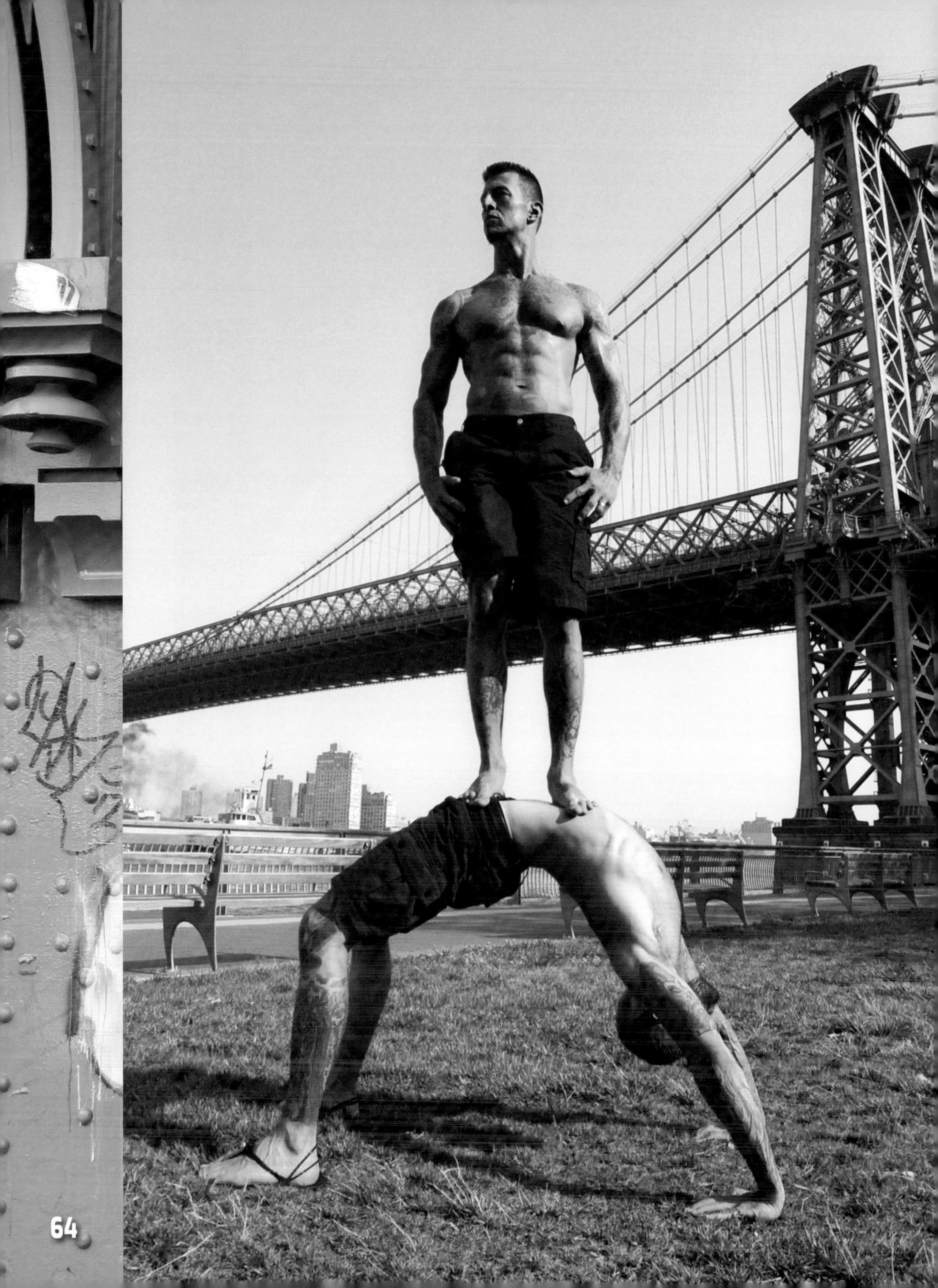

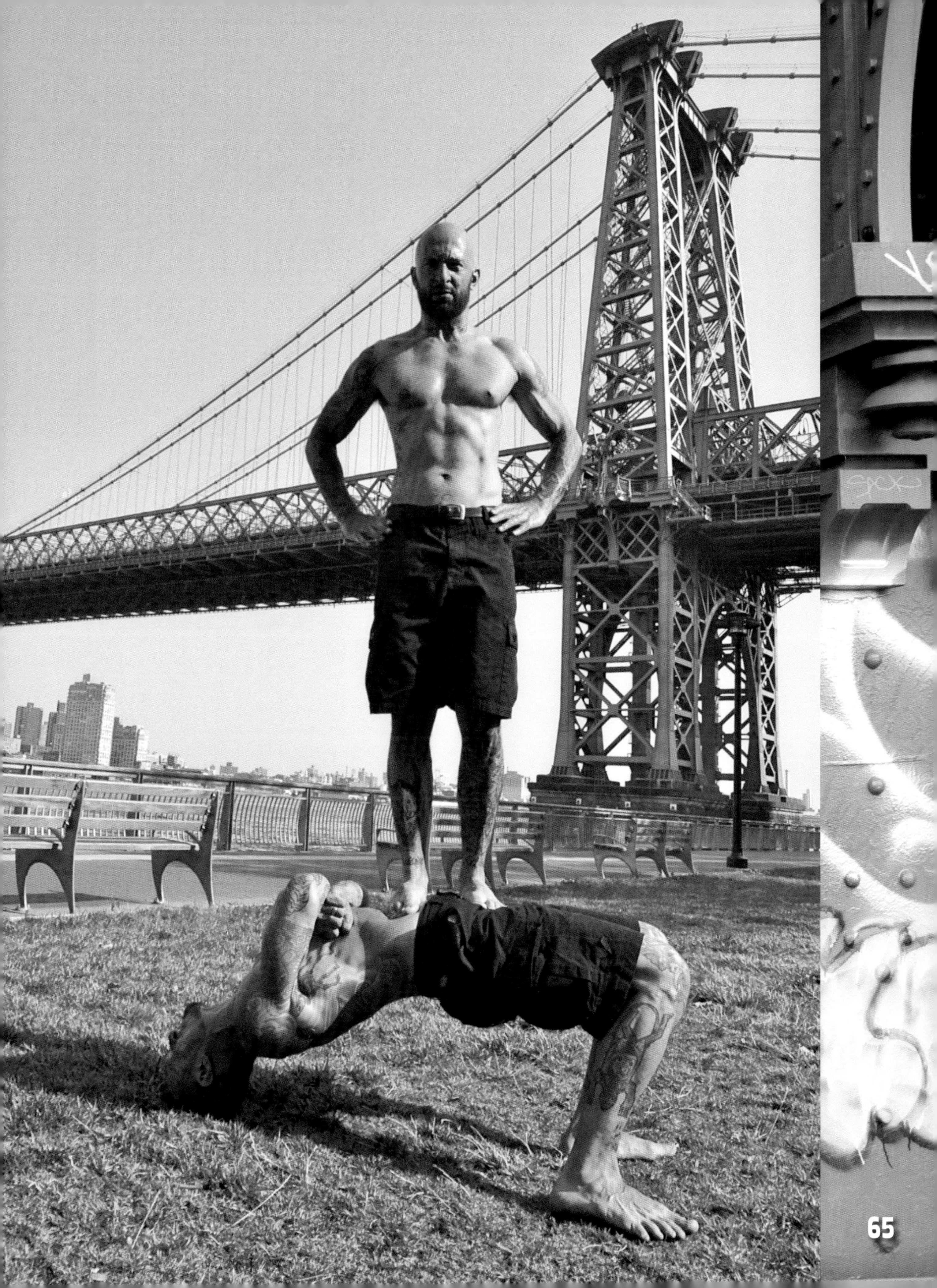

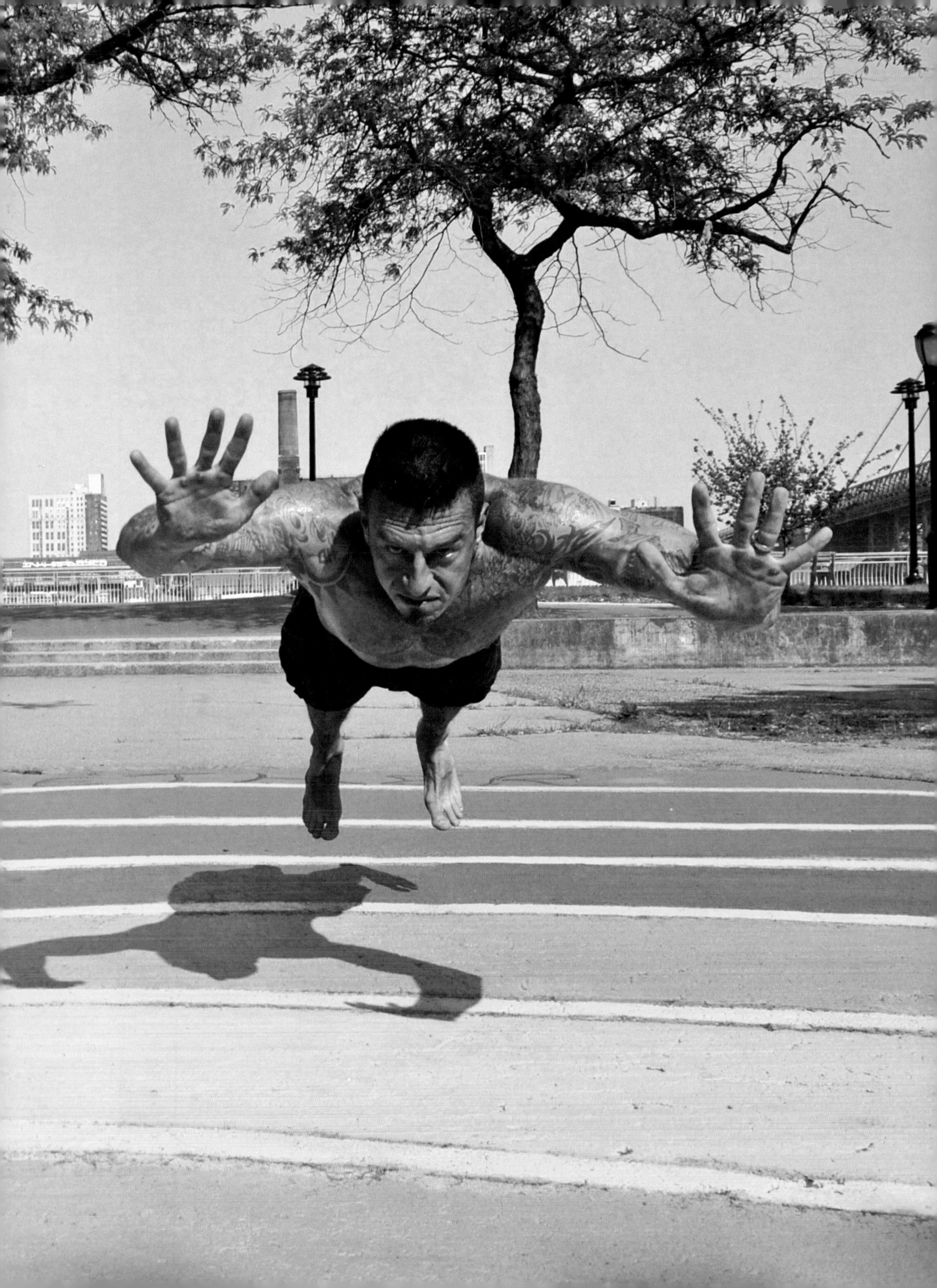

Chapter Four:

Advanced Push-ups

There are a lot of different variations on the push-up. Every time I think I've seen them all, a video pops up somewhere on the internet with someone busting out something new! I've done my best here to focus on the most common (or at least the most essential) variations on the push-up, though I urge you to explore the boundaries of where you can go with this exercise.

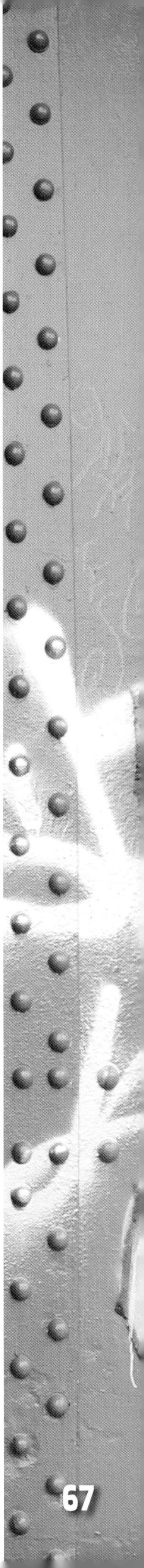

Diamond Push-up

Generally speaking, the closer you keep your hands during push-ups, the harder the exercise is going to be, it's simply a matter of leverage. The classic "diamond push-up" is probably the most well known of the close grip push-up variations. Before you start working on these, make sure you can do at least twenty standard push-ups. In fact, don't do any of the exercises in this chapter until you can do those twenty.

A diamond push-up involves keeping your hands close enough to touch the tips of your index fingers and thumbs to each other, making a diamond-like shape of those four digits. Be careful not to flare your elbows out when you perform diamond push-ups, as doing so can be troublesome for your joints and less effective for your muscles. You've gotta keep your elbows right by your sides. I actually find it preferable to keep my hands in more of an arrowhead shape with my thumbs tucked in, rather than a traditional diamond. This makes angling my elbows closer to my torso more natural.

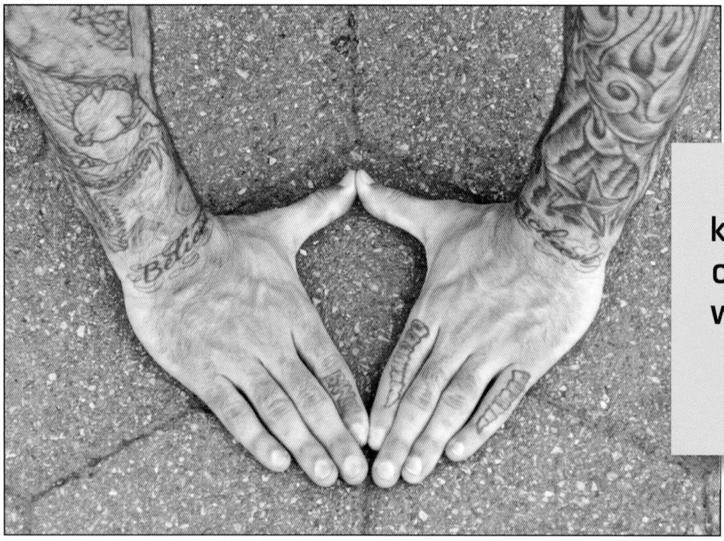

I find it preferable to keep my hands in more of an arrowhead shape with my thumbs tucked in, rather than a traditional diamond.

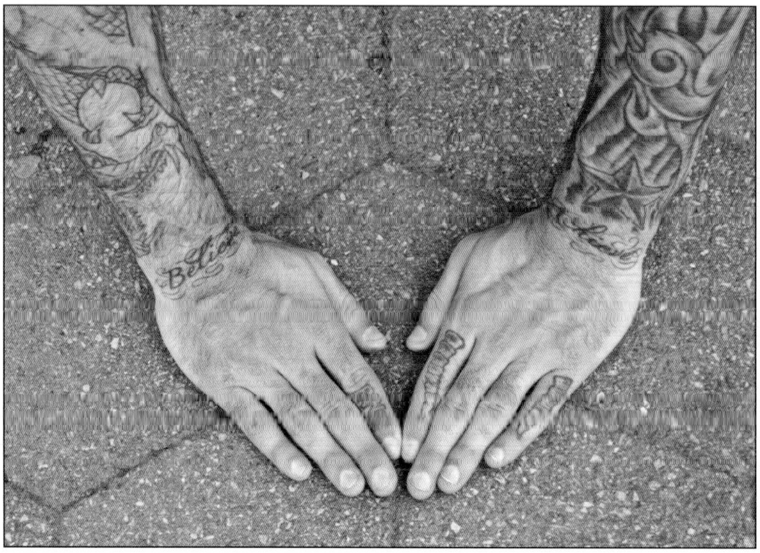

When performing diamonds (or arrowheads), make sure to go all the way down until your hands touch your chest with your forearms grazing your ribs at the bottom. It's also important to stay aware of your alignment. It's common for people to leave their hips too low when performing this exercise. I recommend doing the mirror drill from Chapter One when you are beginning with diamond push-ups. When you do the drill with your hands close together, your feet should line up with your hands in the mirror. Keep your abs, legs and glutes tight. Remember, a push-up is always a moving plank.

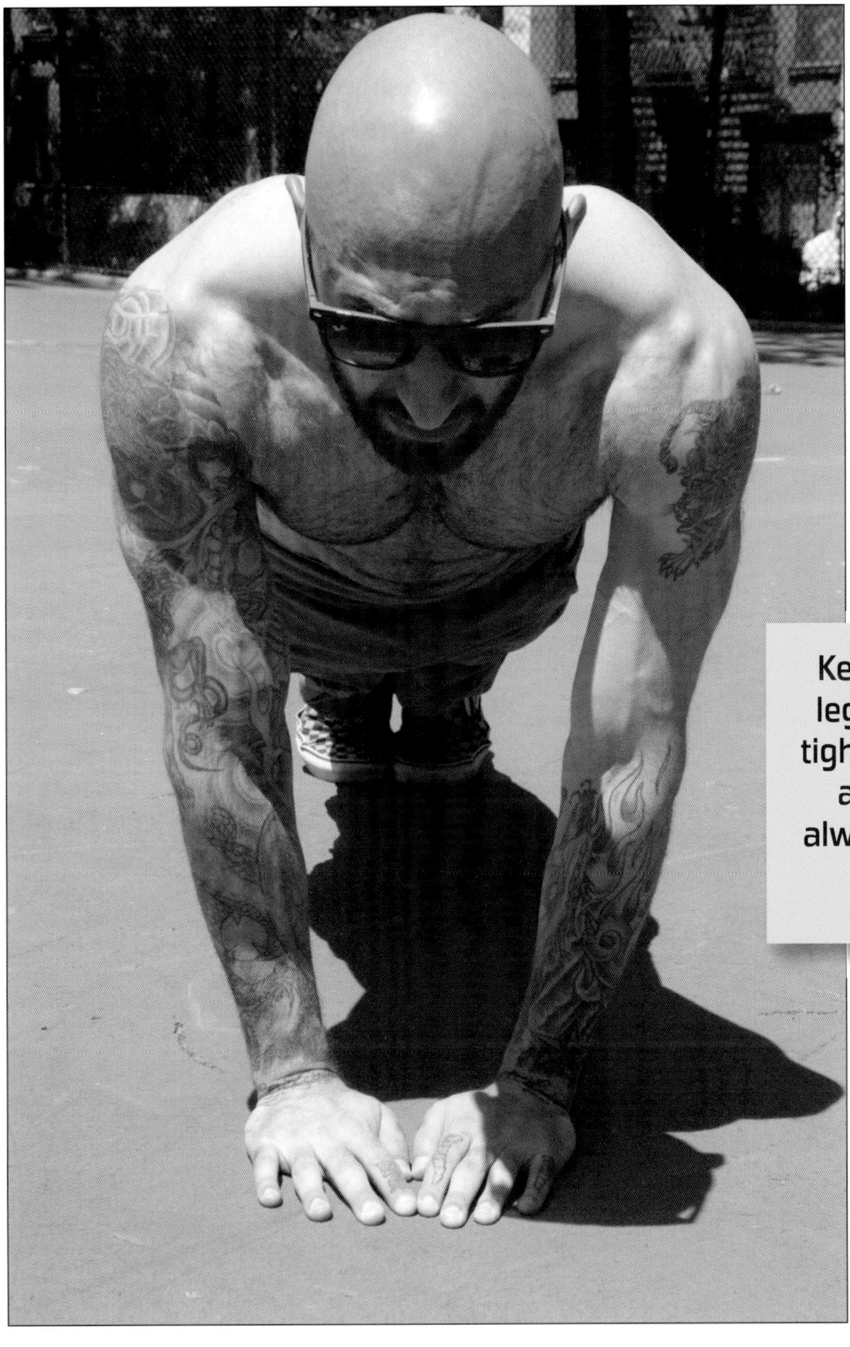

Keep your abs, legs and glutes tight. Remember, a push-up is always a moving plank.

Yoga Push-up

Another variation on the close grip push-up involves keeping your elbows in by your ribs like a diamond push-up but with your hands at shoulder width instead of right next to each other. This is a yoga style push-up or "chaturanga" as yogis call it. It can be a slightly easier variation for beginners before going for a full diamond or arrowhead push-up.

If you can do 20 standard push-ups, but attempting a diamond is giving you too much trouble, try yoga push-ups first. They're not as difficult for your muscles and they're also a bit easier on the wrists.

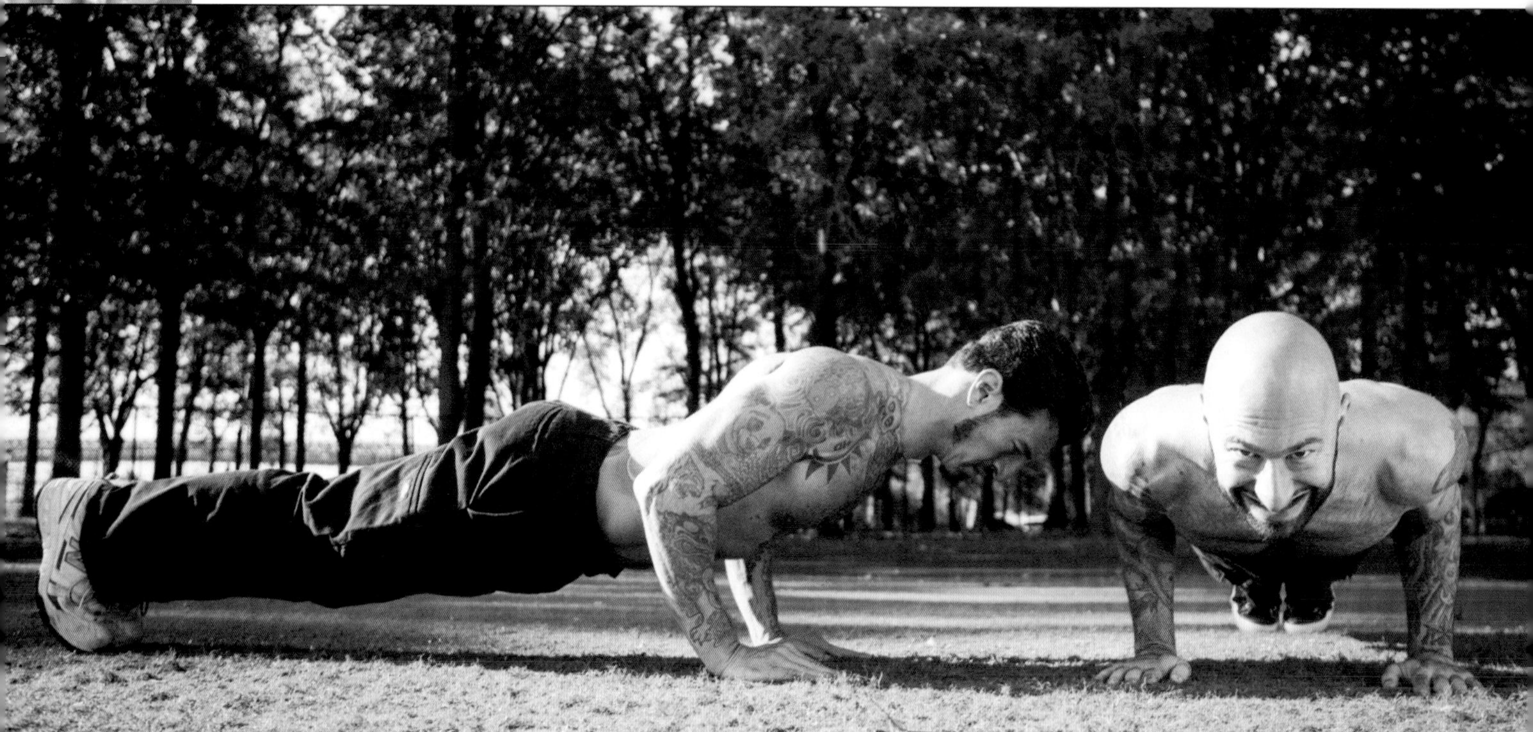

Hinge Push-up

A hinge push-up is a great way to add a unique stability challenge to your push-up while also increasing the range of motion. Begin in a standard push-up position, then lower yourself to the ground. Instead of pressing yourself back up from there, however, shift your weight onto your elbows at the bottom. You'll wind up in a forearm plank with your palms flat on the floor in front of your shoulders. From here, tighten up your body, pull your elbows off the floor, slide forward and press yourself back to the top. Your toes and feet will need to flex back and forth as you slide in and out. The hinge push-up requires a lot of trunk stability, so remember to keep your abs, back and glutes engaged throughout.

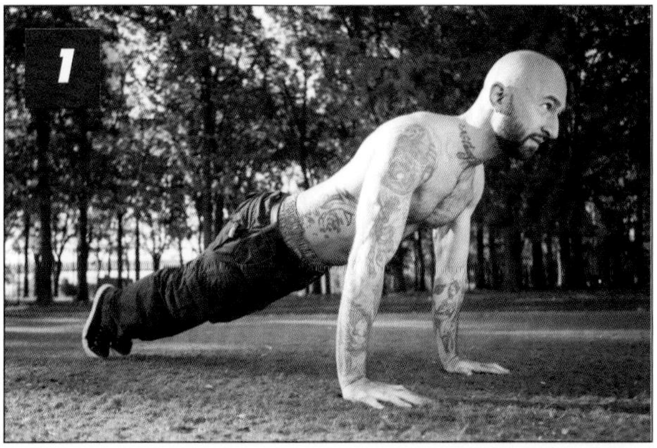

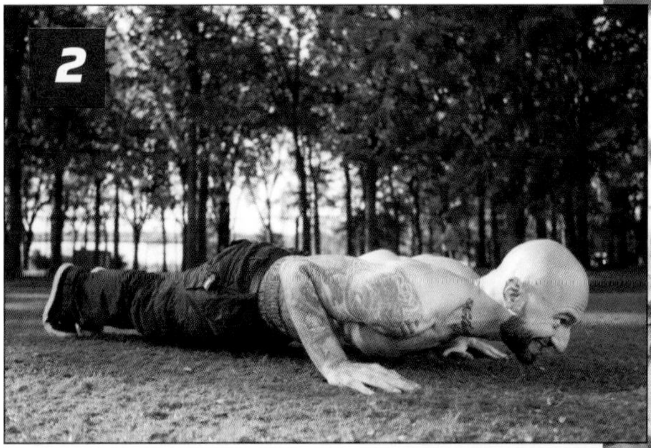

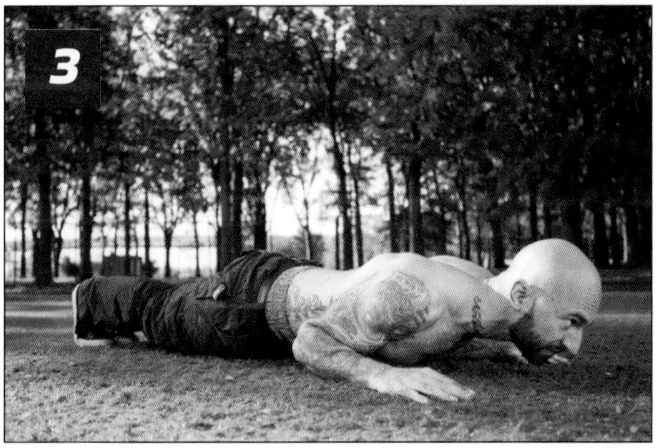

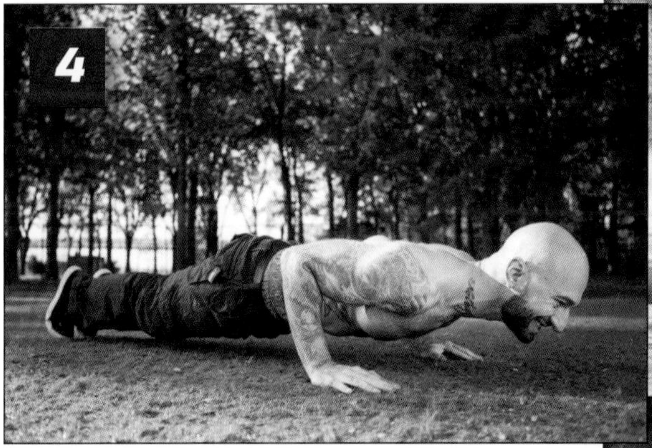

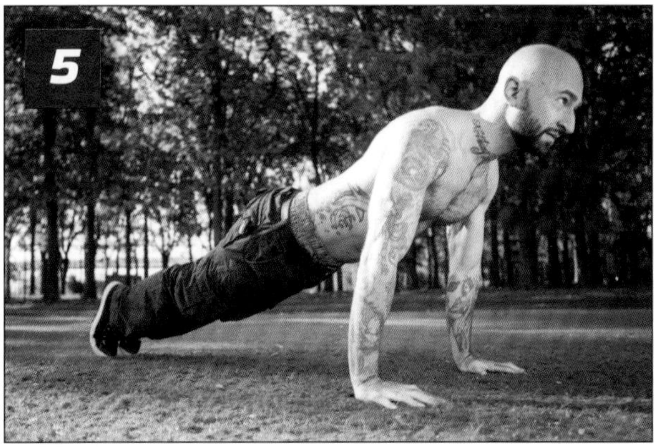

The hinge push-up requires a lot of trunk stability, so remember to keep your abs, back and glutes engaged throughout.

Feet Elevated Push-up

Just like I told you how you can make a full push-up easier by angling your body with your hands against a wall or other inclined surface, the opposite holds true as well. If you want to make your push-up more difficult, you can try elevating your feet. The higher up you put your feet, the harder the exercise becomes. Eventually if you walk up far enough you'll be doing a handstand push-up!

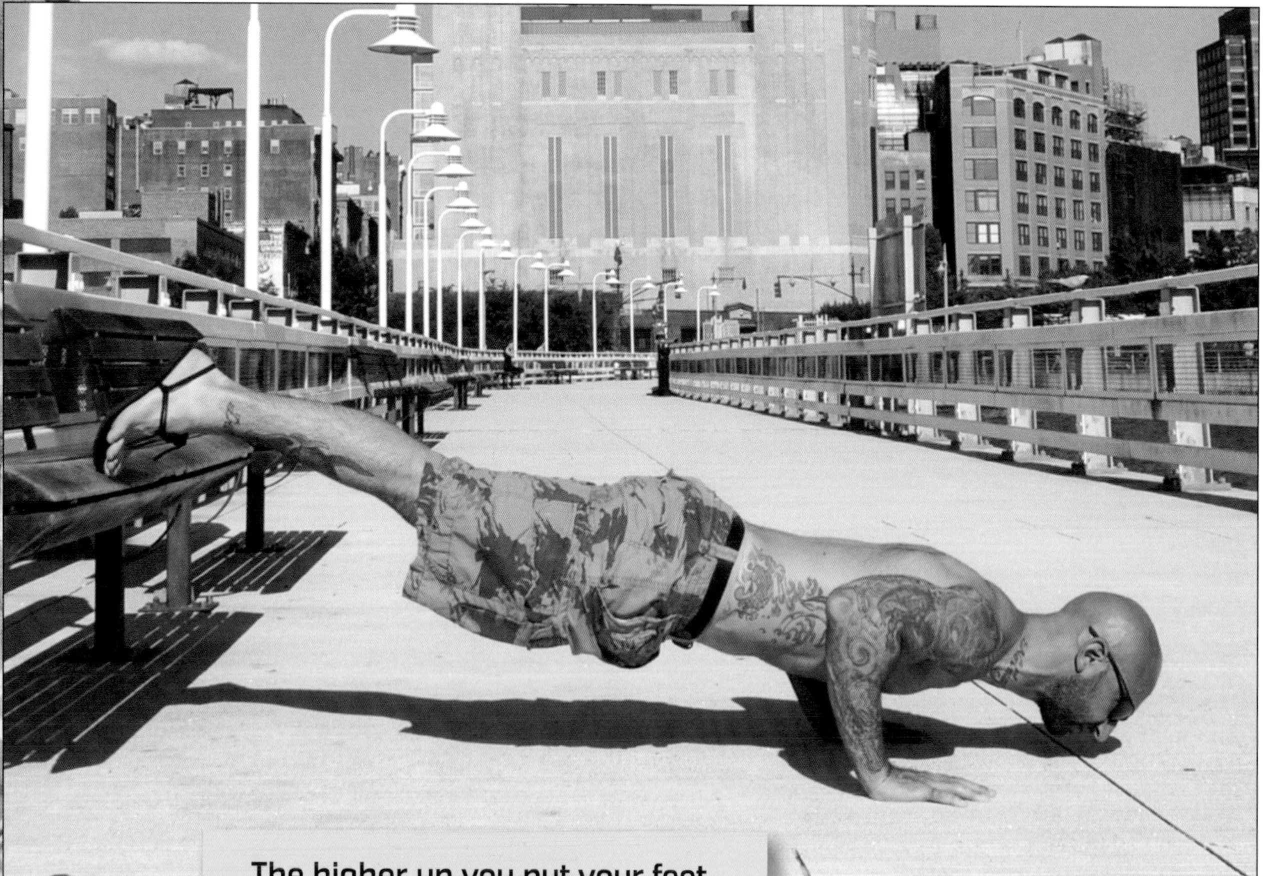

The higher up you put your feet, the harder the exercise becomes.

Knuckle Push-up

Doing push-ups on your fists is totally badass, plus knuckle push-ups allow for a bigger range of motion than flat palm push-ups. That extra few inches of depth can make repping out a lot more challenging.

While some people's wrists may need time to acclimate to the extra work required to maintain stability during a knuckle push-up, for others, the neutral wrist position can actually make the push-up less stressful than having the wrists bent back. The skin on your hands may be sensitive when starting out, so the simple discomfort of supporting your weight on your knuckles might be an additional obstacle. You may want to start out practicing on a soft surface for this reason.

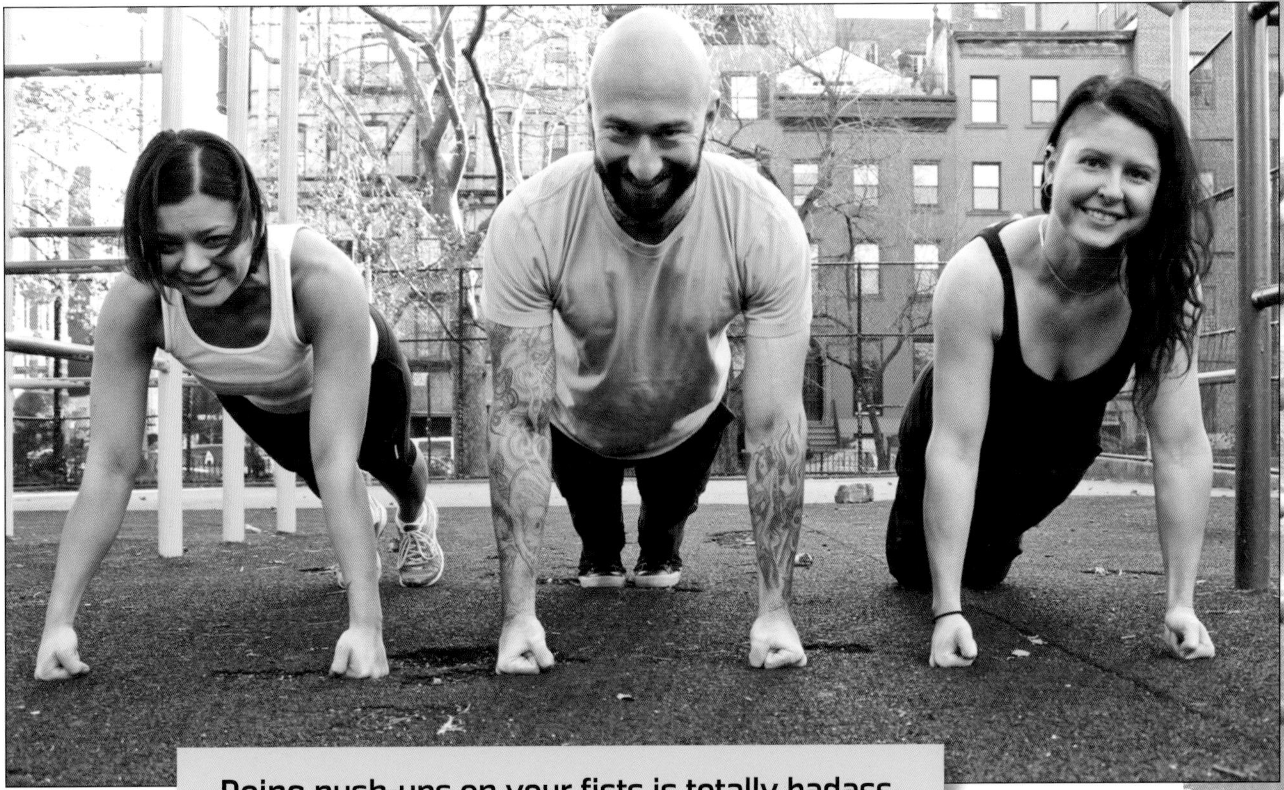

Doing push-ups on your fists is totally badass, plus knuckle push-ups allow for a bigger range of motion than flat palm push-ups.

Fingertip Push-up

Hand strength is some of the most functional strength you can have. From carrying groceries to opening jars and packages, we use our hands in day to day activity more than any other part of our body. If you want strong hands, fingertip push-ups are an essential exercise. As the hands are a key component of so many exercises, practicing fingertip push-ups can help your training across the board.

If you don't have the strength to do fingertip push-ups yet, I recommend practicing the isometric plank position on your fingertips. Start with a few seconds at a time — eventually you should be able to build to a 10 second fingertip plank. Once you've achieved that, you'll be ready to start practicing fingertip push-ups. Begin with just a few reps, slowly adding more over time.

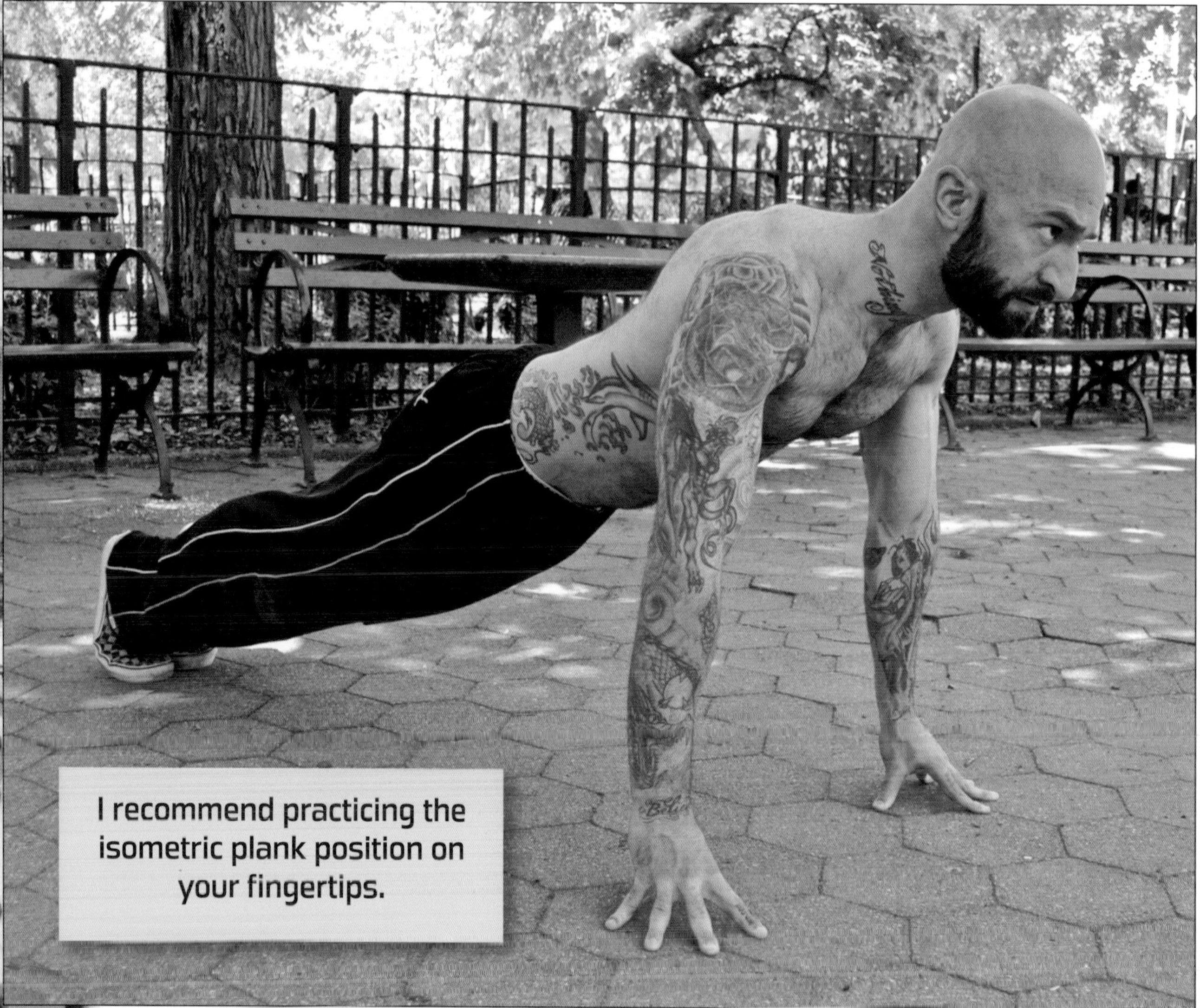

I recommend practicing the isometric plank position on your fingertips.

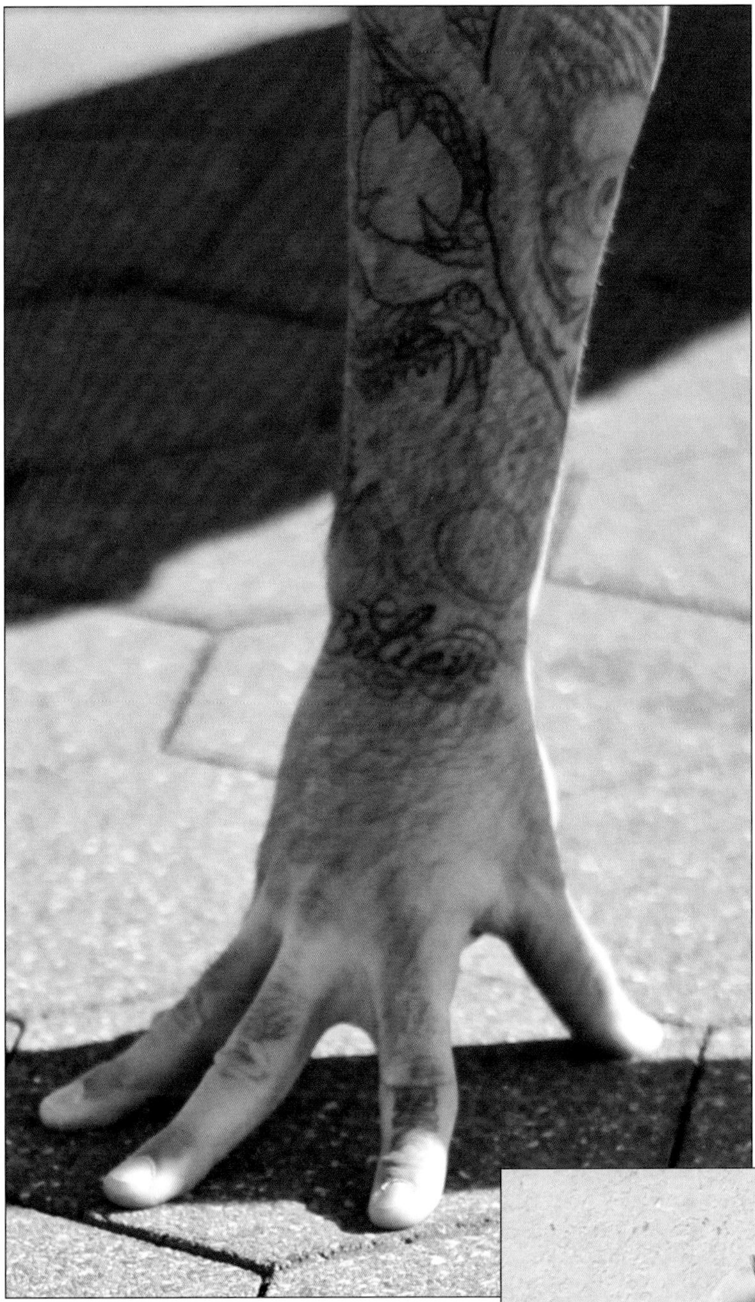

It's important to note that the term "fingertip push-up" is a bit of a misnomer. You don't actually want to be all the way on the tips of your fingers, but rather on the pads of them with the tips slightly bent back. Some people's digits will wind up bending back more than others. This is not a huge deal. Just don't allow any part of your palm to touch the ground if you want it to be legit.

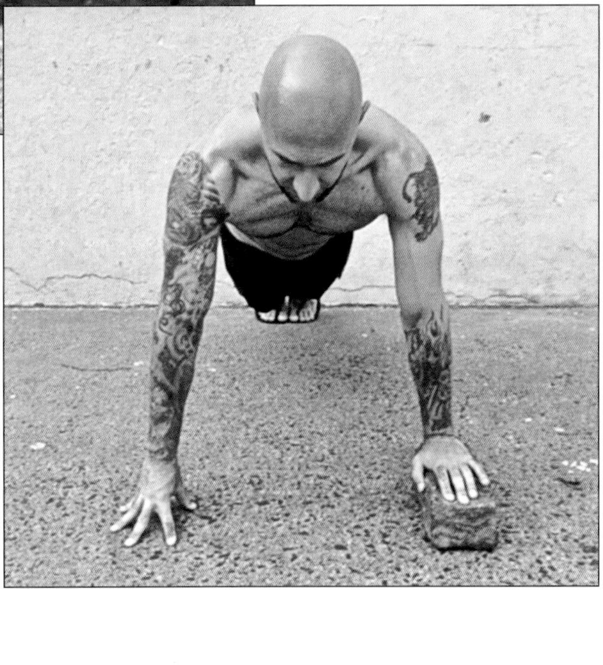

If you aren't able to hold the plank on your fingertips, try placing one hand flat on a slightly elevated object while the opposite hand is supported on the fingertips. Hold for several seconds, then switch hands.

Wrist Push-up

Wrist push-ups, aka back of the hand push-ups, have been helping athletes perform better for quite some time. Martial artists, gymnasts and other people looking to take their body to the limit of its physical potential have long been known to benefit from training wrist push-ups. Though this can be a potentially hazardous exercise, with increased risk can come increased benefits. Just like knuckle push-ups, I recommend training on a soft surface, as the skin on the backs of your hands will likely feel sensitive and chafe easily when starting out. In time you can condition yourself to performing them on pavement, but you have to give your body time to adapt to new stimuli. With that in mind, the most you'll want to work on this move in the beginning is once or twice a week. After a while your wrists will adapt and become stronger, then you can add more volume as you see fit.

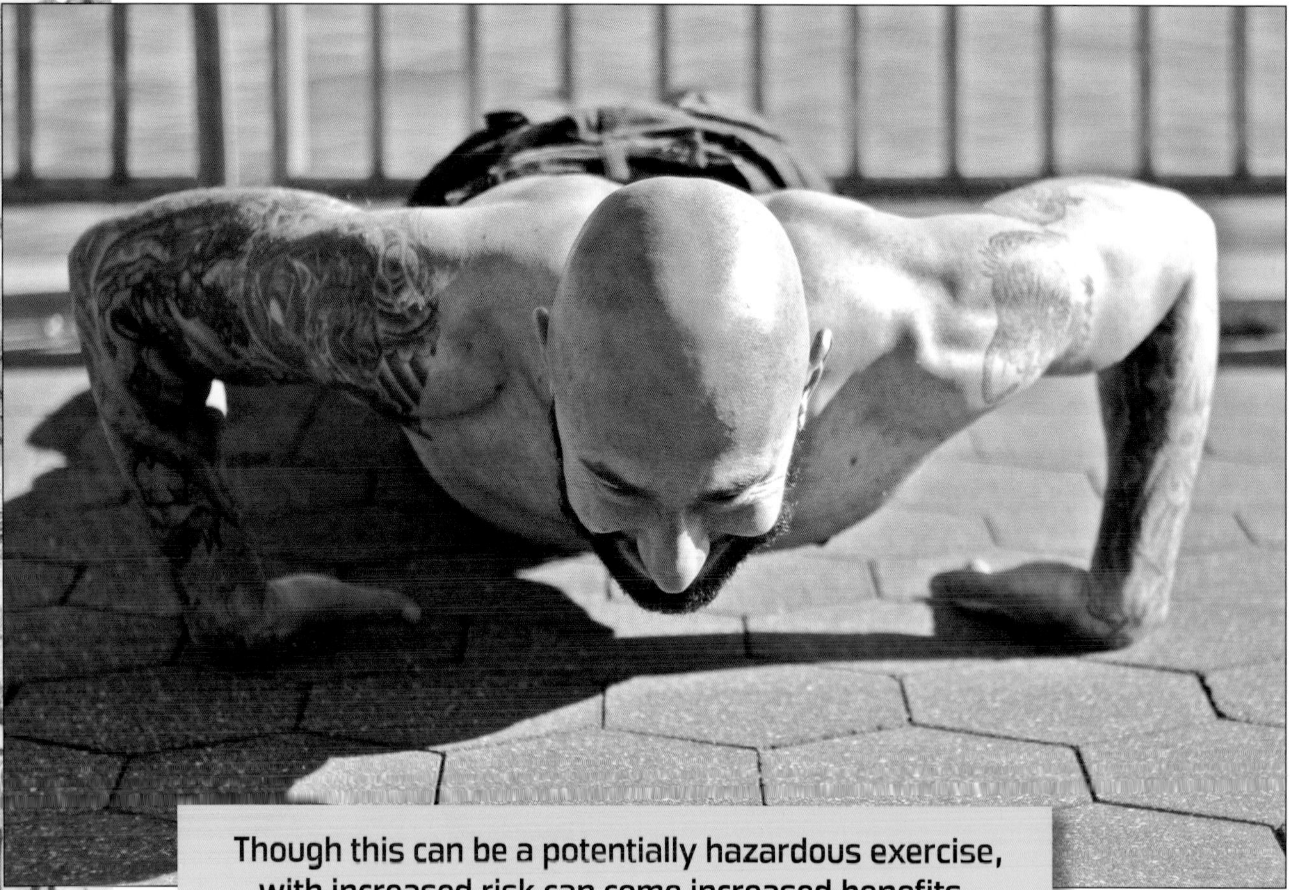

Though this can be a potentially hazardous exercise, with increased risk can come increased benefits.

One And One Push-up

Before going for a full wrist push-up, you might try a push-up with one hand on the palm and the other backwards. I call this a "one and one" push-up. Some people may feel more comfortable with their backward hand facing inward rather than completely upside down (see photo). To keep things balanced, switch which hand is face up on alternating sets. After a couple of sessions (or longer depending on individual conditioning) you may be ready to progress to full back of the hand push-ups.

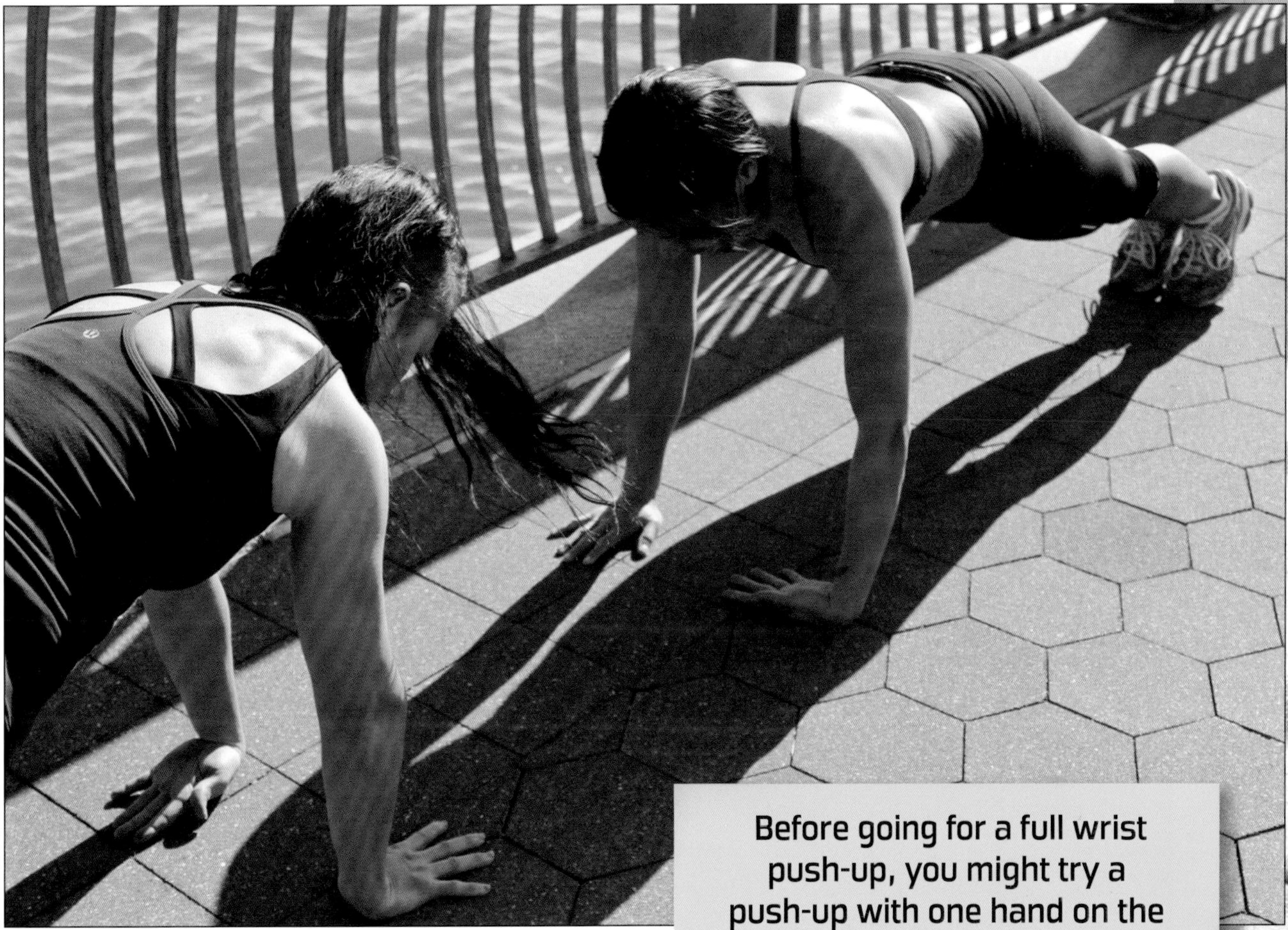

Before going for a full wrist push-up, you might try a push-up with one hand on the palm and the other backwards.

Handstand Push-up

A handstand push-up is almost an entirely different exercise than the standard push-up. While a typical push-up involves pressing in the horizontal plane, a handstand push-up closer resembles an overhead press. The emphasis moves away from your chest and into your shoulders. Additionally, having your body in a vertical position means you are lifting much more of your total body weight than you are with your feet resting on the ground. The handstand push-up is a double whammy — you're lifting more of your weight with a smaller primary muscle group!

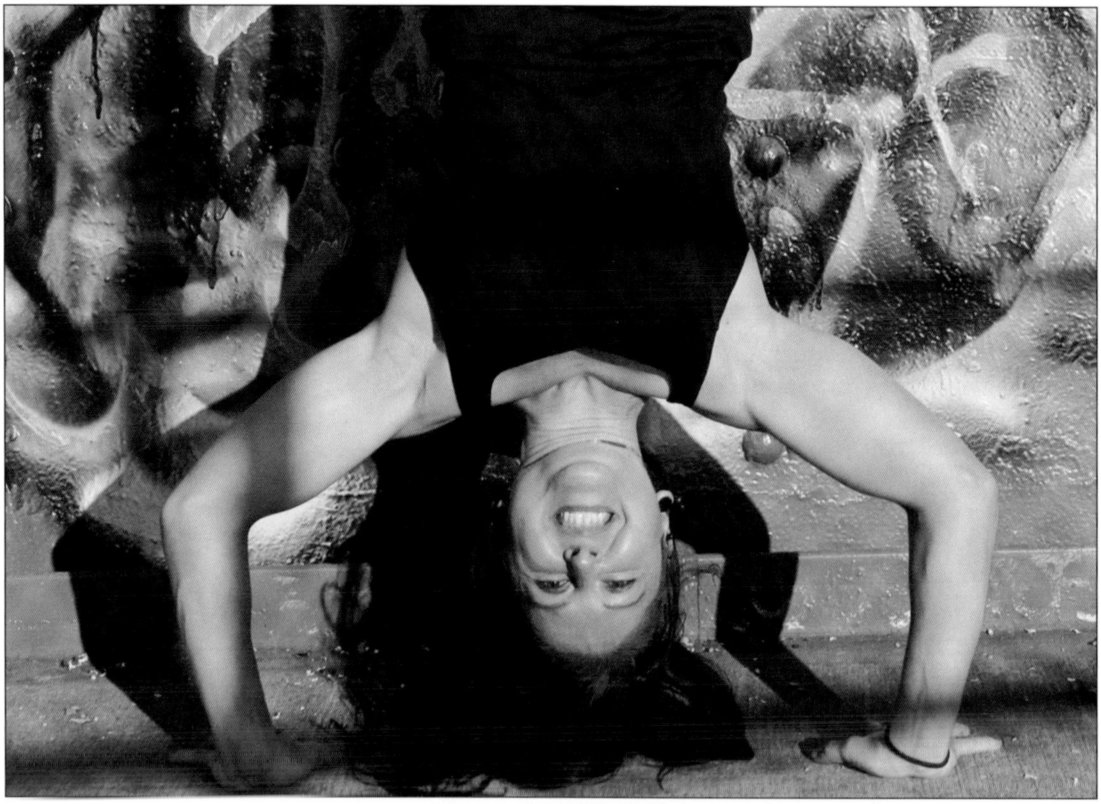

I recommend getting to at least thirty standard push-ups before attempting a handstand push-up (probably more). There's no set number that's right for everyone, but this is not an appropriate exercise for a beginner trainee.

When you are ready to start learning handstand push-ups, practice with your legs resting against a wall. This will help with the balance and it will also improve your leverage, making the move less taxing on your muscles.

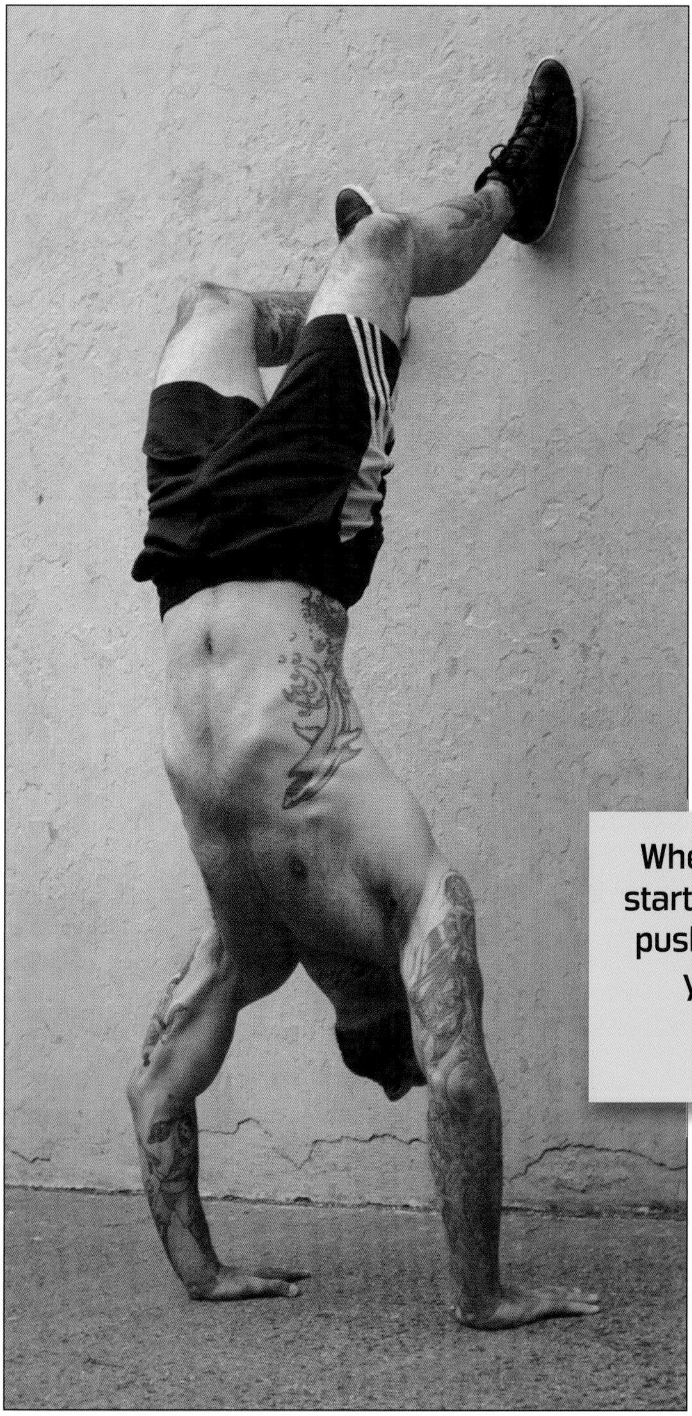

Just like any push-up, it's important not to flare your elbows out to the sides. Keep them pointed behind you instead. I recommend looking a few inches in front of your hands, rather than right in between them as you lower yourself down and press back to the top. If you've ever pressed a barbell over your head, you know that you have to move the bar around your face so you don't smack yourself in the chin or the nose. The handstand push-up is essentially the same movement pattern turned upside down.

When you are ready to start learning handstand push-ups, practice with your legs resting against a wall.

Though I recommend eventually working towards learning this skill freestanding, you should get to the point where you can perform ten consecutive handstand push-ups against a wall before attempting to do so. (*More on handstands in Chapter Six.*)

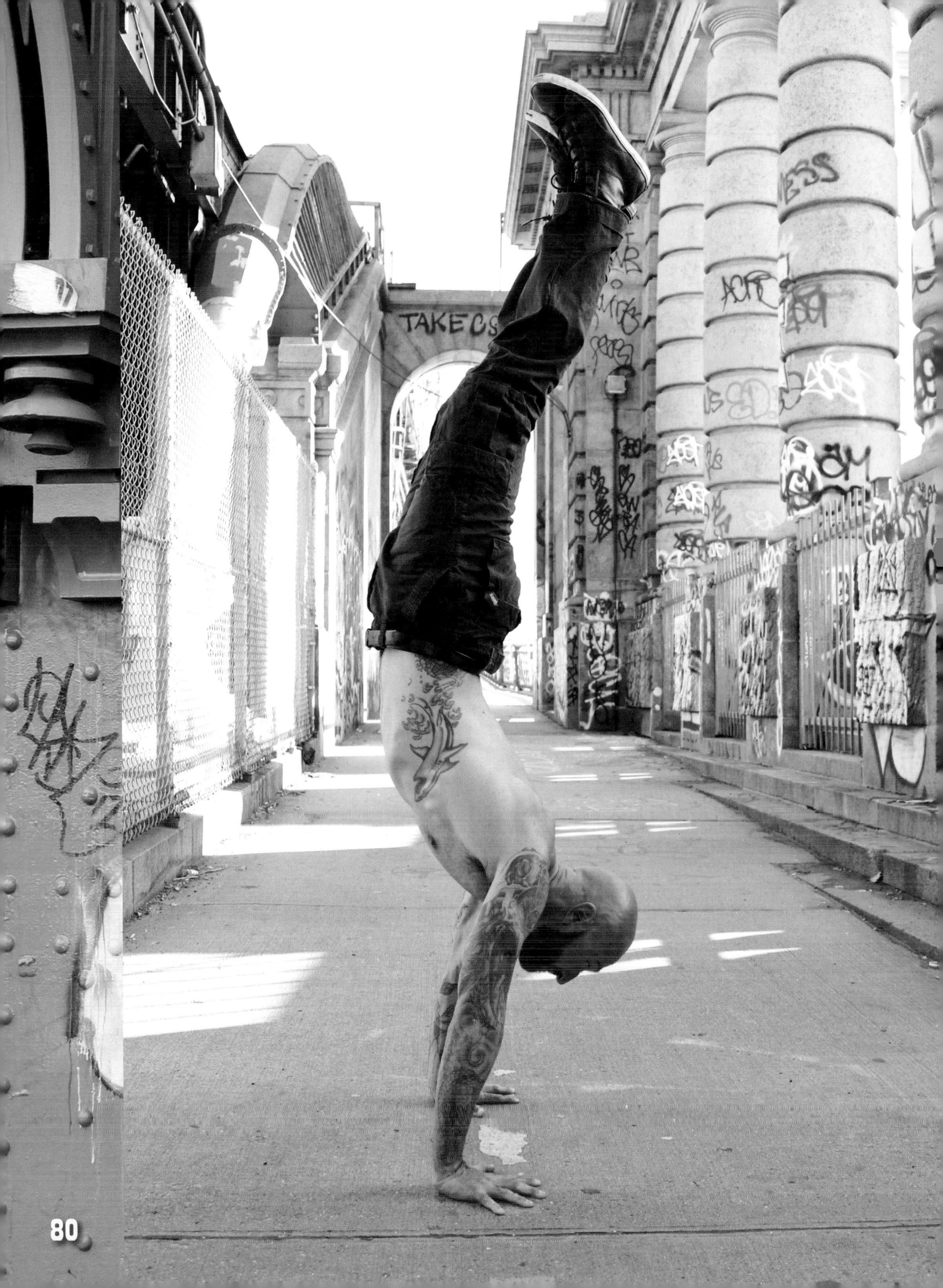
TAKECS

Pushing The Limits!

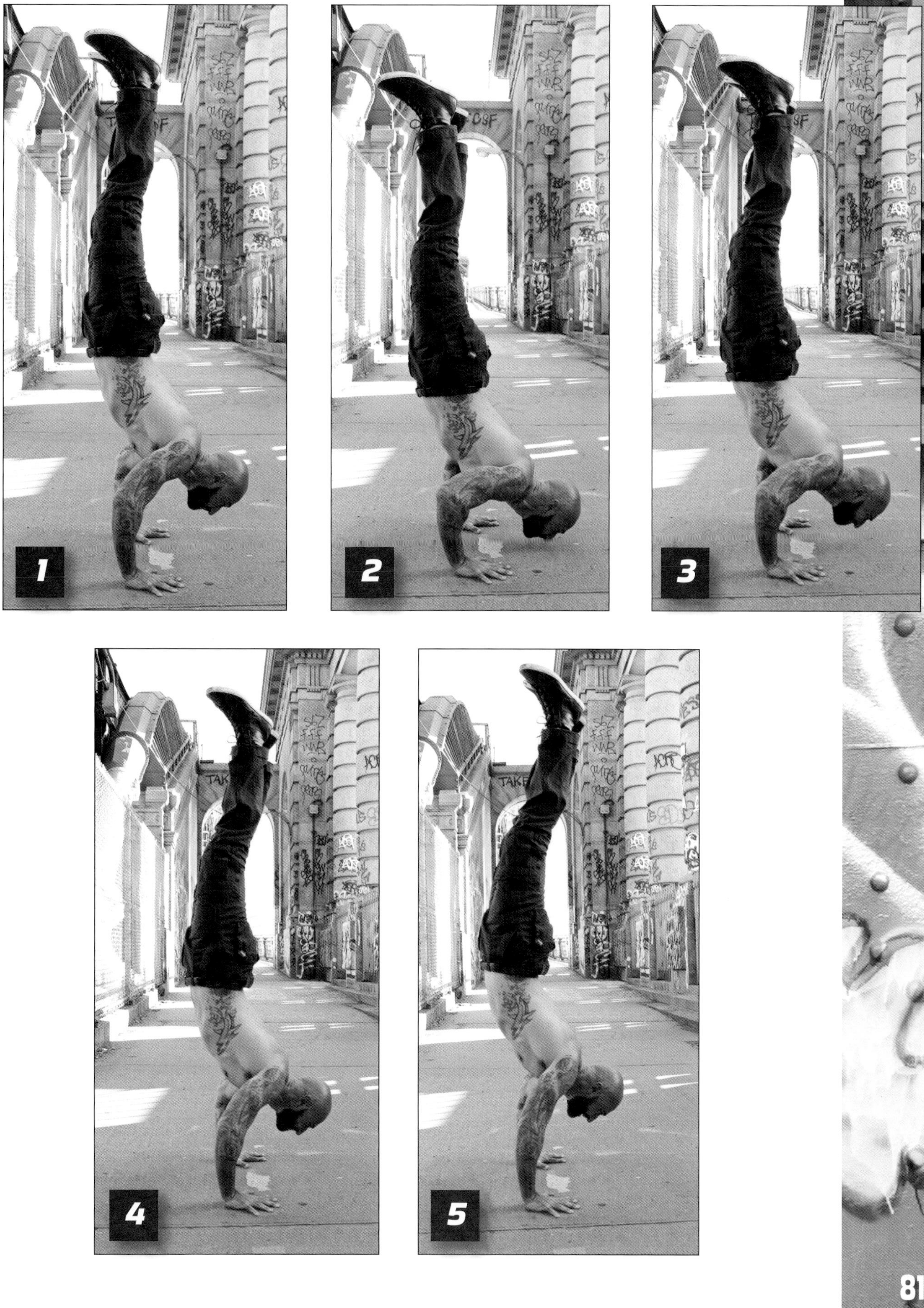

Pike Push-up

Typically I tell people not to let their butt go up in the air when they do a push-up, but there are exceptions to every rule. The pike push-up is a helpful intermediary step between the standard push-up and the handstand push-up, and as the name suggests, you actually want to pike your hips as high as they can go throughout the range of motion. The start position looks just like the yoga pose known as downward facing dog (you should feel a stretch in your hamstrings). From here, lower the top of your head towards the ground, keeping your hips up high, just like they would be in a handstand push-up. Doing this variation with your feet elevated also works well as a precursor to the full handstand push-up.

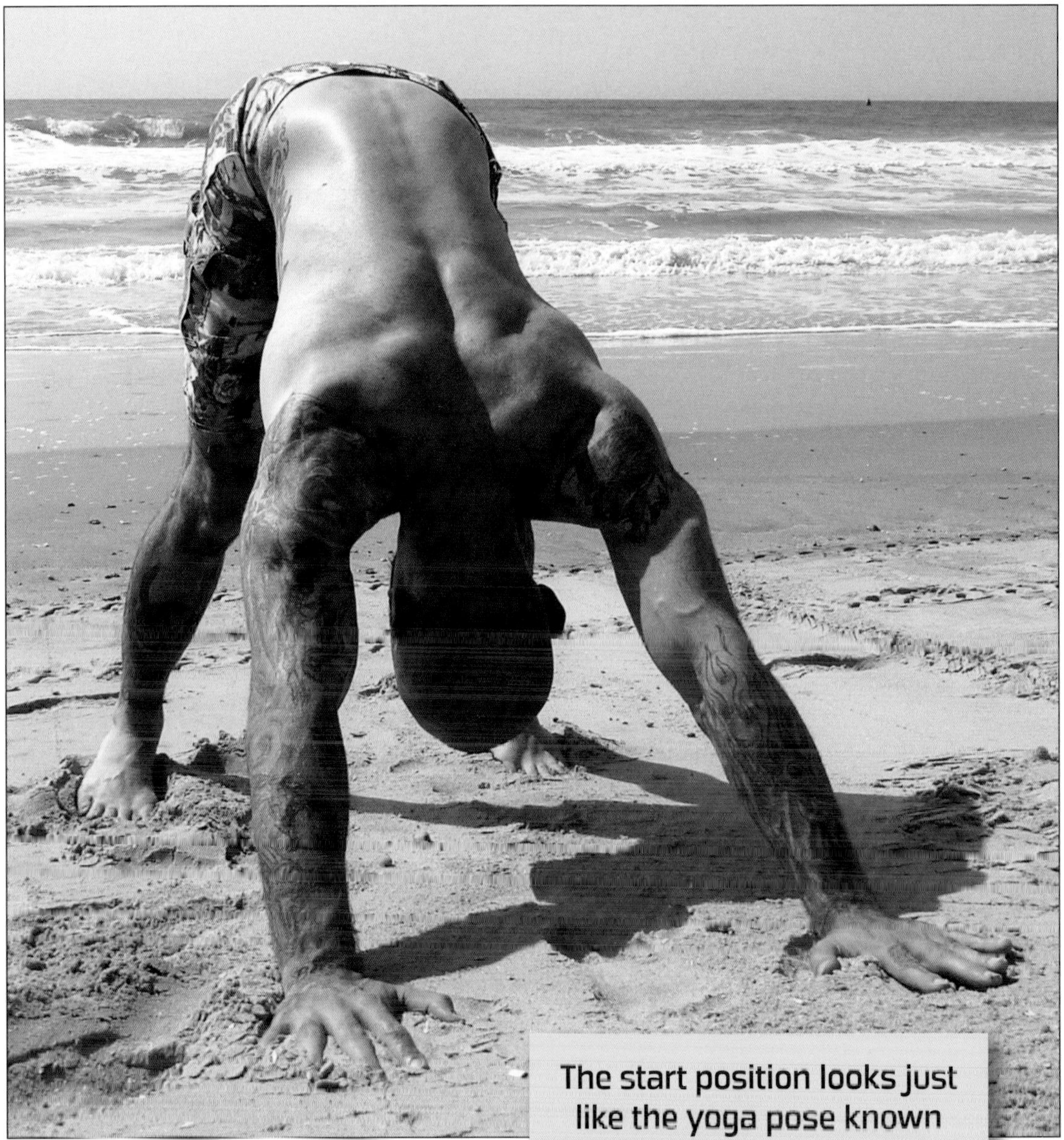

The start position looks just like the yoga pose known as downward facing dog.

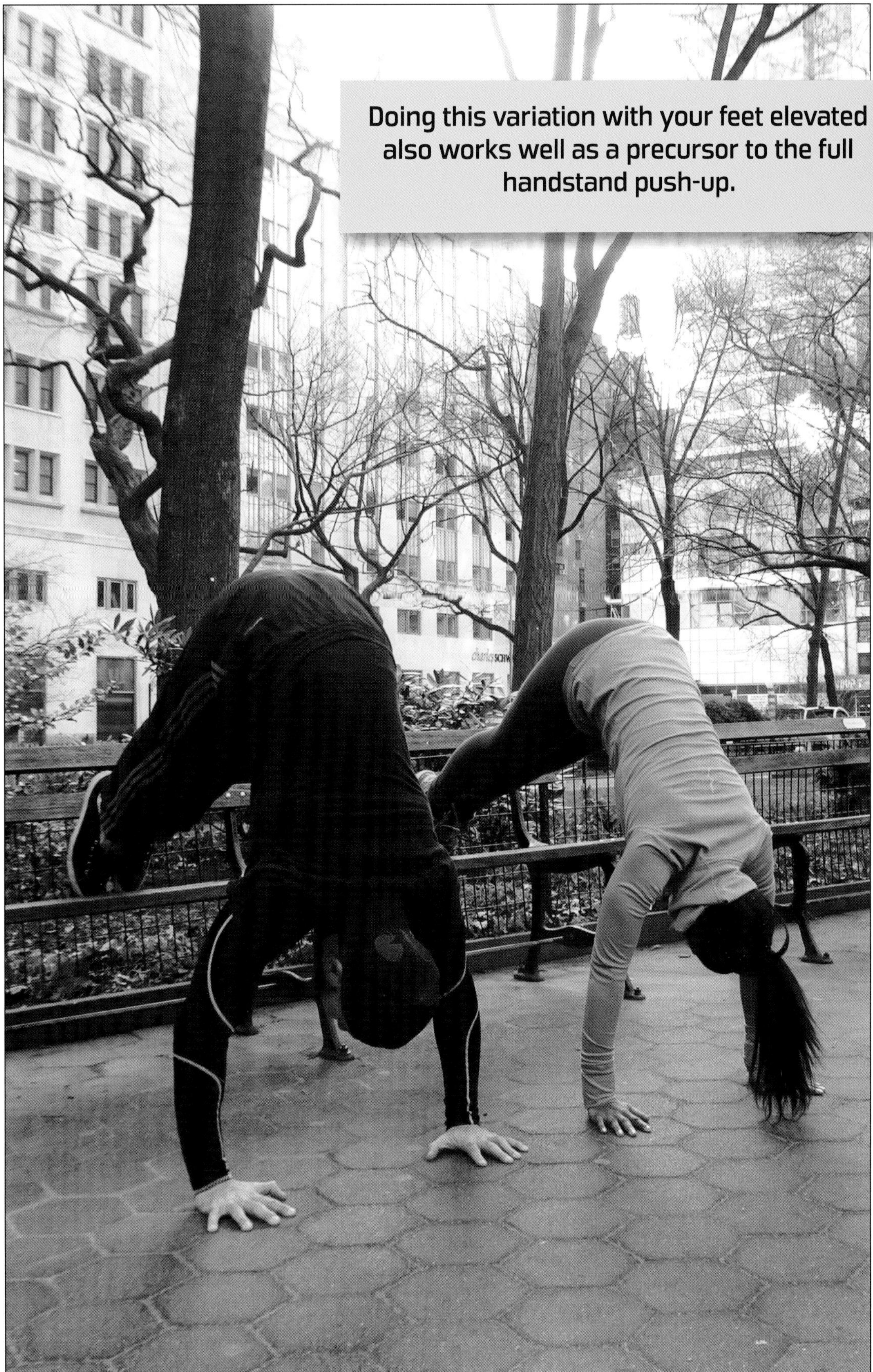

Doing this variation with your feet elevated also works well as a precursor to the full handstand push-up.

Hindu Push-ups and Dive Bombers

Hindu push-ups and dive bombers are two variations that start in the same position as the pike push-up. Once you lower your head to the floor, however, you don't simply press back to the top. Instead, quickly drop your hips, swoop your torso up and look in the air, all in one smooth motion. The bottom position for the exercise looks like the yoga pose known as upward facing dog (you should feel a stretch in your chest, neck and abs). Don't allow your shoulders to shrug.

If you're doing a Hindu push-up, you'll keep your arms straight as you raise your hips back up in the air and push your chest towards your thighs to resume the pike position. If you're doing a dive bomber, you'll reverse the swoop movement to return to the start position. For most people, the dive bomber is the more difficult of the two.

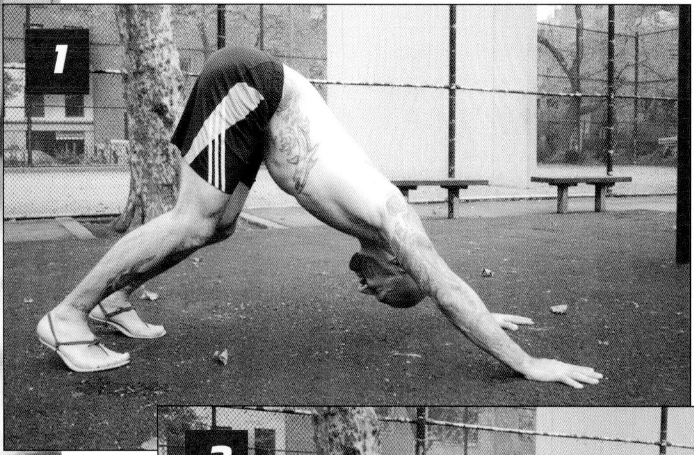

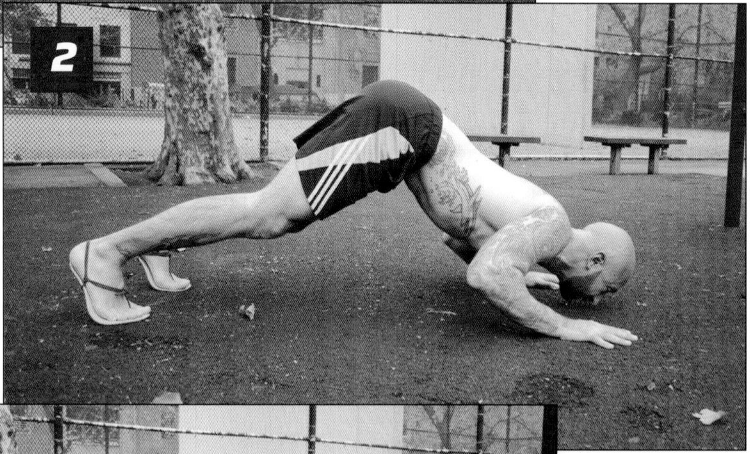

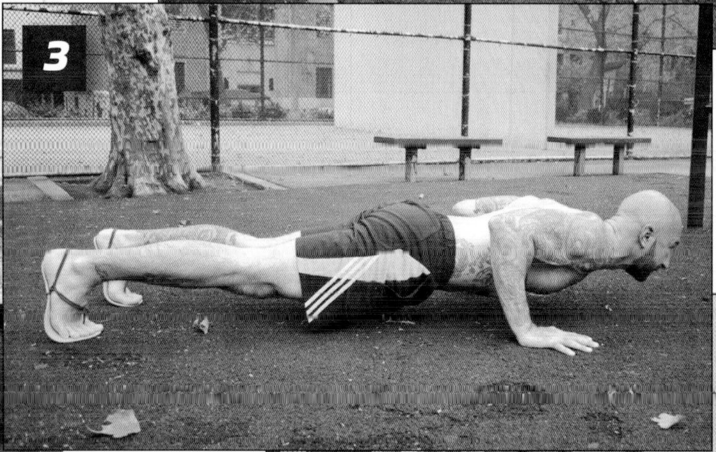

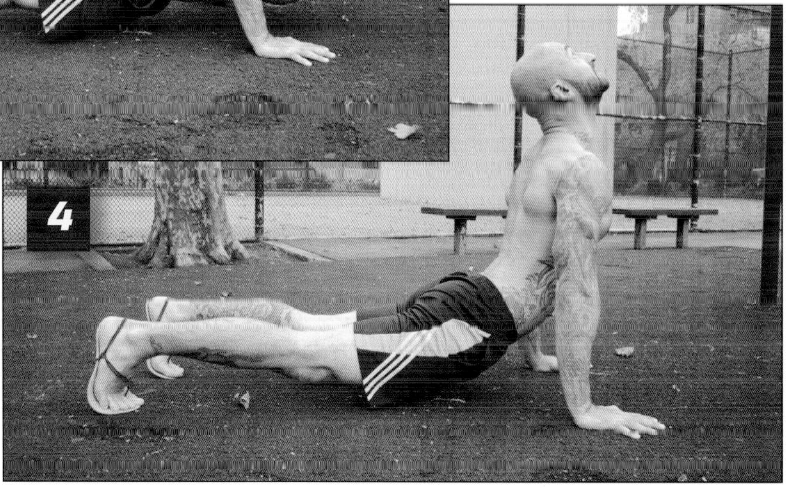

Archer Push-up

The movement of an archer push-up goes from side to side as well as up and down. Begin with your hands much wider than you would for a standard push-up, then slide yourself toward one side while you extend your opposite arm. Push yourself back to the center and then go to the other side. Fee free to play around with gradually moving your arms out farther on each rep to allow for a full range of motion. The position you'll find yourself in at the bottom should look almost like an archer drawing a bow and arrow. This is one of the first techniques you can use to eventually build toward a one arm push-up.

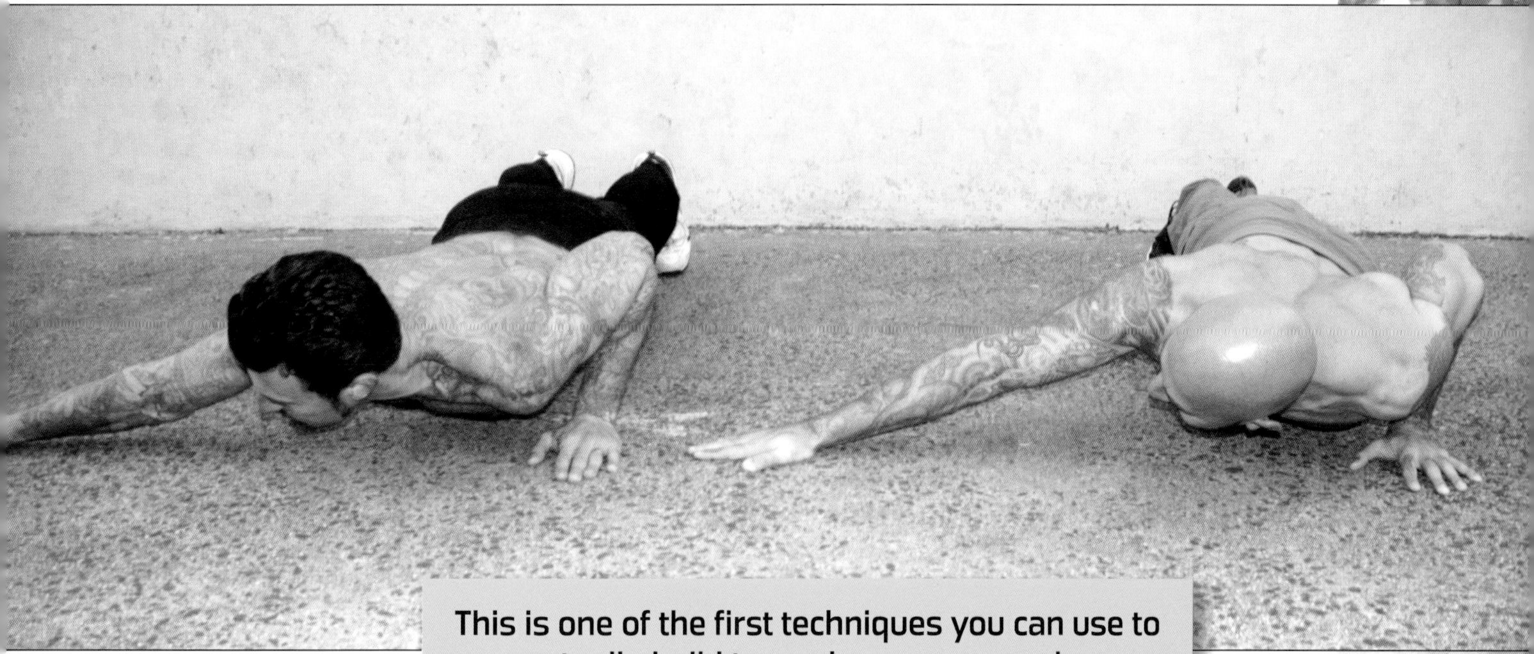

This is one of the first techniques you can use to eventually build toward a one arm push-up.

Uneven Push-up

An uneven push-up involves keeping your hands on two separate surfaces of different heights. You can play around with how much of your weight is placed on the upper arm versus the lower arm. Gradually conditioning one arm to bear most of the weight this way can be another helpful technique to work towards a one arm push-up.

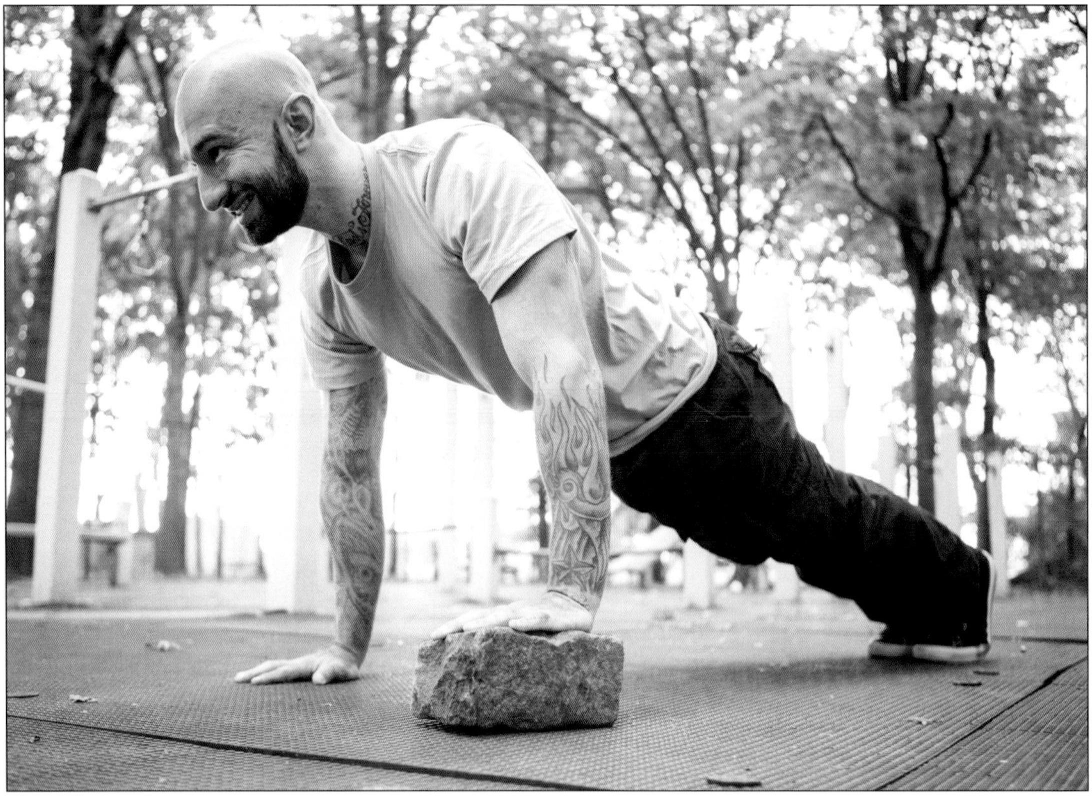

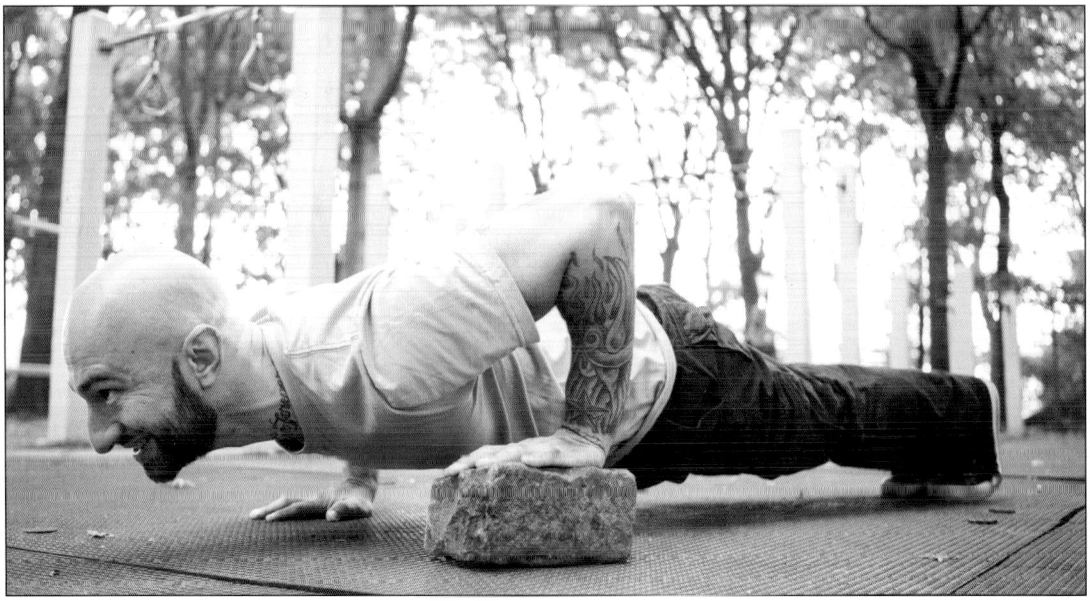

Staggered Push-up

Any type of push-up where you have one hand closer to your body than the other is a staggered push-up. Variations can include one hand in and one hand out or one hand low and one hand high. You can also experiment with staggered foot positions. It is helpful to practice pushing your body weight from many different angles. This way you are unlikely to find yourself in a situation where you cannot utilize your strength effectively.

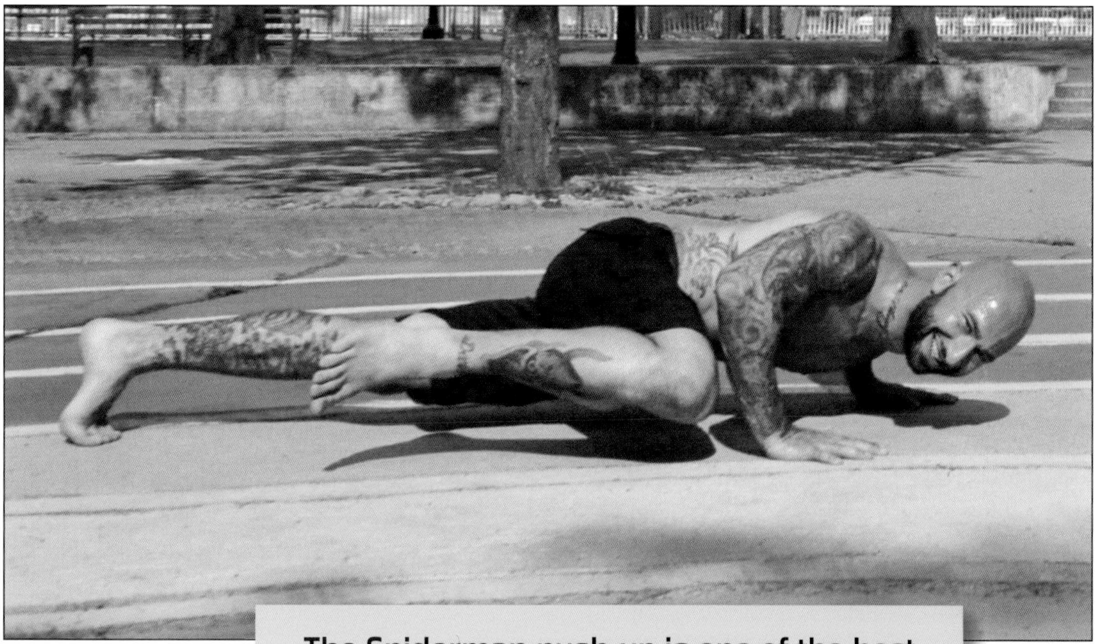

The Spiderman push-up is one of the best known types of staggered push-up.

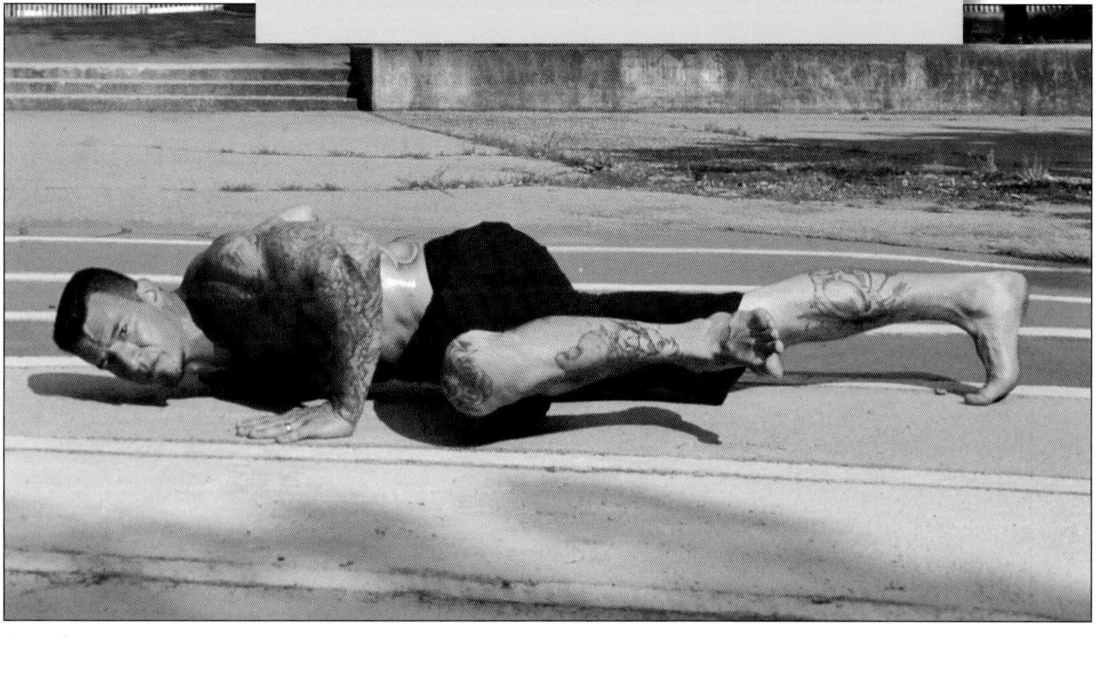

Pseudo Planche Push-up

Just like keeping your hands close together changes the leverage of a push-up, keeping them down by your hips also makes the exercise more difficult. The lower you place your hands, the harder the exercise becomes. In this variation, the hands are all the way down by your hips. Try rotating your wrists out to the sides or backwards if you lack the flexibility to bend them back far enough. You might even try placing the top of your hand on the floor (see photo). When practicing pseudo planche push-ups, you want to put as much of your weight as possible on your arms.

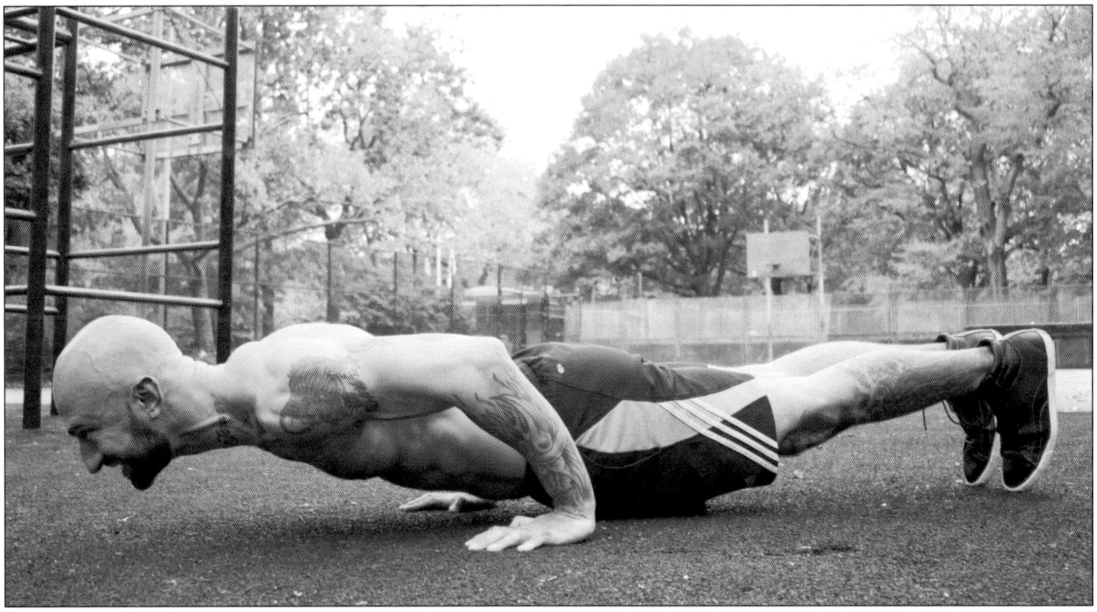

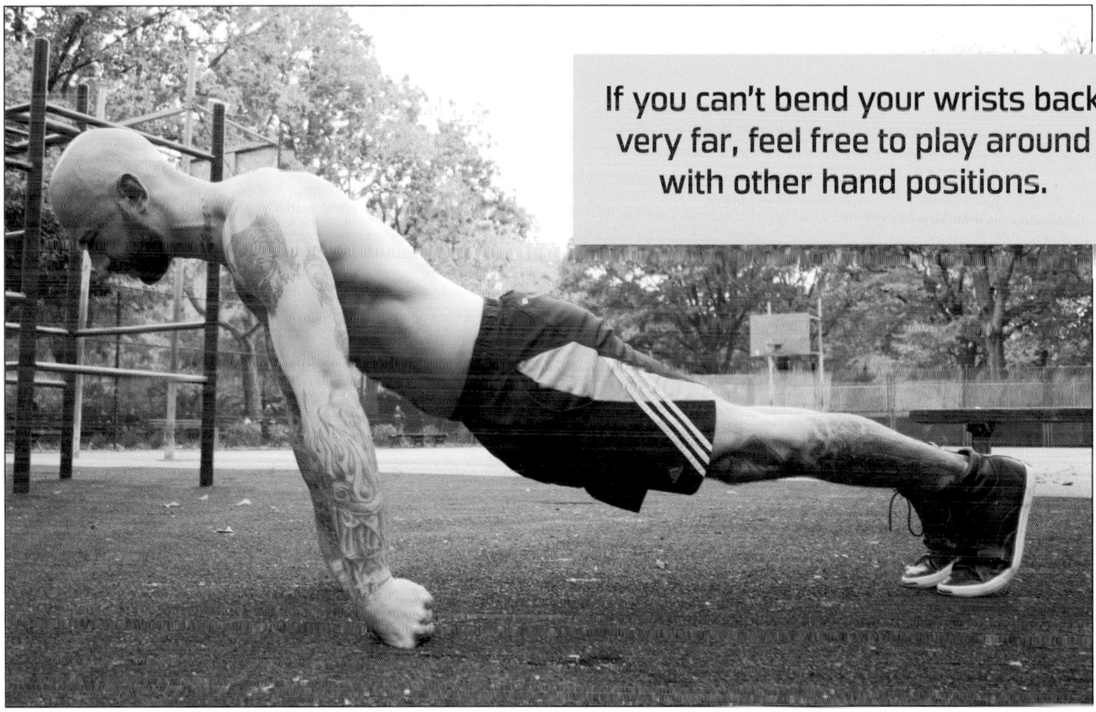

If you can't bend your wrists back very far, feel free to play around with other hand positions.

Planche Push-up

One of the most coveted moves in advanced calisthenics, a planche push-up is a variation on the gymnastics planche, which involves holding the body outstretched above the ground on only the hands. It's like a push-up floating on air! It's one of those moves that always blows people away the first time they see it performed.

While gymnasts will hold the planche with their arms locked out at the elbows the entire time, the planche push-up involves lowering yourself down and pressing yourself back up like you were doing a regular push-up — only without your feet ever touching the ground. This is actually less difficult than holding the top position, as the leverage is more in your favor with the elbows bent. In an ideal planche push-up, the body would remain totally straight, though in practice, it is normal for some arching of the back and bending of the knees to take place.

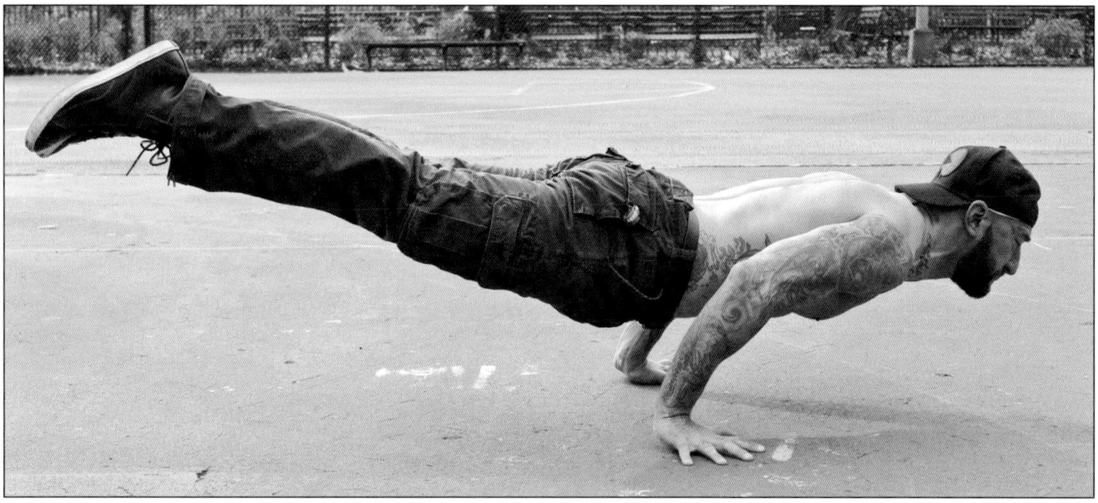

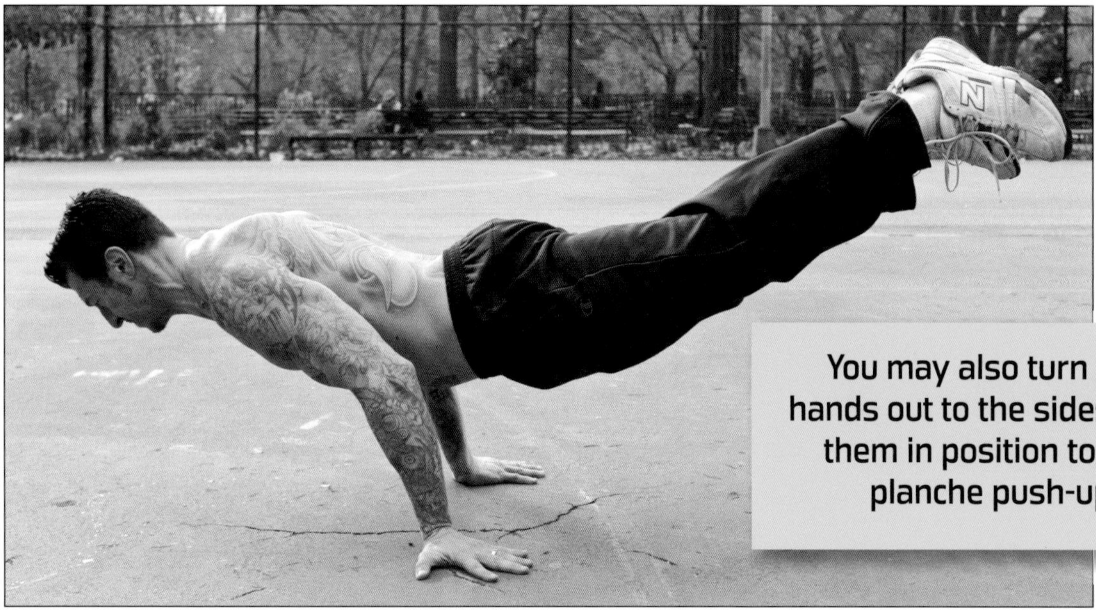

You may also turn your hands out to the sides to get them in position to do a planche push-up.

Plyometric Push-up

The term "plyometrics" is just a fancy way of talking about explosive movements. Any time you get airborne while doing an exercise, it's a plyo. The most common types of plyometrics are jumps (more on them in the next chapter) but you can also catch some air with your arms.

There are many different types of plyometric push-ups, and you need to be very strong to do any of them. The most common type of plyometric push-up is the clap push-up. As

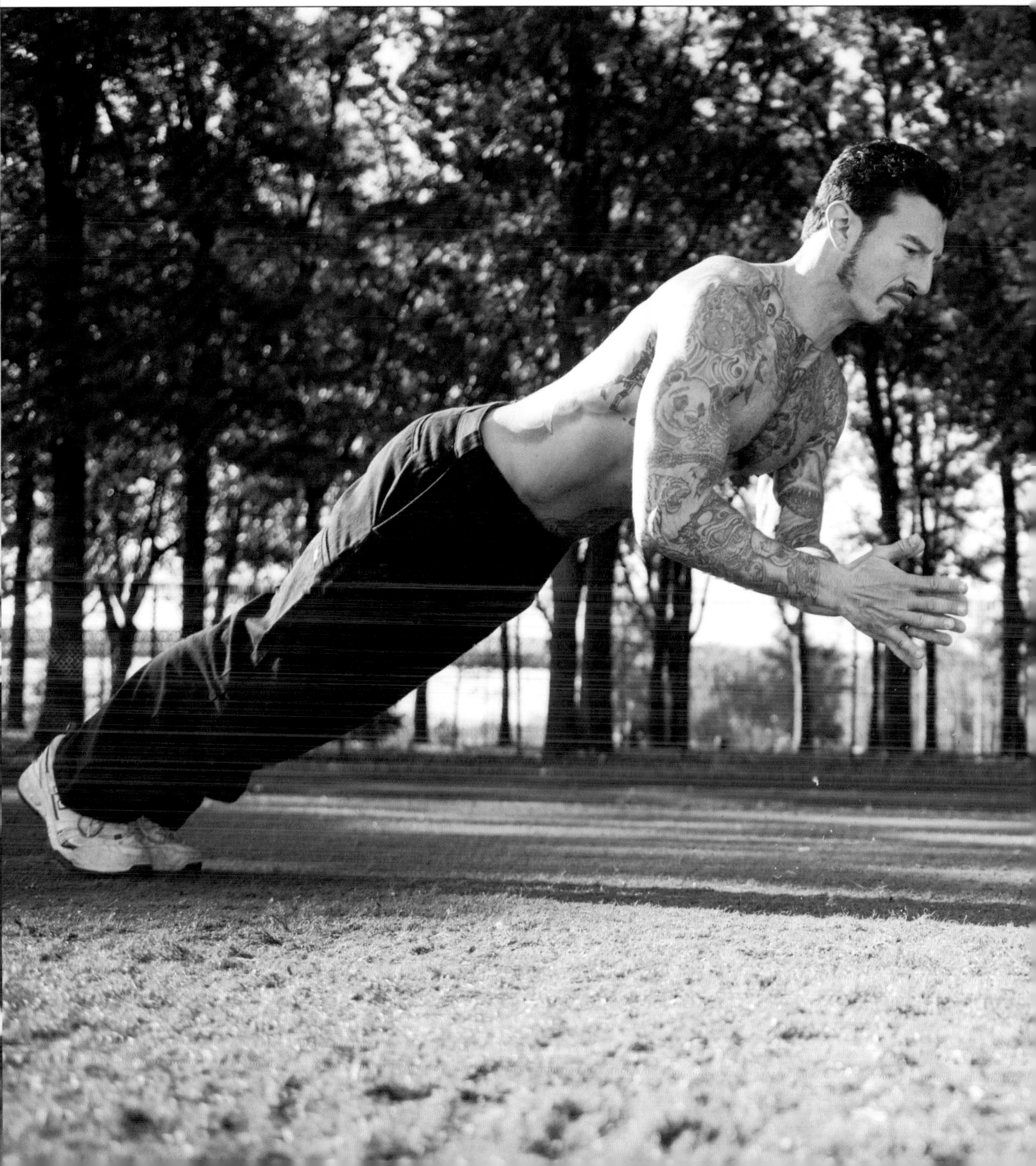

the name implies, the objective is to clap your hands in the air at the top of your push-up and return them to the ground before you fall on your face. But just in case, you might want to practice on a soft surface when starting out. Also be mindful to absorb the impact during the lowering phase and avoid landing with your elbows extended.

When performing plyo push-ups, aim to be as explosive as possible. Your objective should be to push your body as far away from the ground as you can. While speed is an important part of performing a clap push-up, getting your body high enough is what will eventually allow you to perform a behind-the-back clap, double clap or superman push-up.

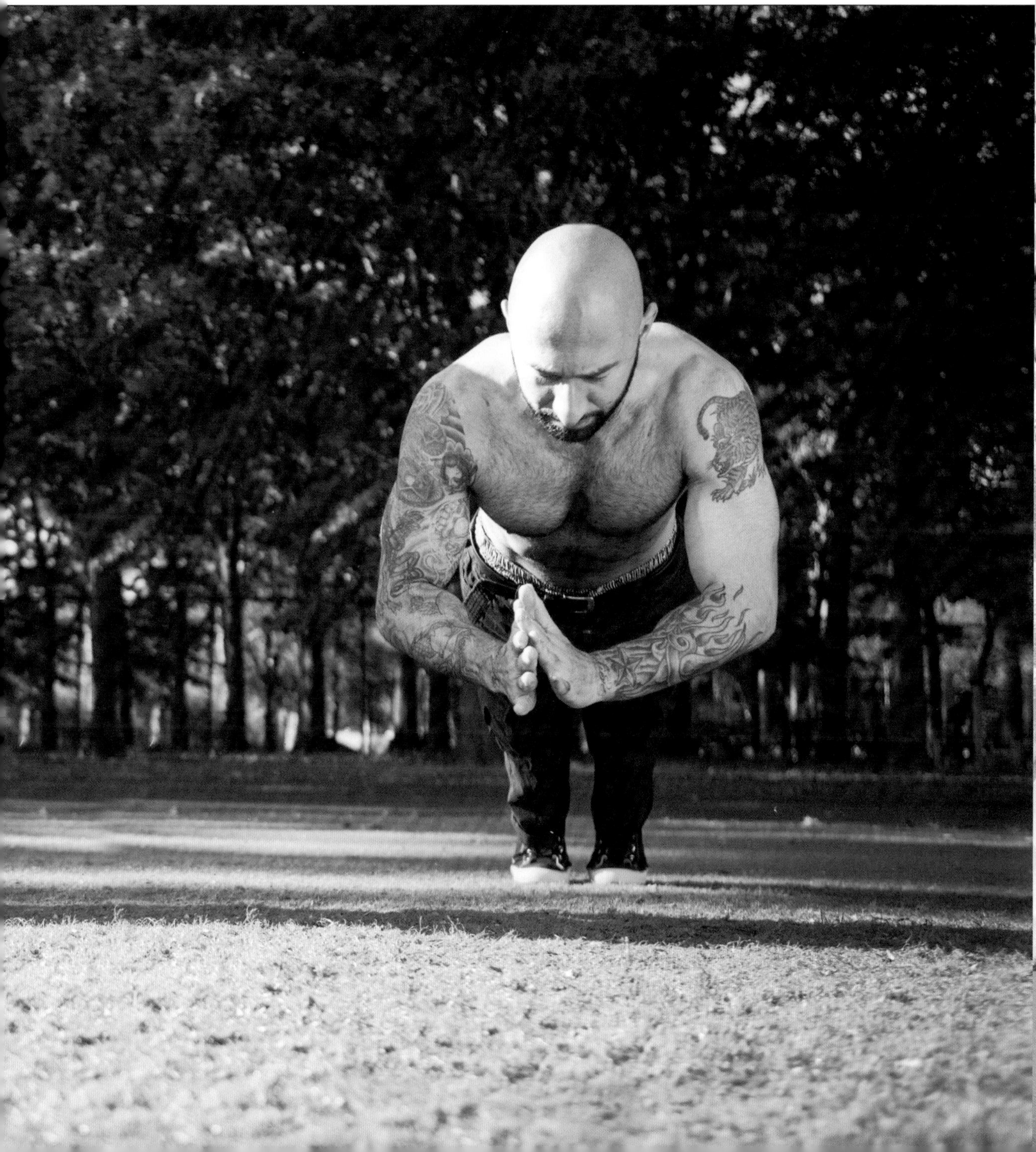

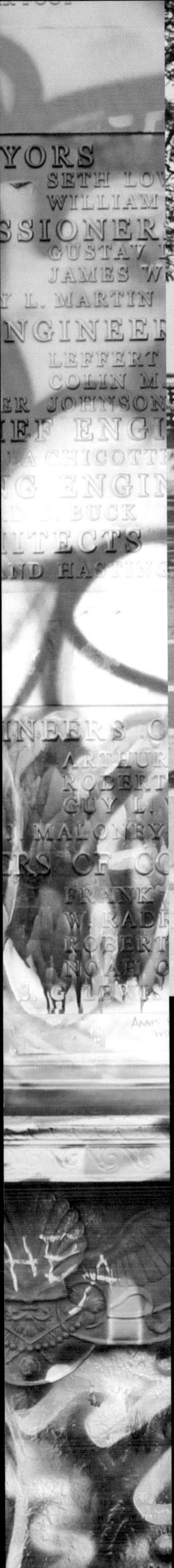
SETH LOW
WILLIAM
GUSTAV
LEFFERT
JOHNSON
BUCK

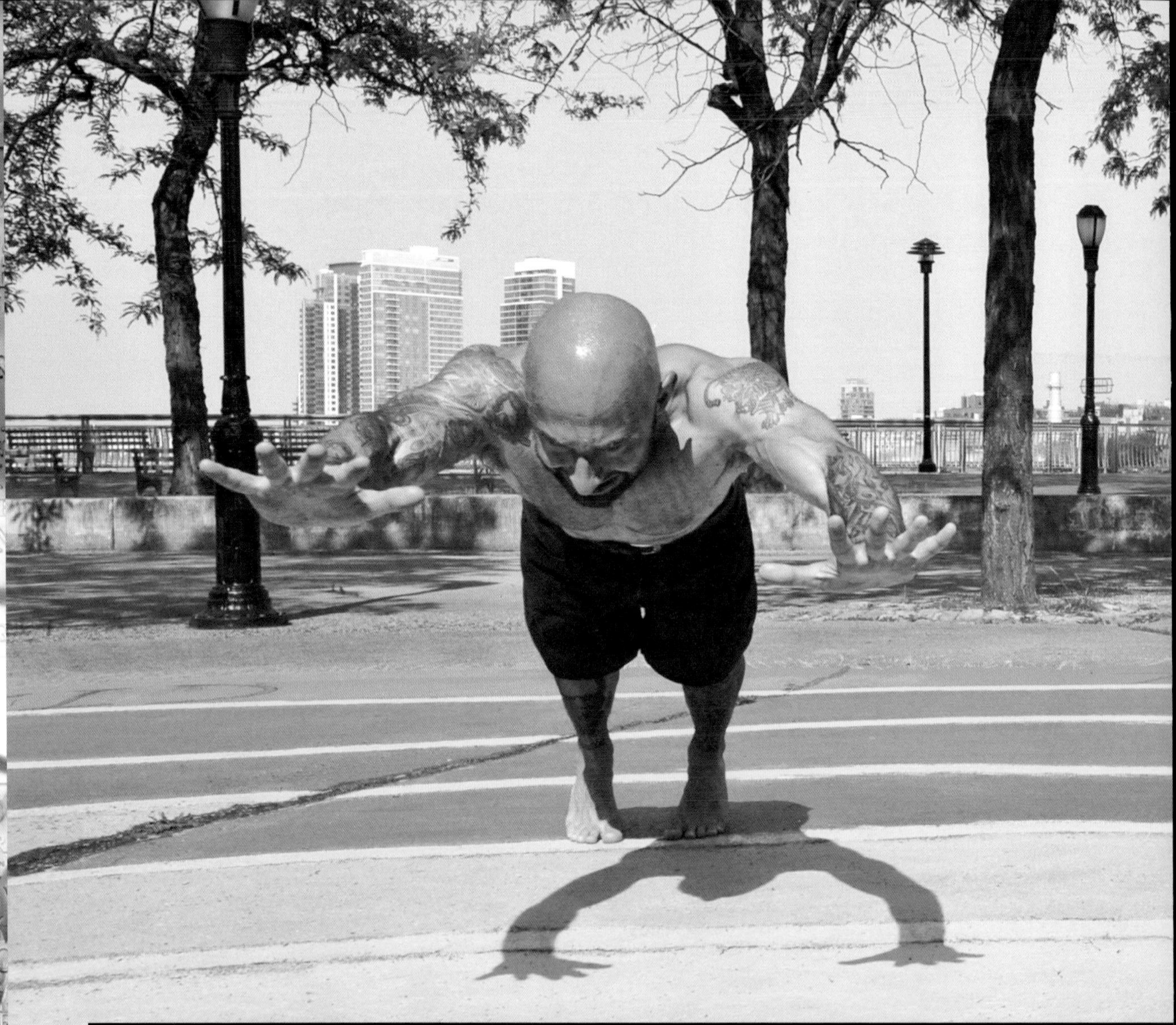

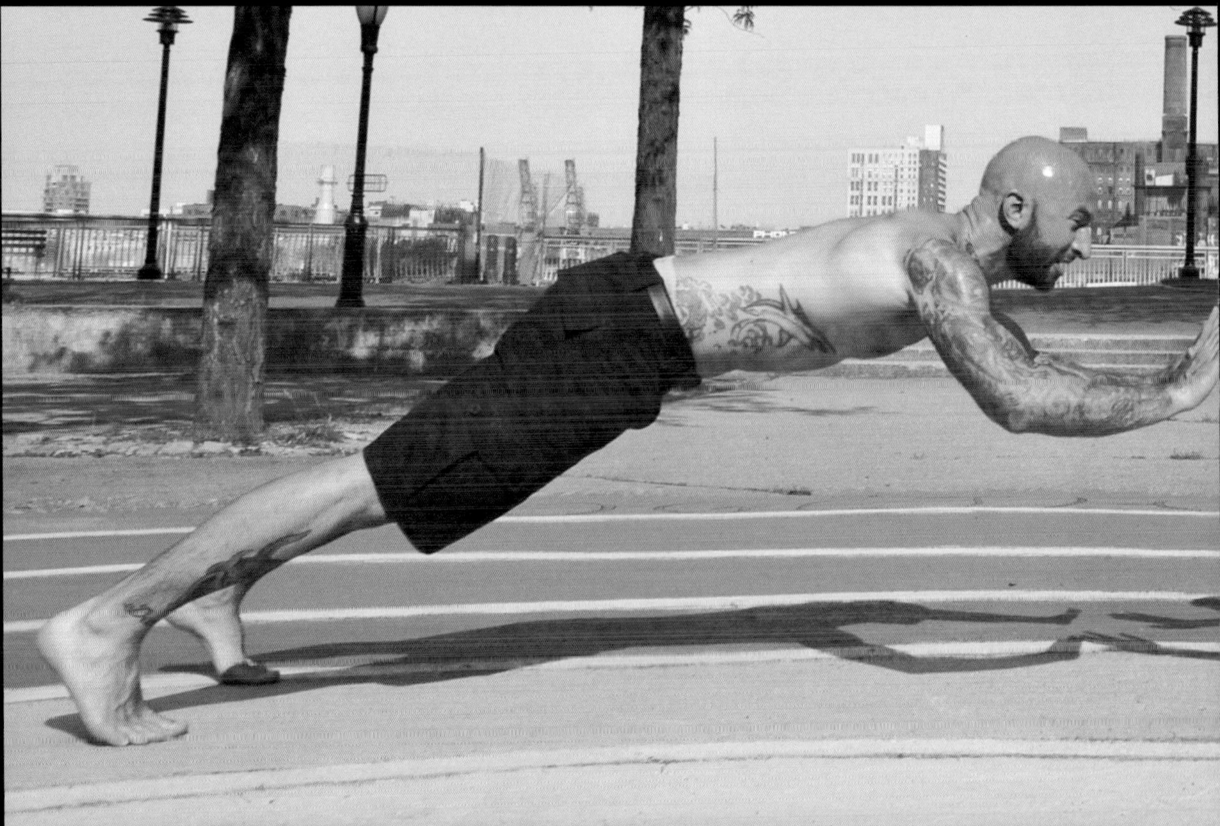

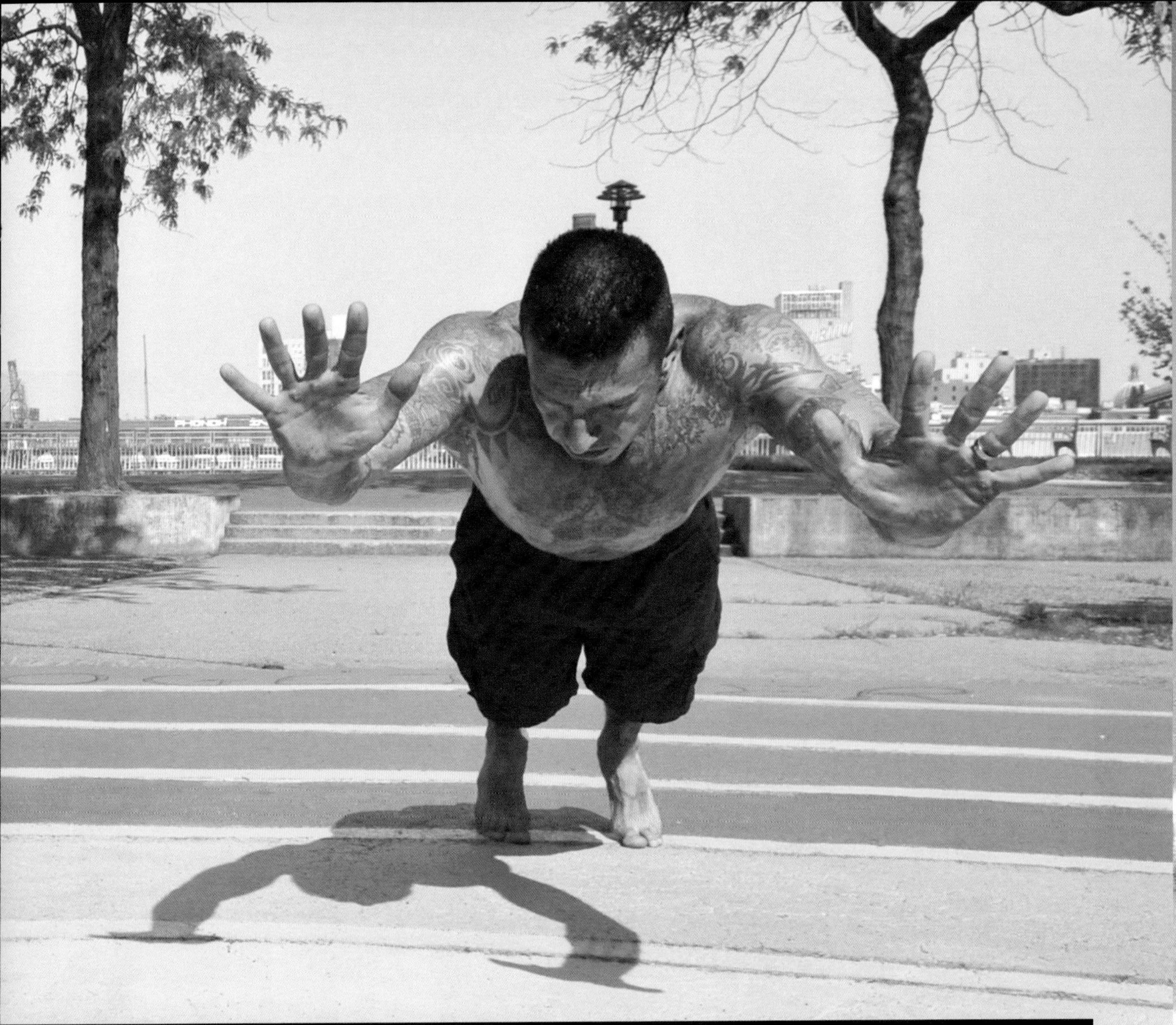

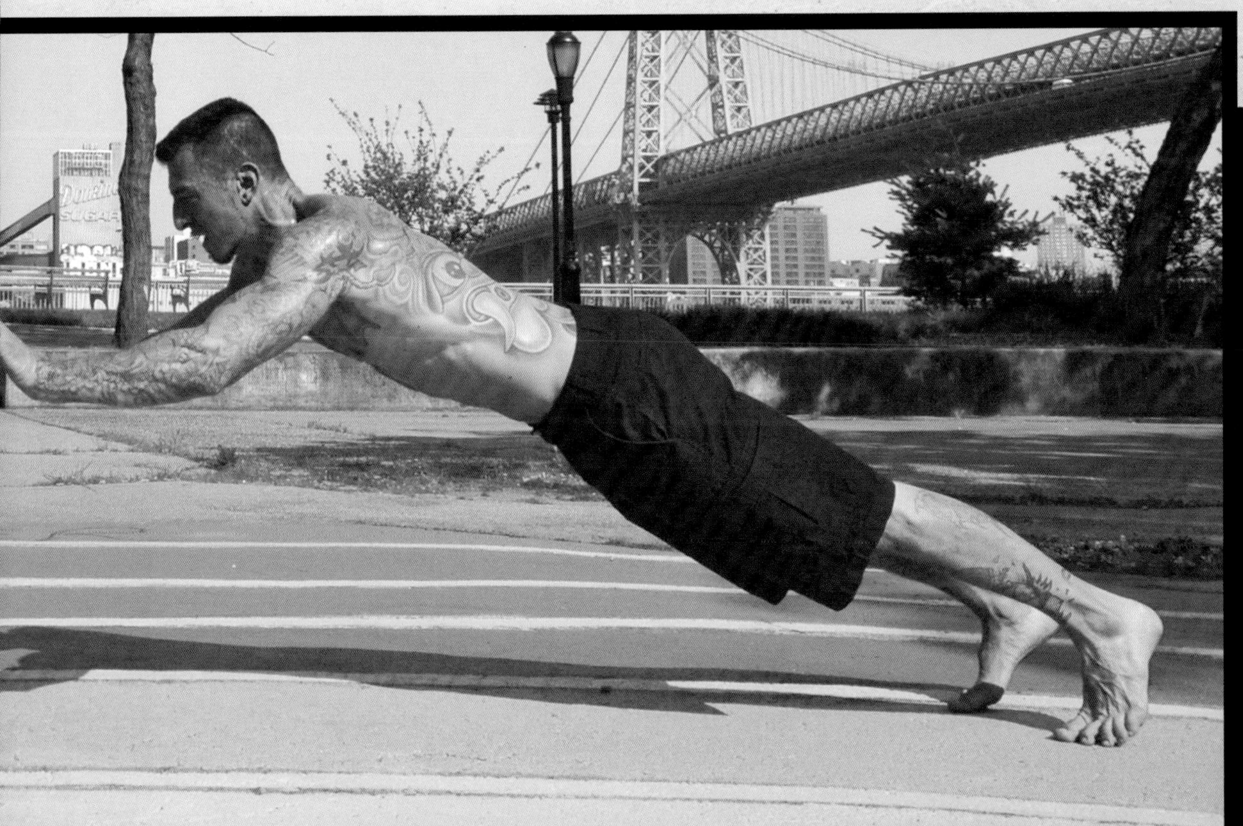

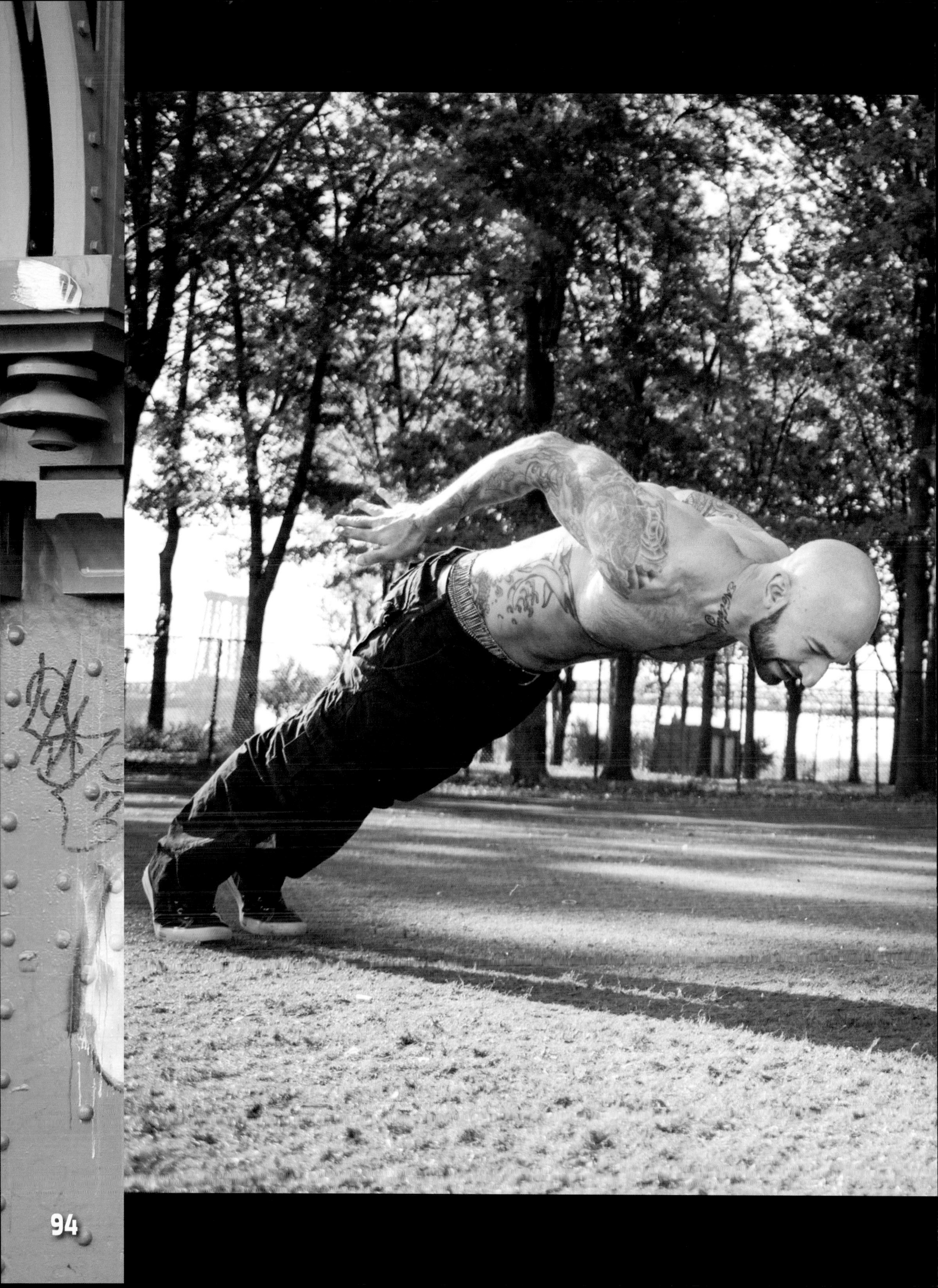

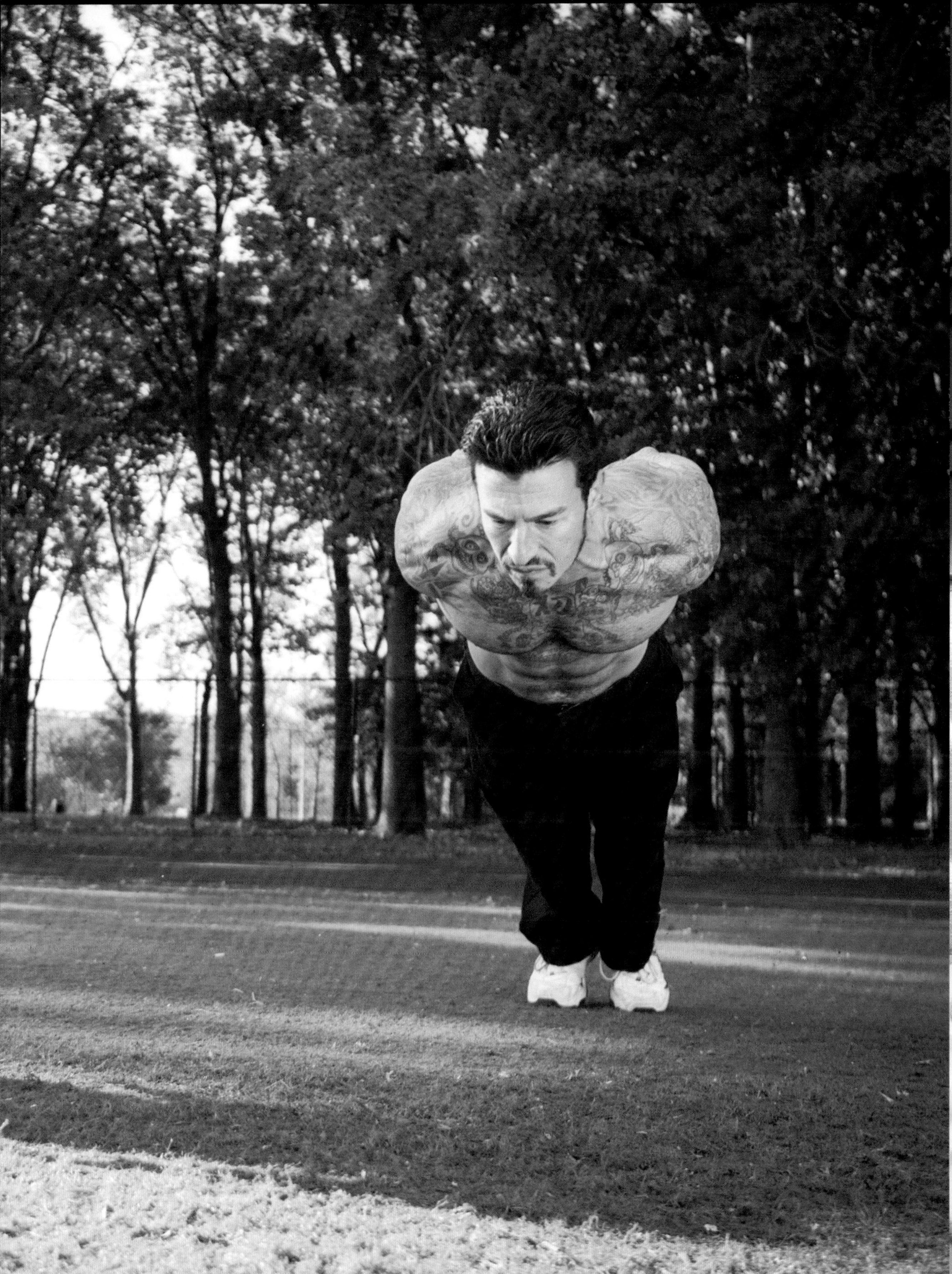

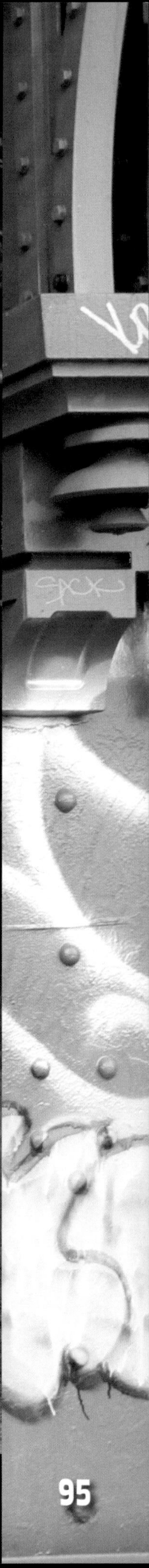

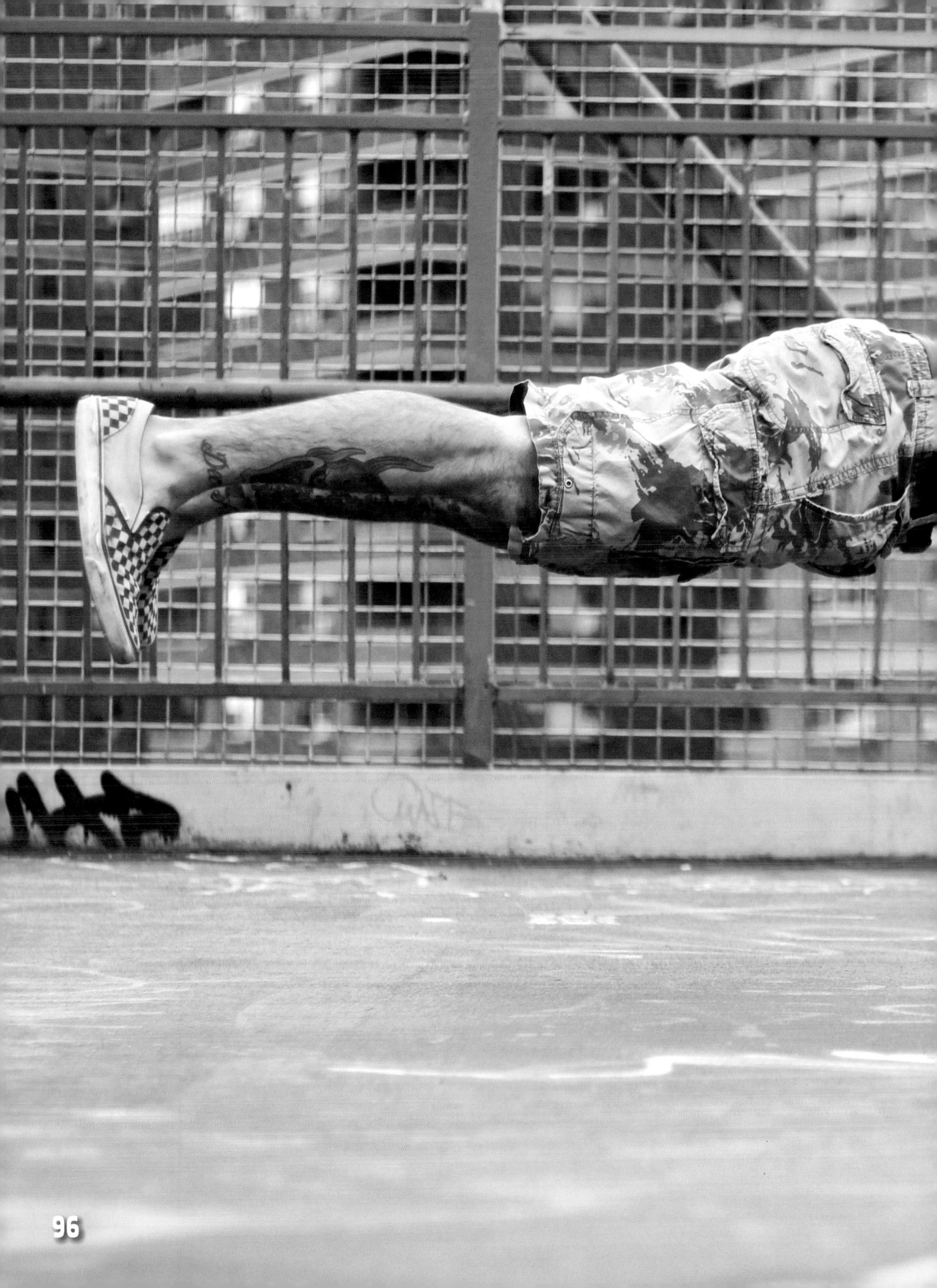

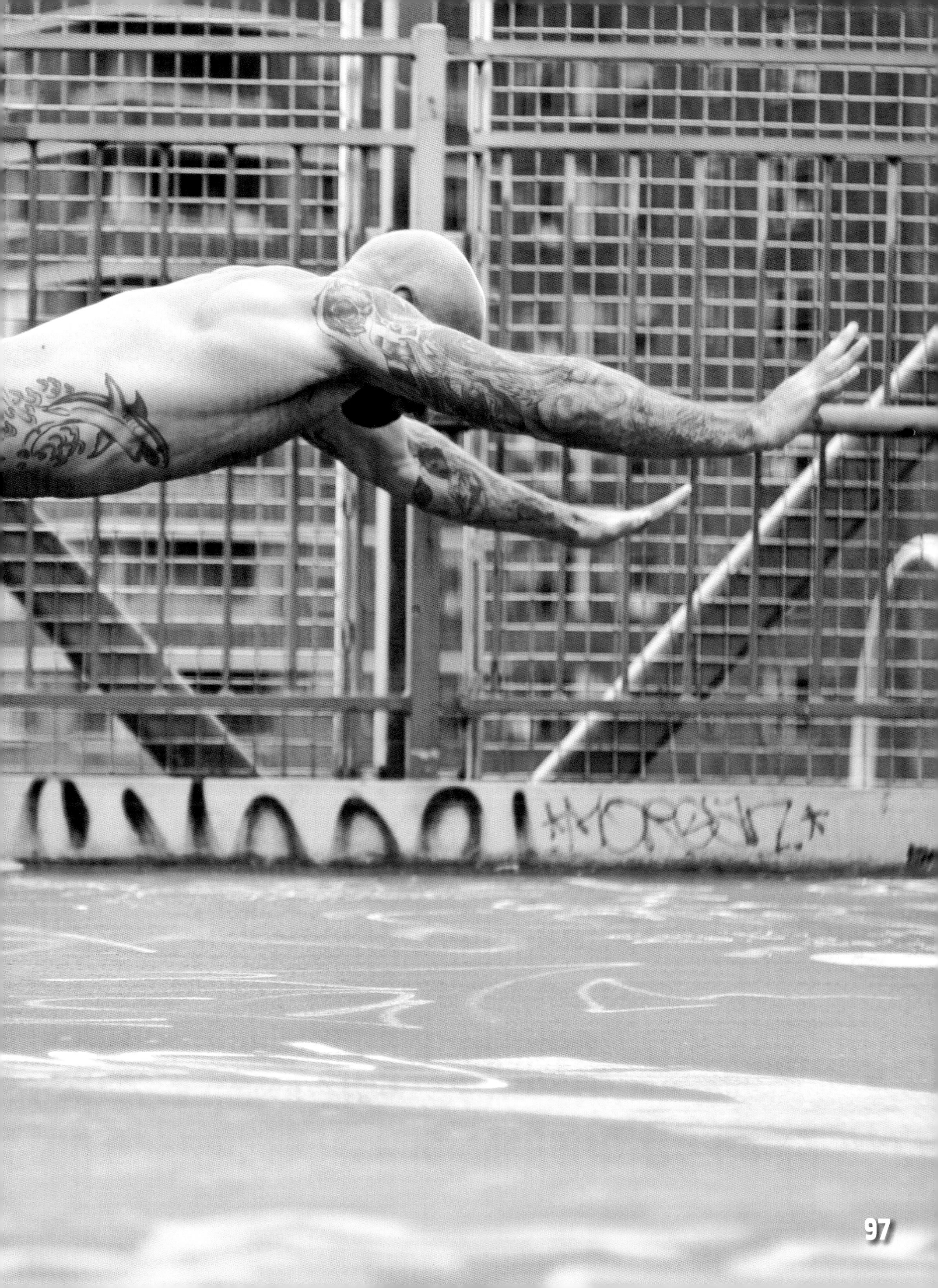

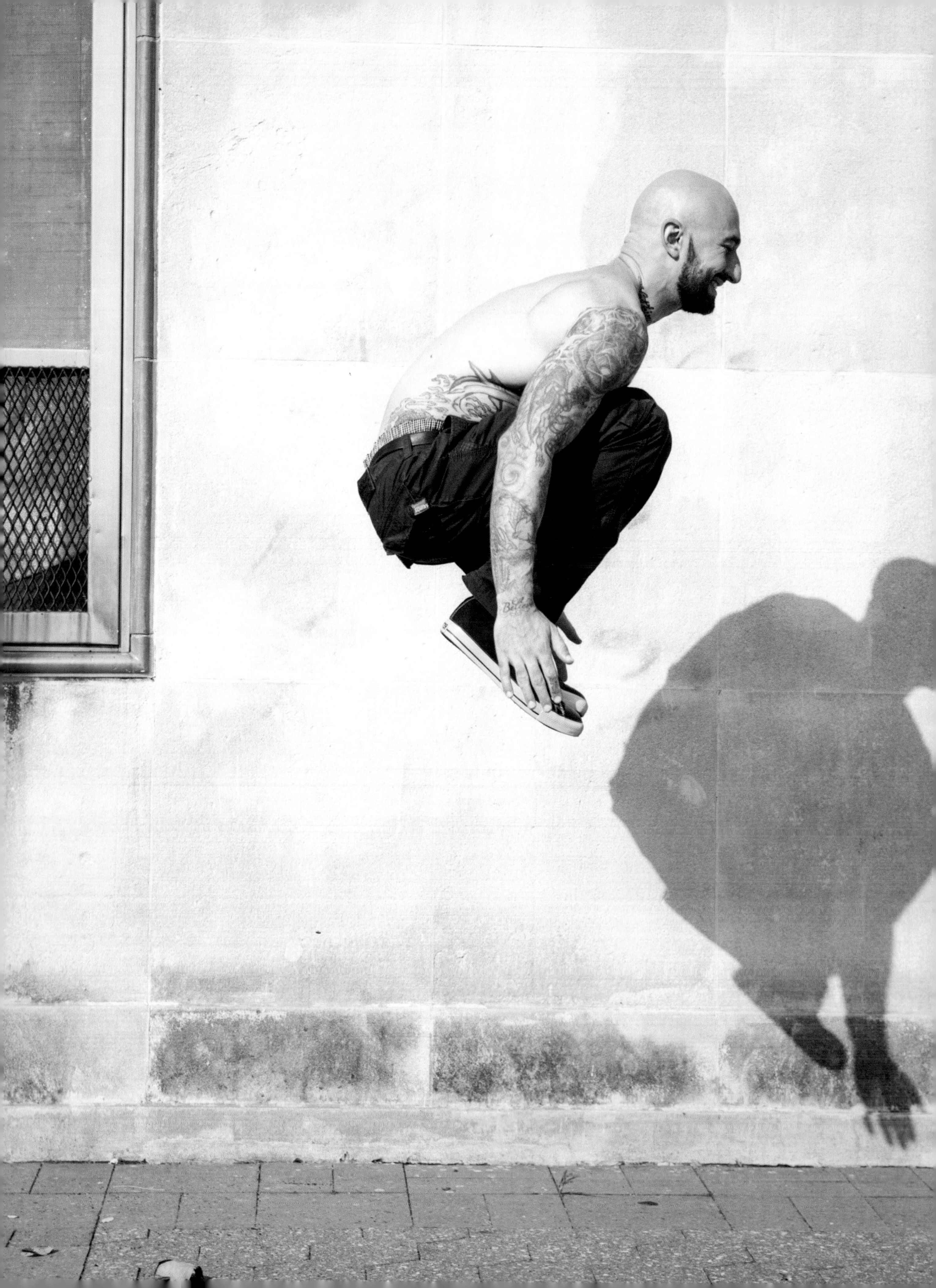

CHAPTER FIVE:

Advanced Squats

The basic squat is a fantastic exercise, though with enough practice you'll eventually get to the point where you can do hundreds of them in a row. Unlike the basic push-up, which will start to get quite challenging for even the fittest guys after 50 reps or so, one could theoretically go on and on indefinitely with bodyweight squats without hitting muscular failure if they had the mental tenacity to deal with the discomfort. Your legs are built to withstand a lot more work than your arms. Hell, even on a recovery day, they still have to carry you around everywhere!

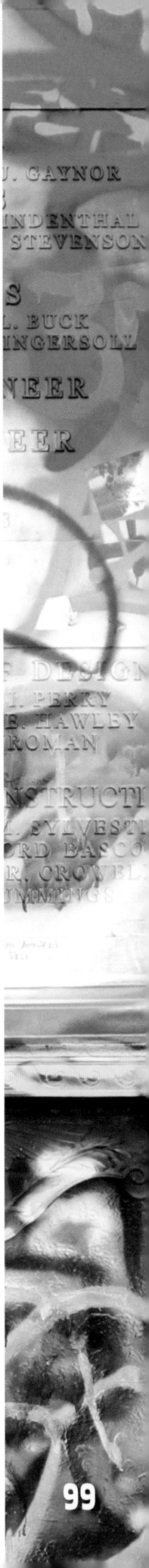

Close Squat

Just like a push-up, bringing your feet closer together can increase the difficulty of a squat. An ideal close squat involves keeping your feet and knees together while squatting all the way down until your hamstrings are pressed against your calves. These can become a wonderful active stretch as well as a serious core exercise when performed properly. As with a standard squat, it may help to start out with a bench behind you to help achieve a full range of motion. You can also work towards narrowing your feet over time in order to get from the traditional shoulder-width stance into a heels-together close squat.

An ideal close squat involves keeping your feet and knees together while squatting all the way down until your hamstrings are pressed against your calves.

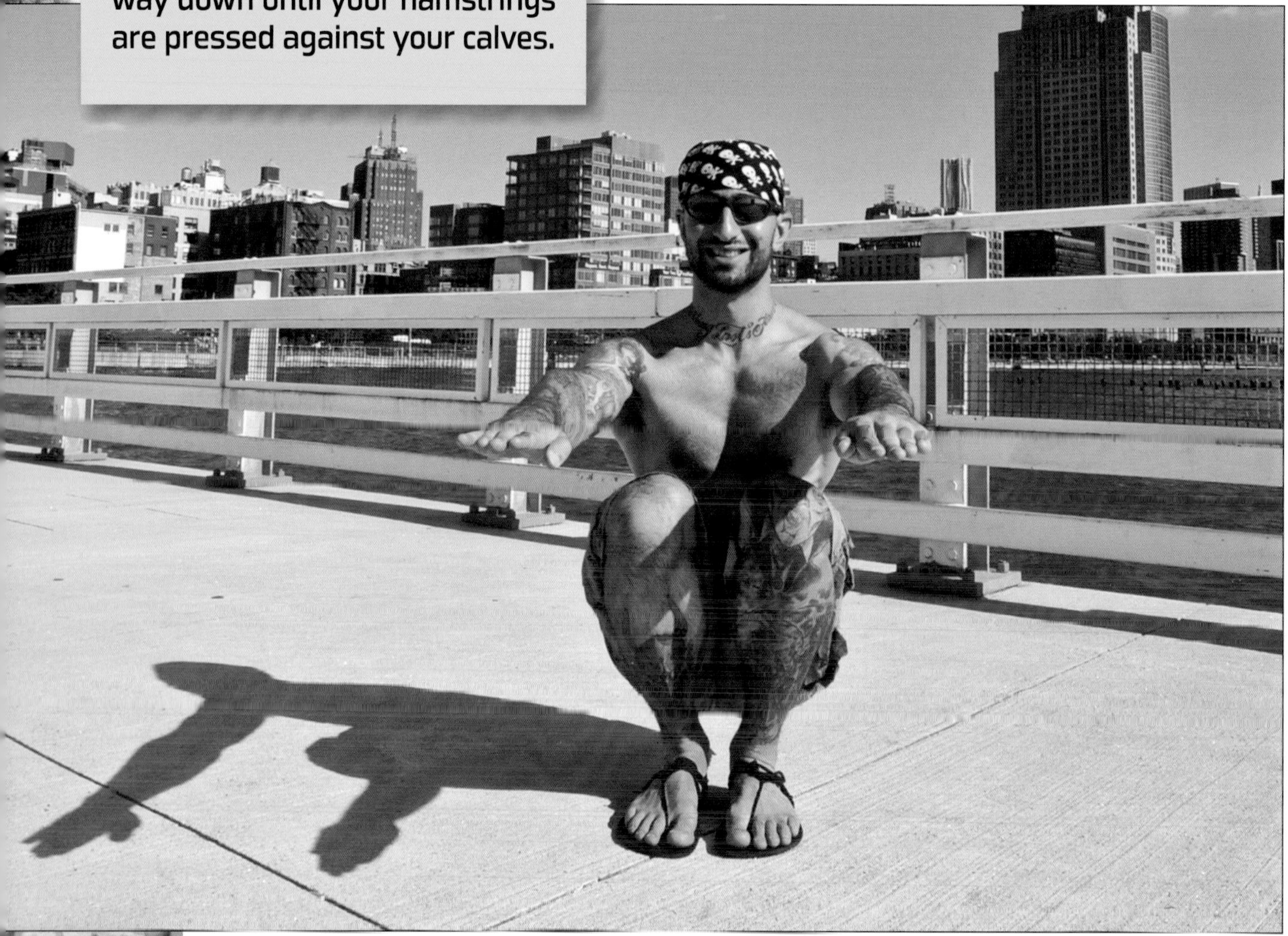

Bulgarian Split Squat

Manipulating leverage is the key to varying the intensity of bodyweight exercises. By elevating your rear foot while performing a split squat, you not only change the leverage of the exercise, you also turn it into an active stretch for the hip flexors and quads of your elevated side, as well as the hamstrings of the lower leg. Make sure your stance is deep enough to keep the heel of your front foot planted on the ground through the whole range of motion. As it places most of your weight on your front leg, the Bulgarian split squat is a great introductory exercise toward eventually doing a one legged squat. Like a normal split squat, do your best to stay upright when you perform this variation

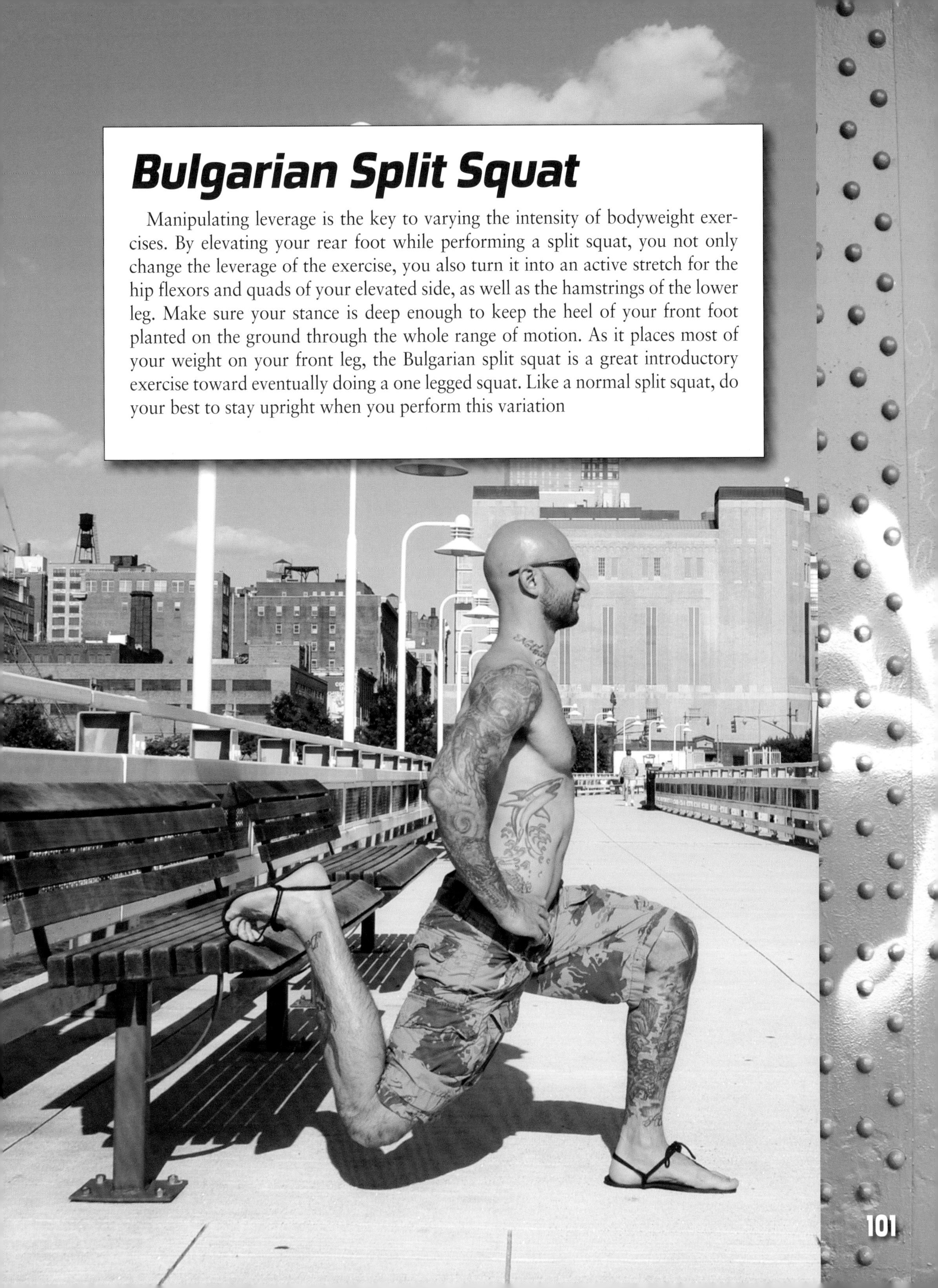

Side-to-Side Squat

Also known as the "cossack" squat, the side-to-side squat is a strength and stability challenge as well as a fantastic active stretch. As one leg winds up taking on most of the load, side-to-side squats are also a helpful precursor to one legged squats.

Begin in an exaggerated wide stance squat position with your toes turned out. Slowly shift your weight towards your left foot while bending from your hips and your left knee. Your right leg will stay straight and your right foot will roll onto the heel with your toes pointed up. You should feel a stretch in your groin when you get to the bottom. The more you focus on pointing the toes of your straight leg up, the deeper you will be able to get into the squat on the opposite side. Like any type of squat, your intention should be to get down as low as you can without sacrificing your posture (no shrugging). Keep your abs tight, reach your arms in front for balance, and make sure the heel of your squatting leg stays down the whole time. When coming up, press into that heel to activate your glutes.

The side-to-side squat is essentially the lower body equivalent of the archer push-up, though due to the nature of the hip joint, it is more of a flexibility challenge. Like archer push-ups, I like to do side-to-side squats alternating legs, but you may do one side at a time if you are trying to give one of your legs some extra attention.

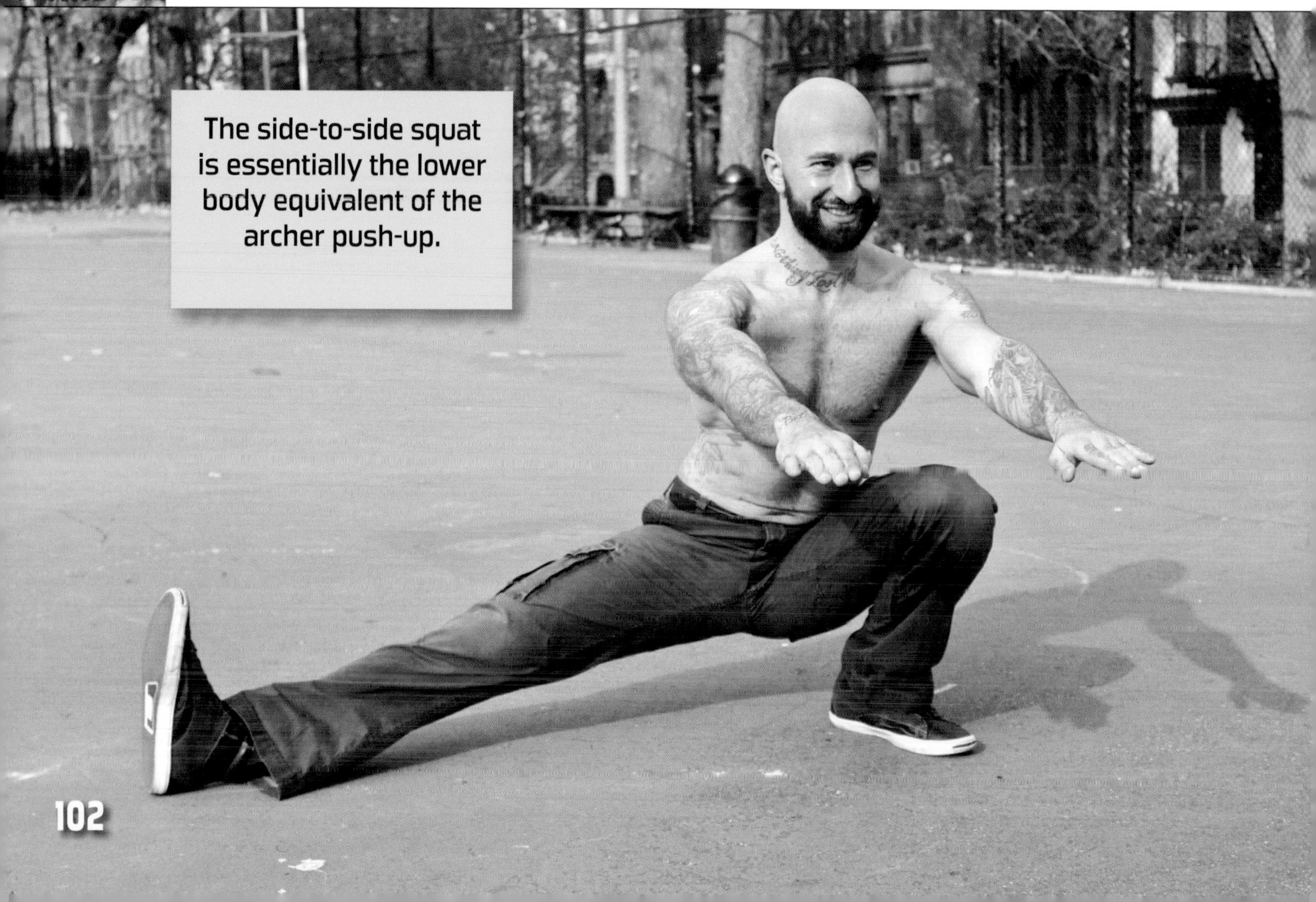

The side-to-side squat is essentially the lower body equivalent of the archer push-up.

Tuck Jump

Plyometric squats can build tremendous strength and power in your legs as well as provide you with a cardiovascular effect similar to sprinting. 20 consecutive tuck jumps will get anyone's heart racing. Just typing it is making my pulse rise!

When you do a tuck jump (or any other type of jump squat), you don't need to go all the way down at the bottom. This is one instance in which I am cool with people doing partial range of motion on their squats. Just get down a few inches, jump as high as you can and tuck your knees to your chest. Though your legs obviously do most of the work, tuck jumps can be a full body exercise, so use your arms to generate momentum. Remember to stay light on your feet and avoid landing with locked out knees.

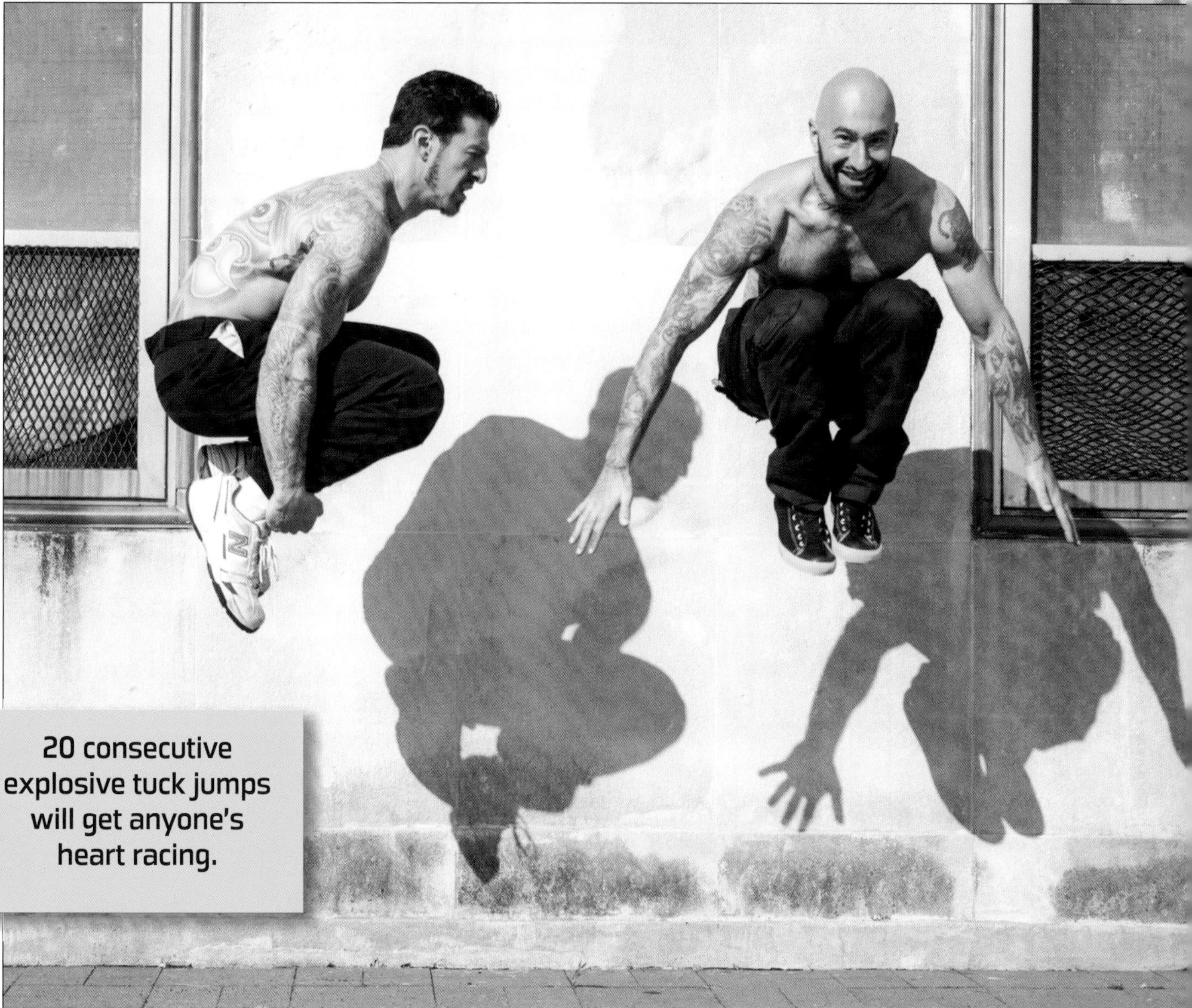

20 consecutive explosive tuck jumps will get anyone's heart racing.

Box Jump

A box jump is another great lower body plyometric exercise. It's similar to the tuck jump except you are jumping onto a box or other object as opposed to just leaping into the air. (This exercise does in fact require something other than the floor, but if you don't have anything to jump on, you'll do just fine with tuck jumps.) As with the tuck jump, make sure you land with your joints soft to minimize the impact.

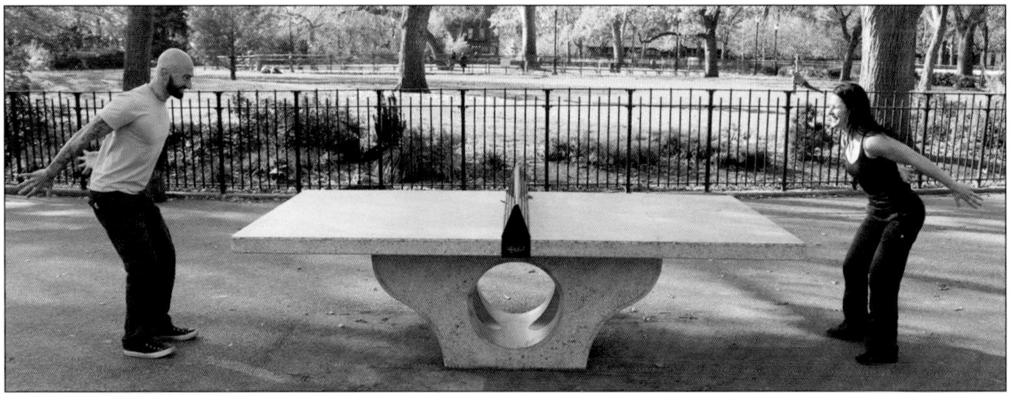

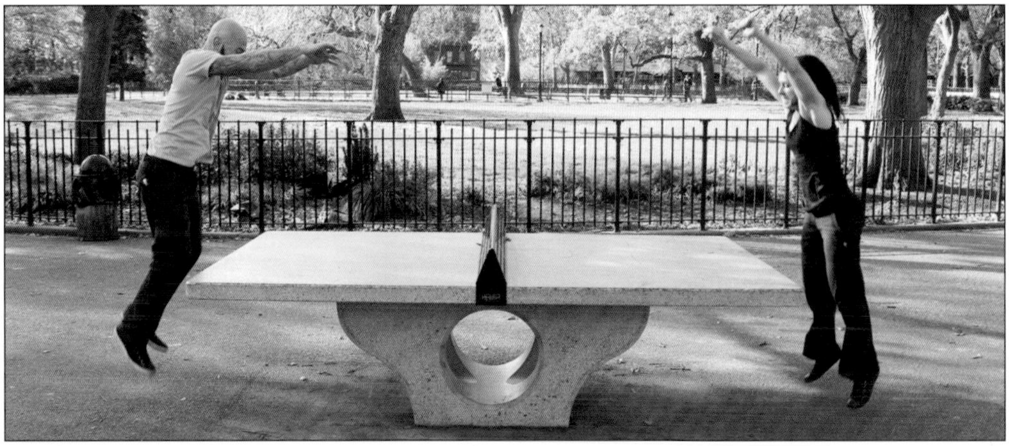

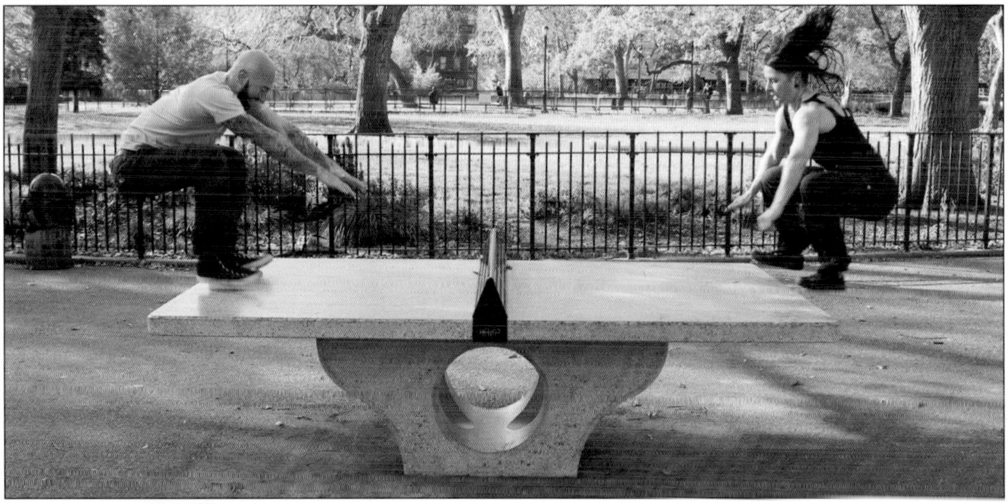

Jump Lunge

Lunges are one of my favorite leg exercises, but like everything in life, you don't want your leg routine to become, well, routine.

Start out with a stationary jump lunge by lowering yourself down into a split squat and jumping up at the top, gently landing back into the bottom position with your knees bent. Do several in a row, then switch legs.

The cycle lunge is a more advanced jump lunge. It starts out the same as the stationary jump lunge, but once you're in the air, you'll have to quickly switch your legs before landing. Continue to alternate legs with each rep, going from one right into the next. You can swing your arms for momentum or keep them at your sides. It might take a little practice to land comfortably without losing your balance.

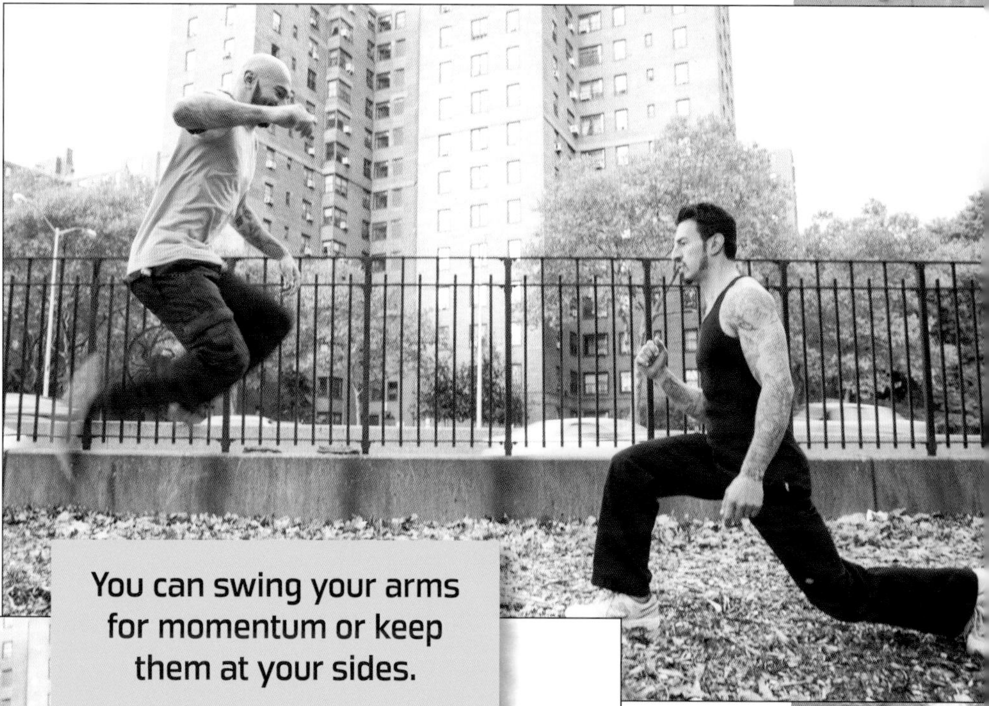

You can swing your arms for momentum or keep them at your sides.

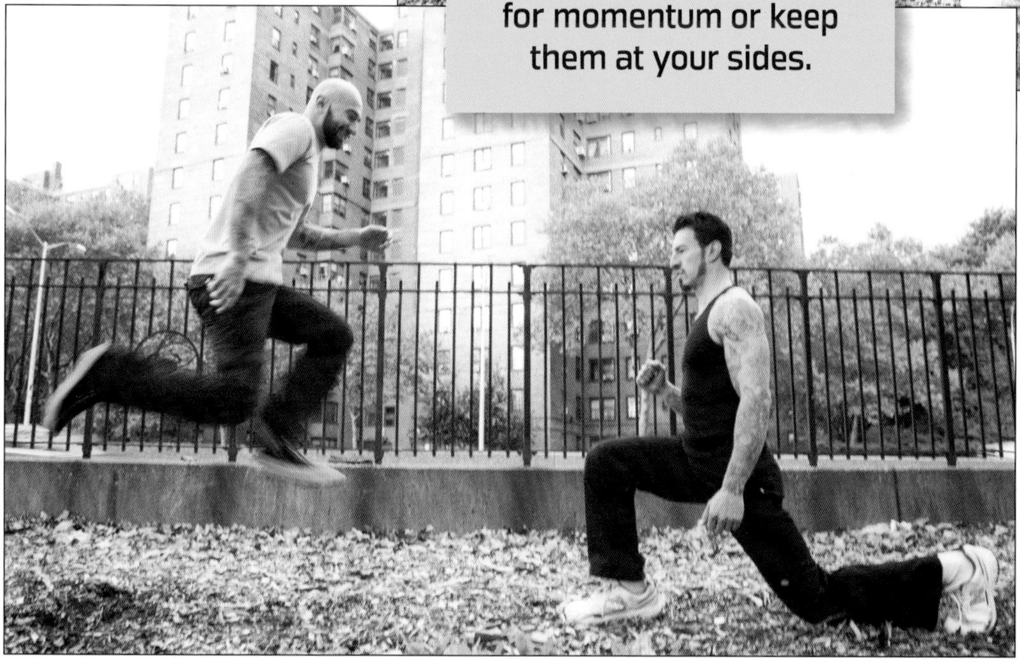

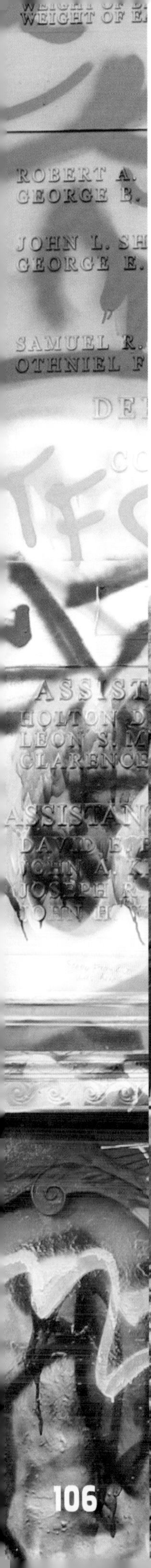

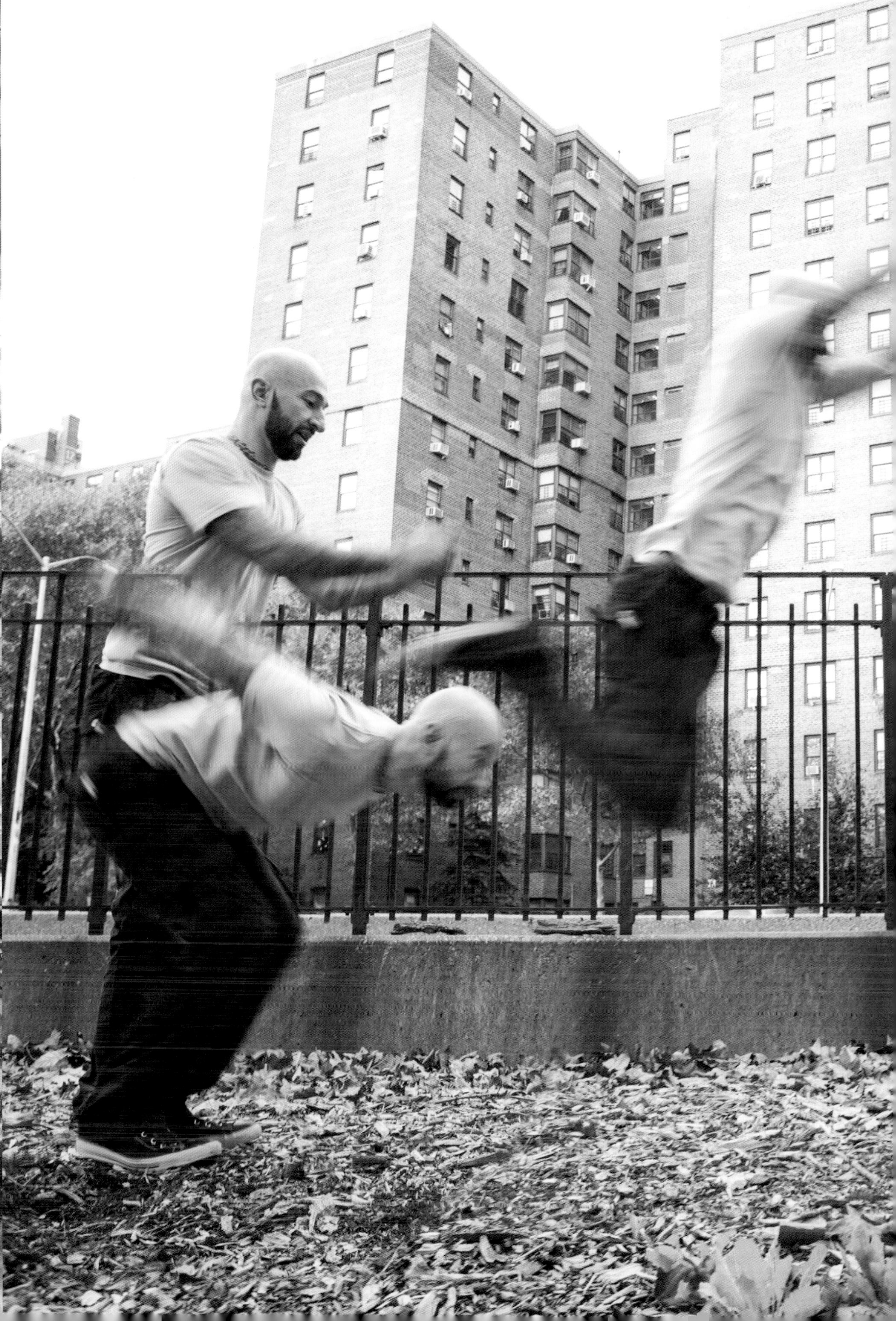

Broad Jump

Another fun plyometric squat variant, the broad jump is essentially the same as the tuck jump except you are jumping forward, not upward. You still want to lift your legs high as you jump, however, as this will help you clear more distance. Leaving your legs dangling isn't as aerodynamic. You'll need a lot of space to practice broad jumps — I recommend a park or field.

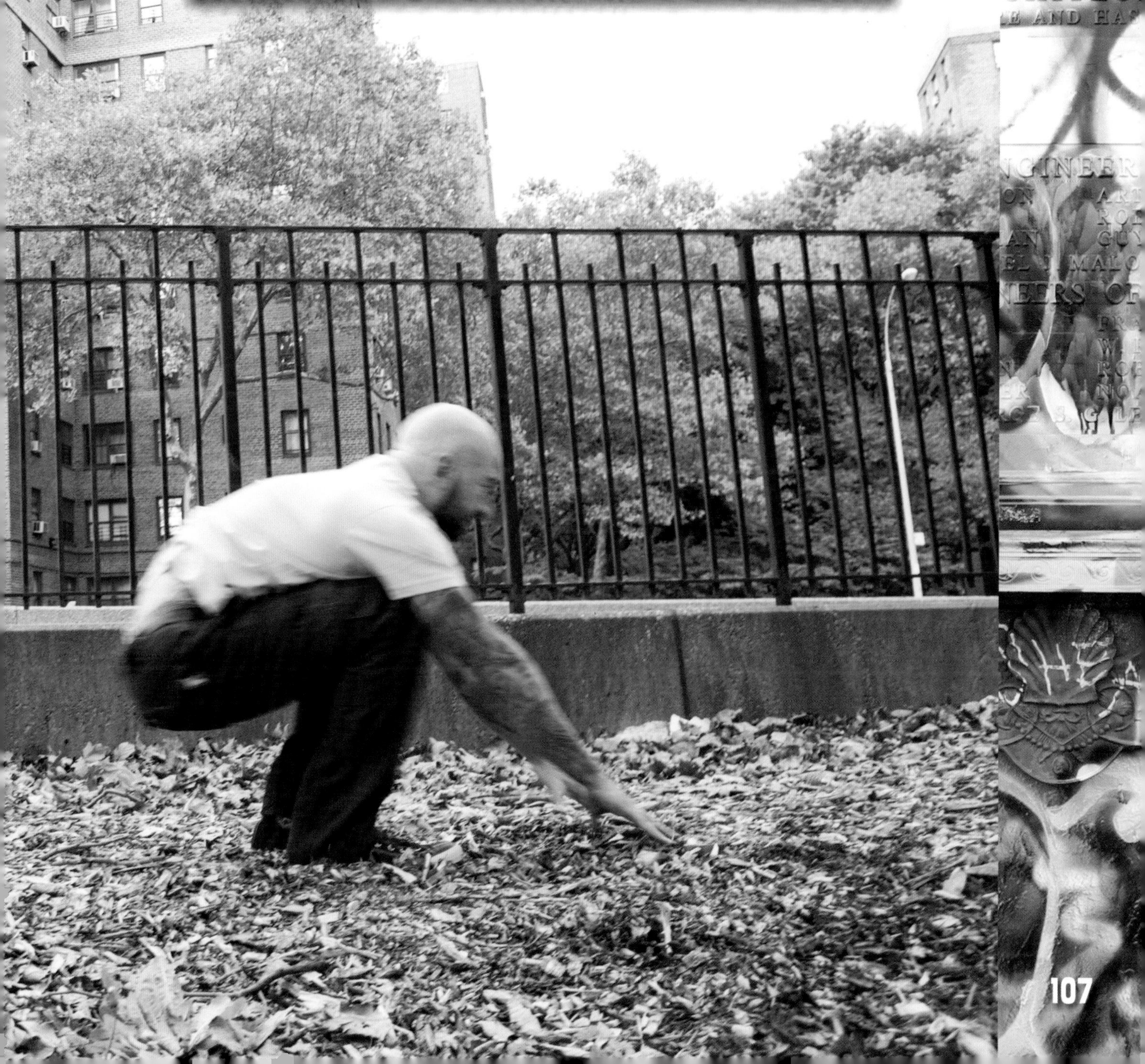

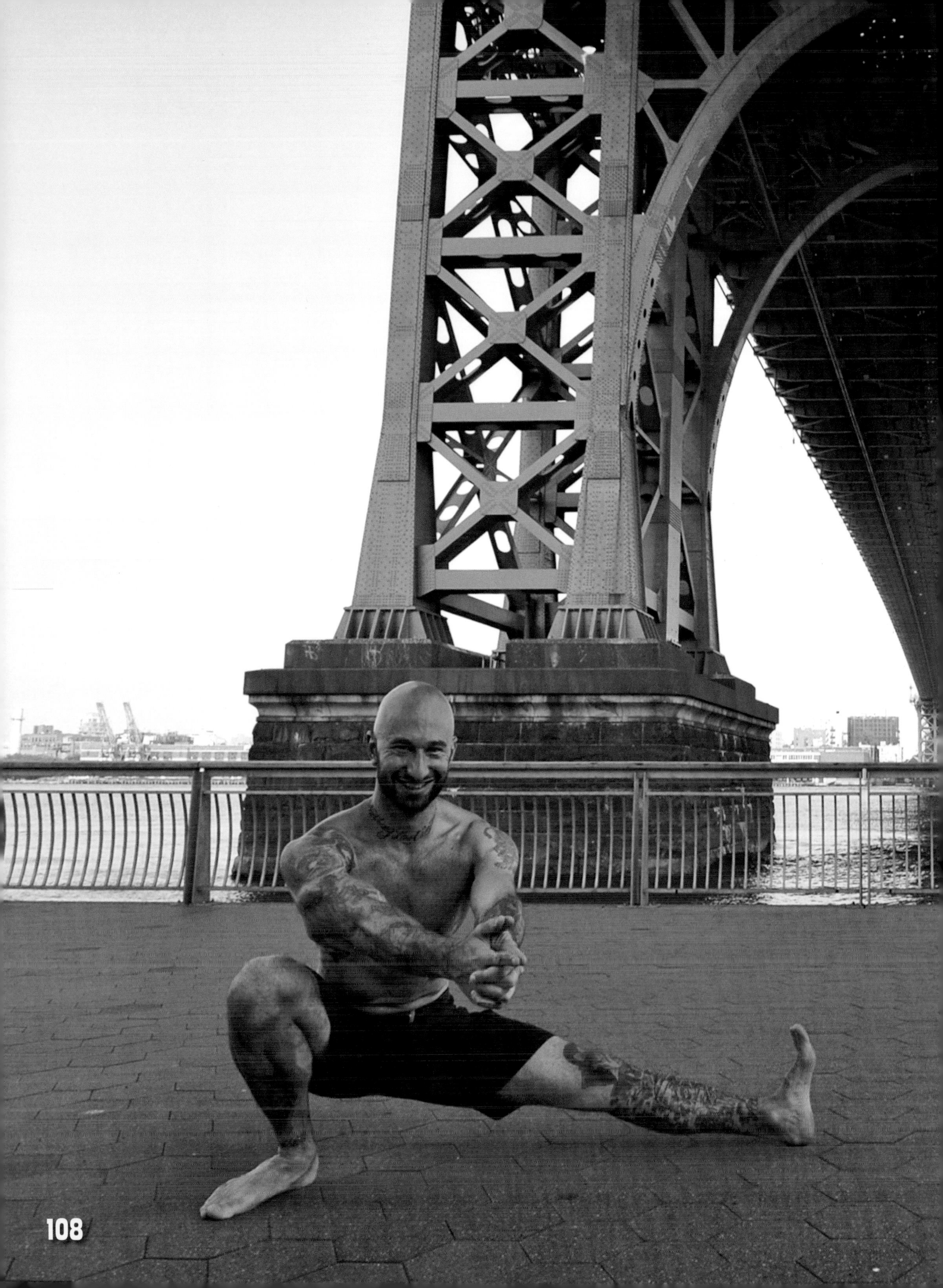

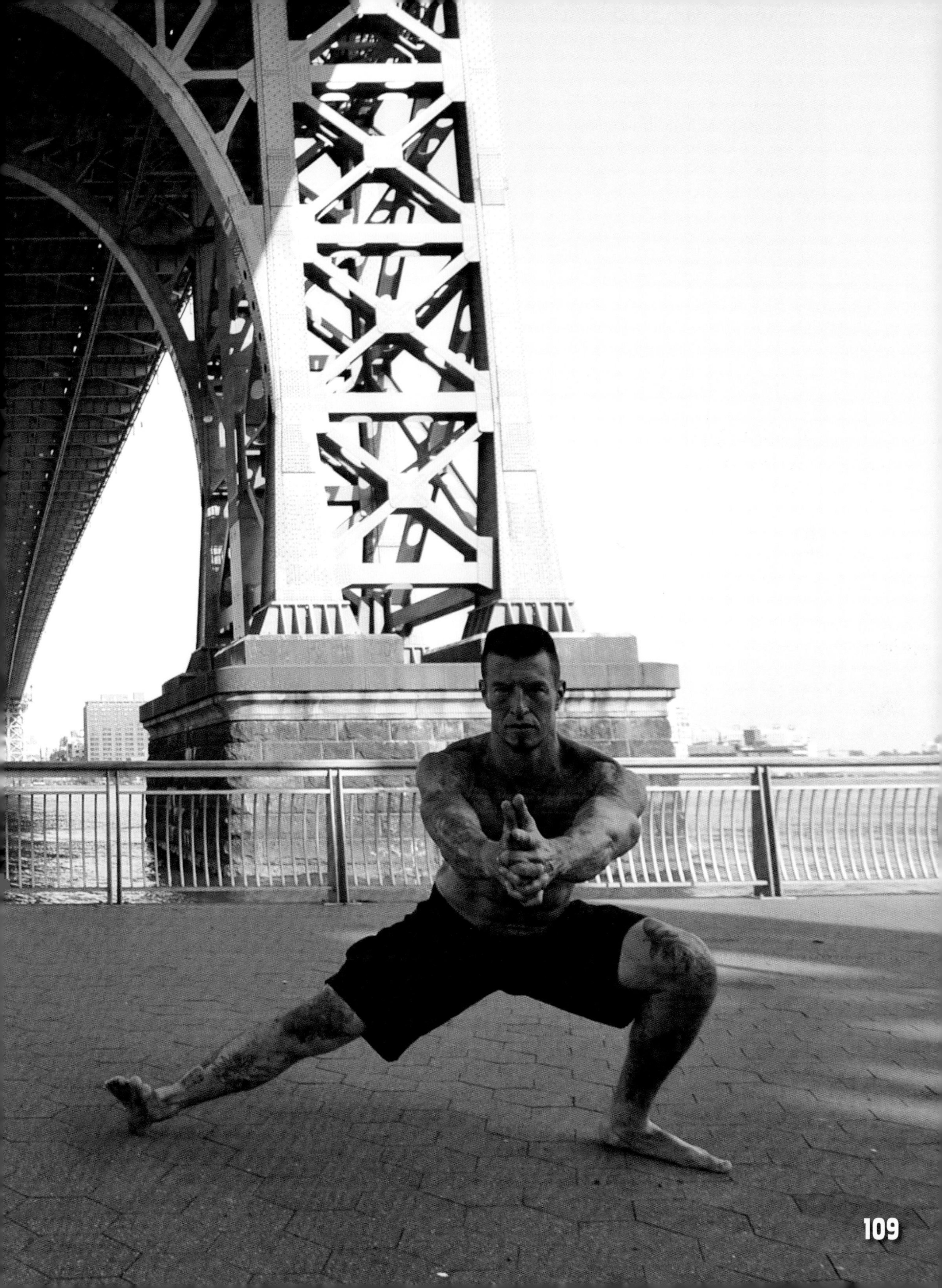

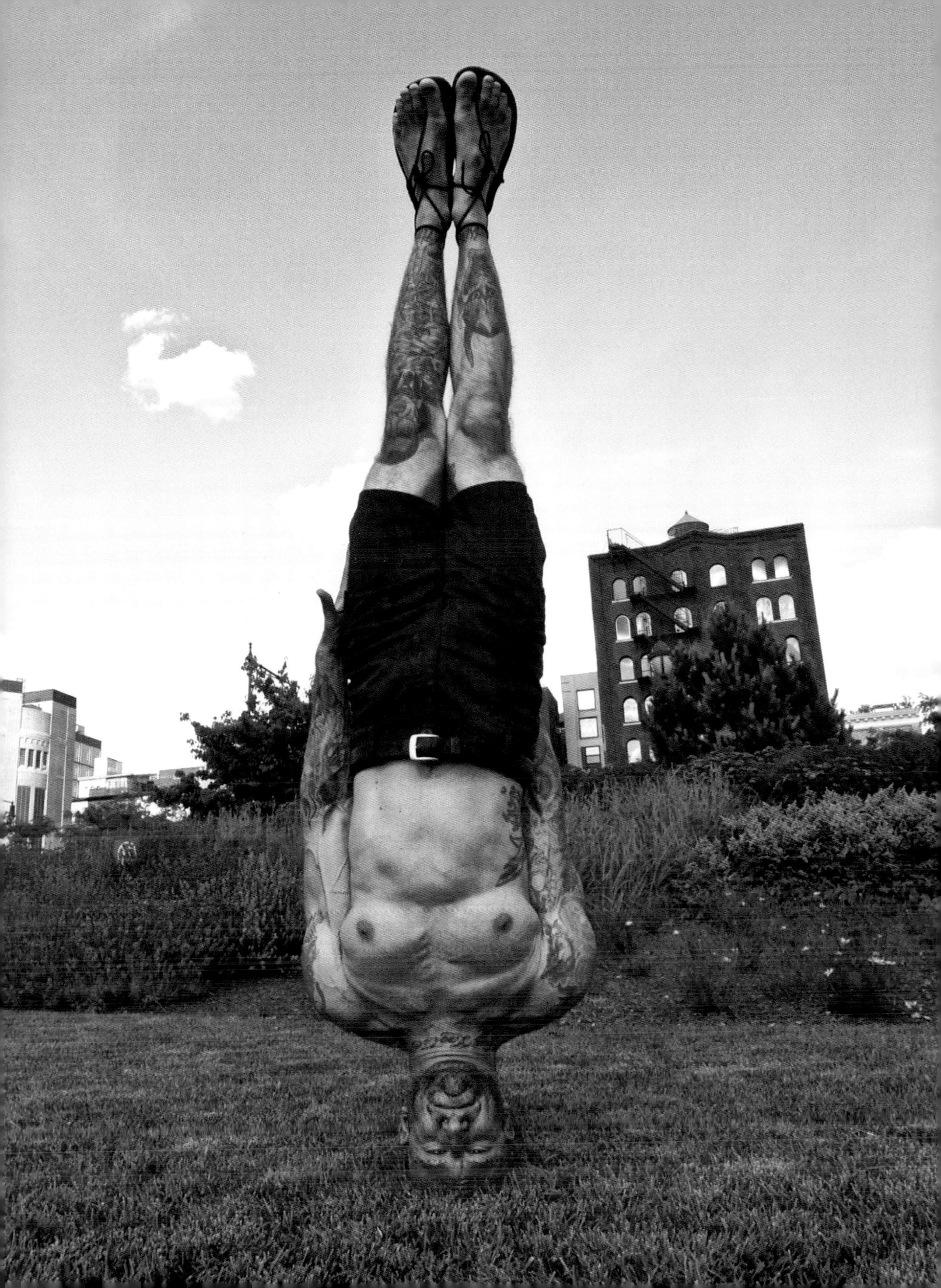

Chapter Six:

Full Inversions

True bodyweight mastery means being able to control your muscles and maintain your bearings in any position. Full inversions open up a whole new playing field for bodyweight training without involving any equipment at all. Since gravity only works in one direction, it's good to sometimes turn yourself upside down to work your muscles from the opposite end.

We've already been over the bridge, which is arguably the most important inversion in terms of building strength and flexibility, but full inversions with your legs off the ground are important for building proprioceptive awareness, balance and core strength. Inversions also benefit the body's circulatory system. Though there are many different types of inversions, I've chosen to focus on the positions that I find most useful for building strength, body awareness and alignment.

In addition to the physical challenge, full inversions can often be psychologically overwhelming for beginners. It's scary to turn yourself upside down at first! Tackling this fear can be very empowering, however. Once you start to get the hang of these exercises, your increased confidence can carry over into other aspects of your life. With that in mind, tread slowly and listen to your body.

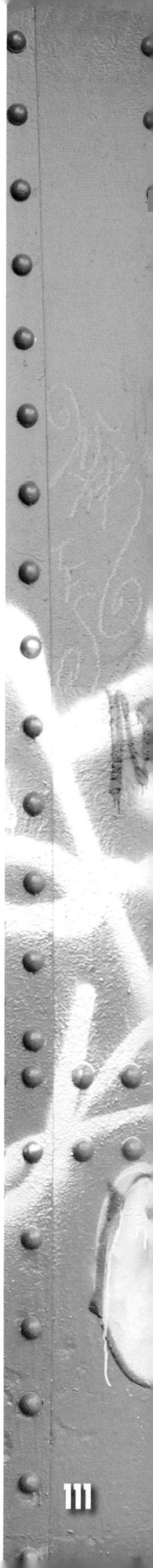

Shoulder Stand

The shoulder stand is the most basic inversion and the easiest for most people to learn. Begin by lying on your back, then pull your legs to your chest and try to get your hips in the air. You're going to need to grab your lower back and gradually wiggle your body to an upright position. It might be a deep stretch on the back of your neck; do not push if there is pain. Ease in and breathe deeply. Think of lengthening your entire body while tightening your abs and extending your legs. You may not be able to achieve a perfectly straight shoulder stand at first, but with practice, it should eventually become a relatively easy move.

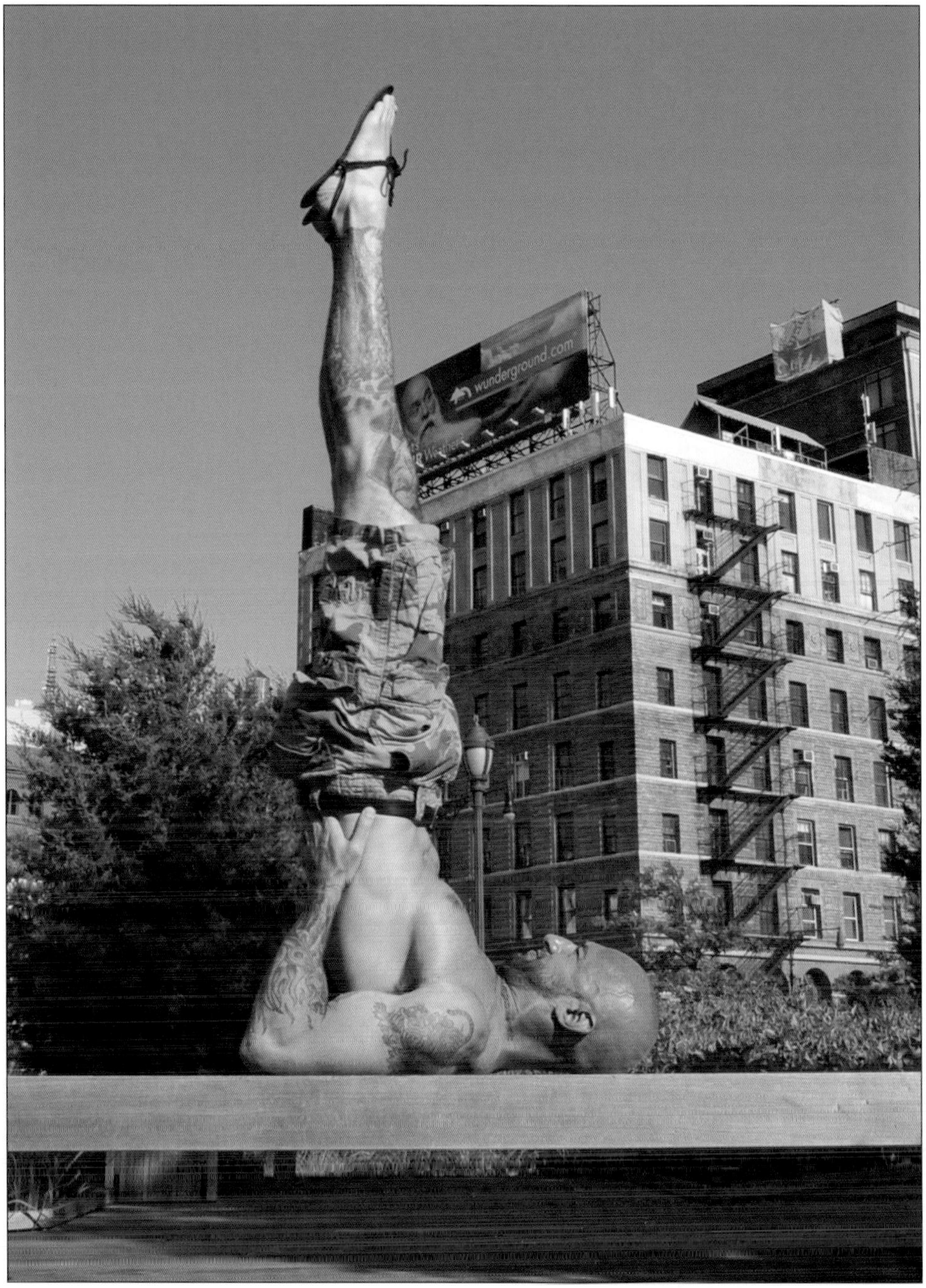

Tripod

Once you can get the feel for the tripod, the headstand will soon follow. To practice, kneel down and place your palms on the floor below your shoulders. Now rest your head on the floor a few inches above your hands. You'll want to make contact with the ground on the top of your head, not the back of the head or forehead. Rise up onto your toes and slowly try to lift your feet and bring your knees to rest on the backs of your arms.

When you do a shoulder stand, you have five points of contact with the ground: two elbows, two shoulders and the back of your head (plus the backs of your arms, I suppose). The tripod allows you just three contact points: the top of your head and your hands (hence tripod). Some people may have a challenge getting acclimated to the feeling of being upside-down. Nonetheless, I still consider it a beginner exercise. Pardon the pun, but if you're worried about being upside down, it's probably all in your head!

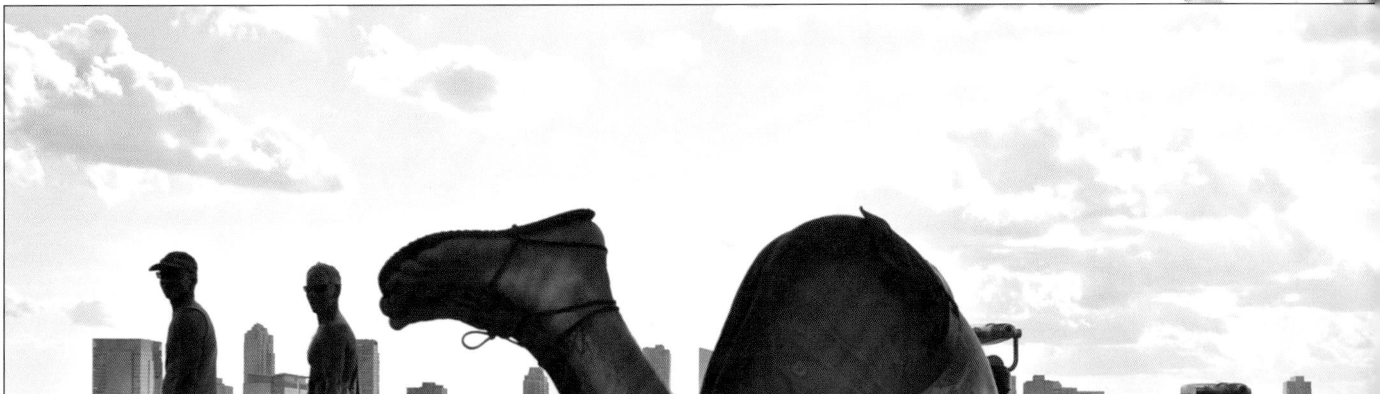

The tripod allows you just three contact points: the top of your head and your hands.

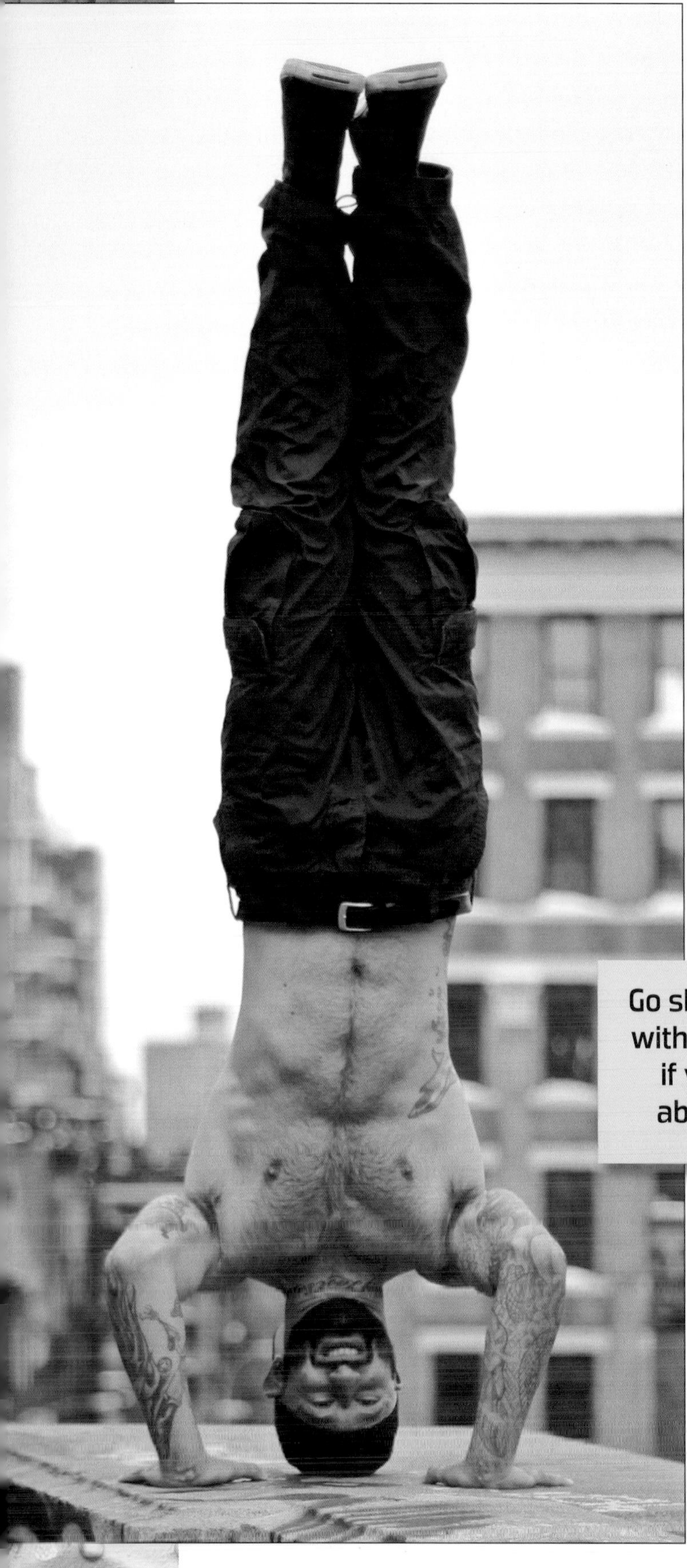

Tripod Headstand

The easiest type of headstand for most people is the tripod headstand. From the tripod position, you'll need to align your hips directly over your shoulders. Then it's simply a matter of lifting your knees off your arms and reaching your legs up in the air. Go slowly and start out with a wall behind you if you are nervous about tipping over. With practice you'll be able to lift to this position without the need to first place your legs on the backs of your arms. It may also be helpful to open your legs into a straddle to help find the balance.

Go slowly and start out with a wall behind you if you are nervous about tipping over.

Elbow Headstand

Once you get the hang of the tripod headstand you can try an elbow headstand, which is the more commonly seen method. Though some people find it easier than the tripod, the elbow headstand can be more difficult to get into, as you'll have your hands behind your head instead of in front, with your weight resting on your forearms and elbows. You won't be able to start with your legs resting on your arms this way and you won't have as much leeway with spreading the balance out either. If you have the flexibility, you can try getting into position by slowly lifting one leg at a time, otherwise you'll have to kick up with your knees bent before extending your legs upward. Either way, the key to finding the balance in this position is to get your hips centered directly over your shoulders.

The key to finding the balance in this position is to get your hips centered directly over your shoulders.

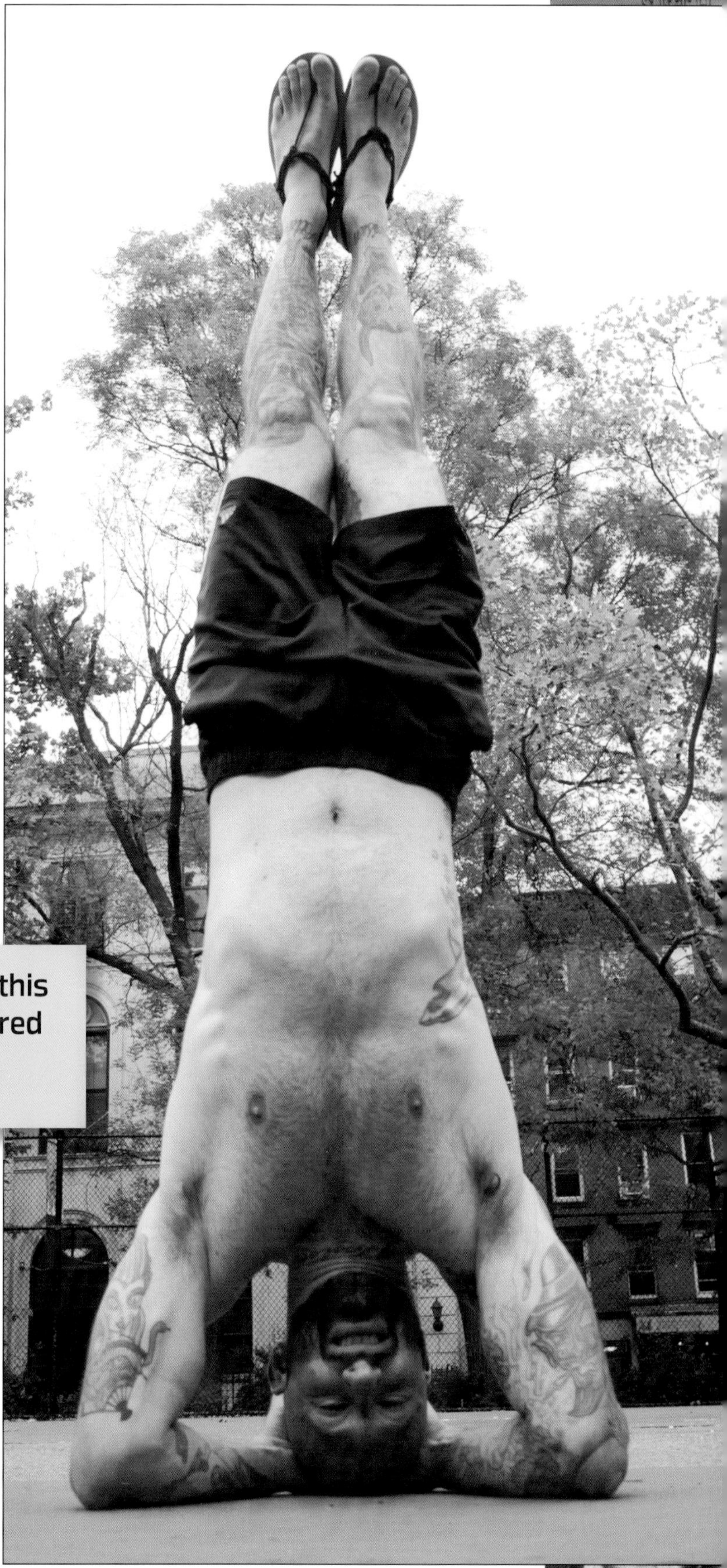

Wrist Headstand

When you've gotten comfortable holding the basic headstands for extended periods of time (at least a full minute), you may try moving onto a wrist headstand, which involves balancing on the backs of your wrists (along with your head) while your arms are extended in front of your body. At first you might try moving into position by starting in either a tripod or elbow headstand and then carefully putting your arms out one at a time, though an advanced practitioner will be able to lift into the full headstand beginning from only their wrists and head.

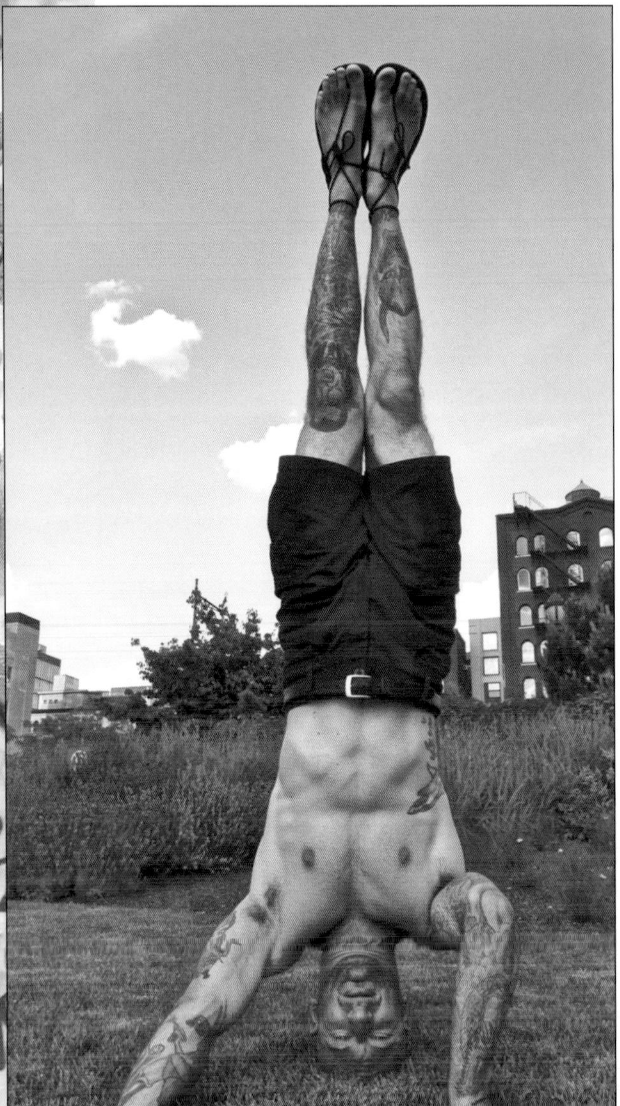

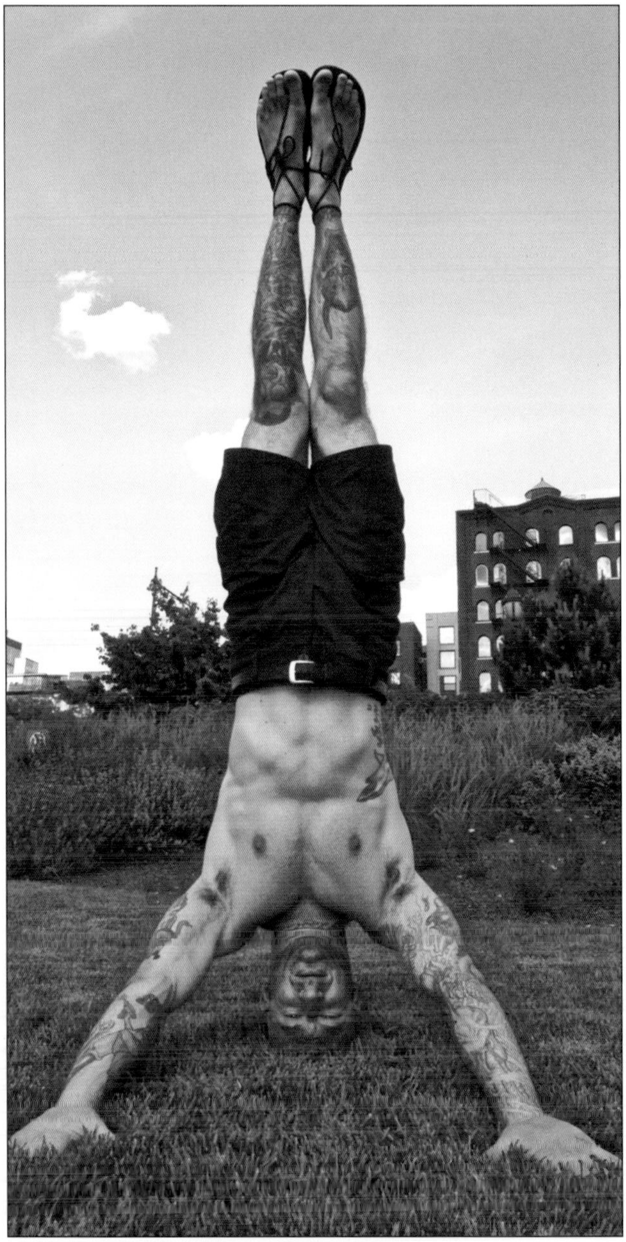

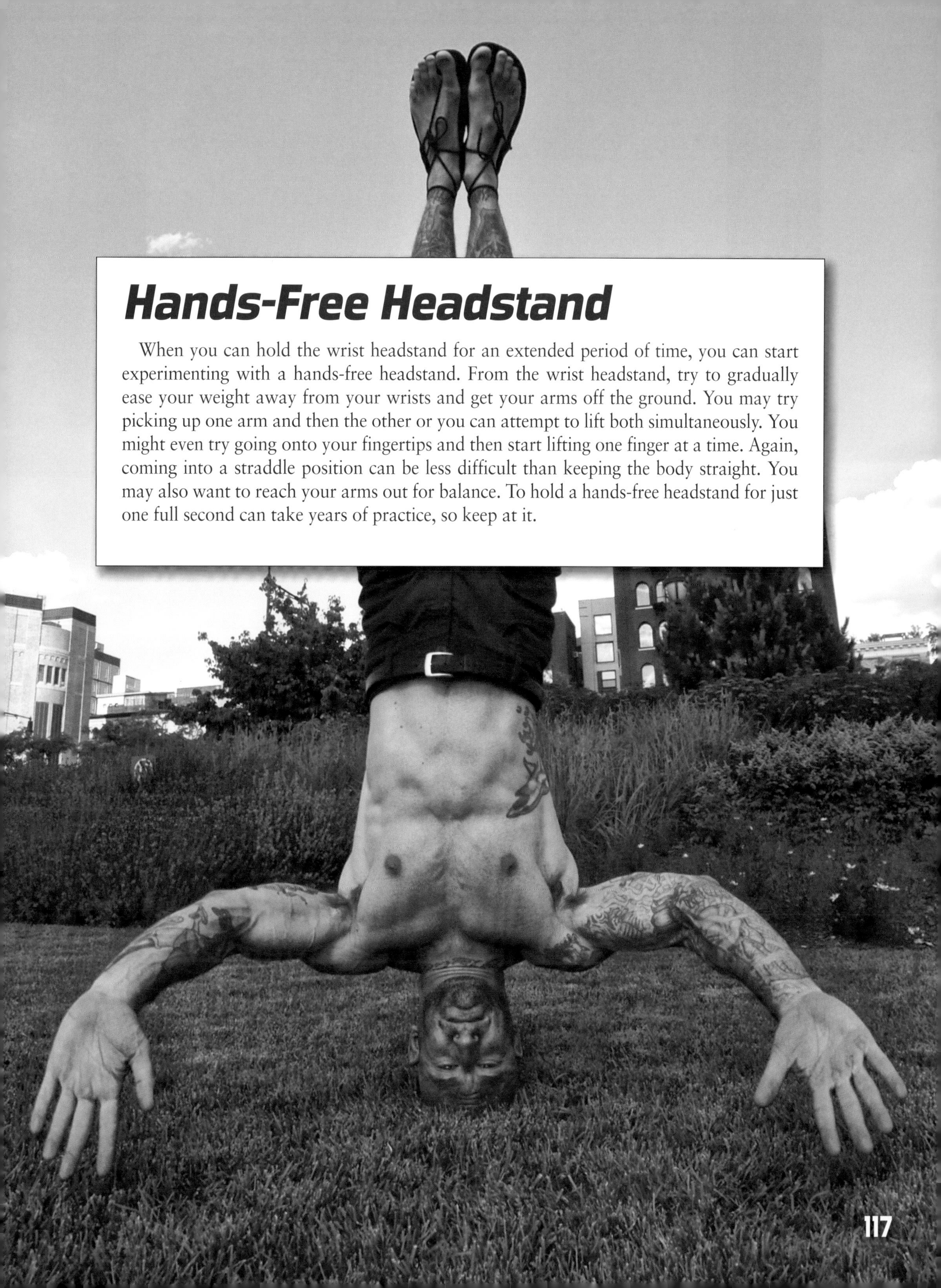

Hands-Free Headstand

When you can hold the wrist headstand for an extended period of time, you can start experimenting with a hands-free headstand. From the wrist headstand, try to gradually ease your weight away from your wrists and get your arms off the ground. You may try picking up one arm and then the other or you can attempt to lift both simultaneously. You might even try going onto your fingertips and then start lifting one finger at a time. Again, coming into a straddle position can be less difficult than keeping the body straight. You may also want to reach your arms out for balance. To hold a hands-free headstand for just one full second can take years of practice, so keep at it.

Forearm Stand

The forearm stand is a great intermediate inversion pose once you've gotten the hang of the basic headstand variations. It requires more upper-body strength than the headstand and the balance can be trickier to find, though it's not quite as elusive as the freestanding handstand. It's almost like an elbow headstand without your head on the ground.

I recommend getting into position by first kneeling down and getting your forearms parallel to each other against the floor. From here you can kick your legs up and try to get your body vertical. It can be helpful to start out practicing with a spotter or a wall behind you. Look in between your hands when kicking up into position while keeping your weight centered between your elbows and hands in order to find the balance. Once you're locked in, you can start slowly straightening your body.

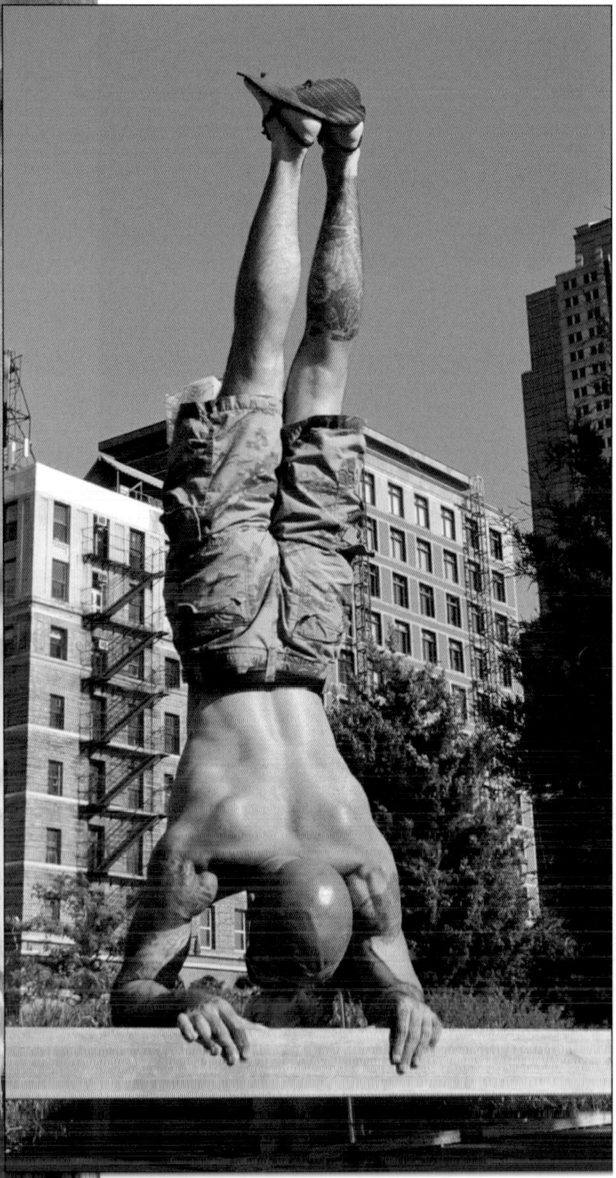

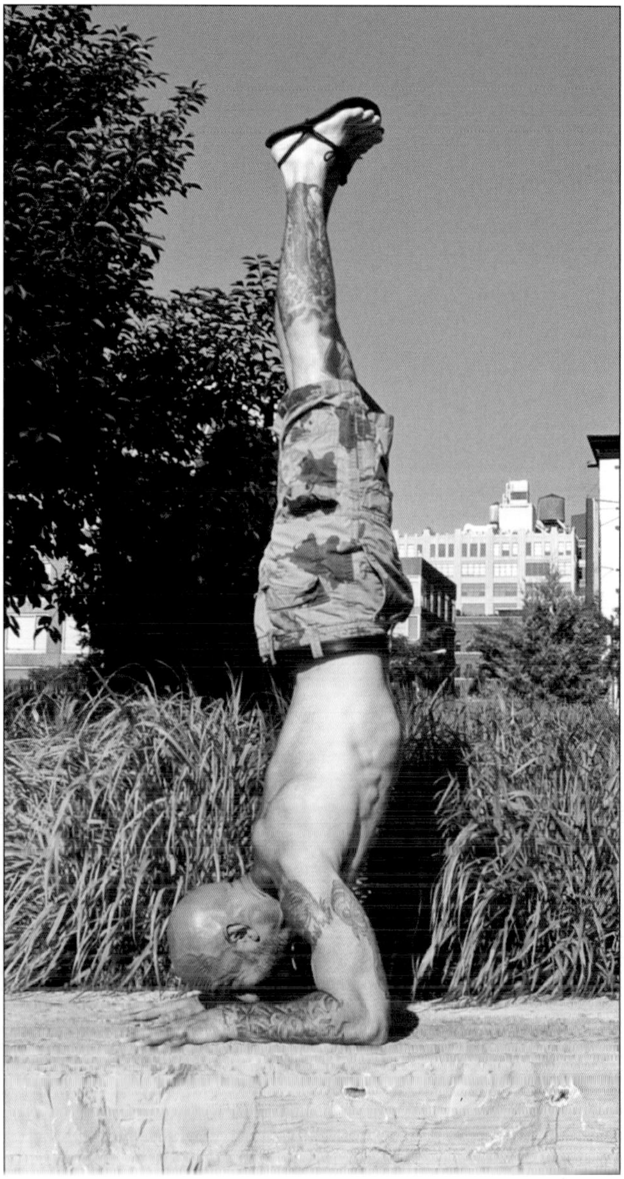

Scorpion

In a traditional forearm stand, the objective is to keep your body straight. In contrast, the objective of the scorpion hold is to create an arc in the body from the forearm balance position. It's almost like combining a forearm stand with a back bridge.

You'll need to let your knees bend while compressing your spine and shifting your center of gravity to prevent from tipping over. Some people may find this pose easier than a straight forearm stand while others will find the balance more challenging with their back arched — we each have our unique strengths and weaknesses.

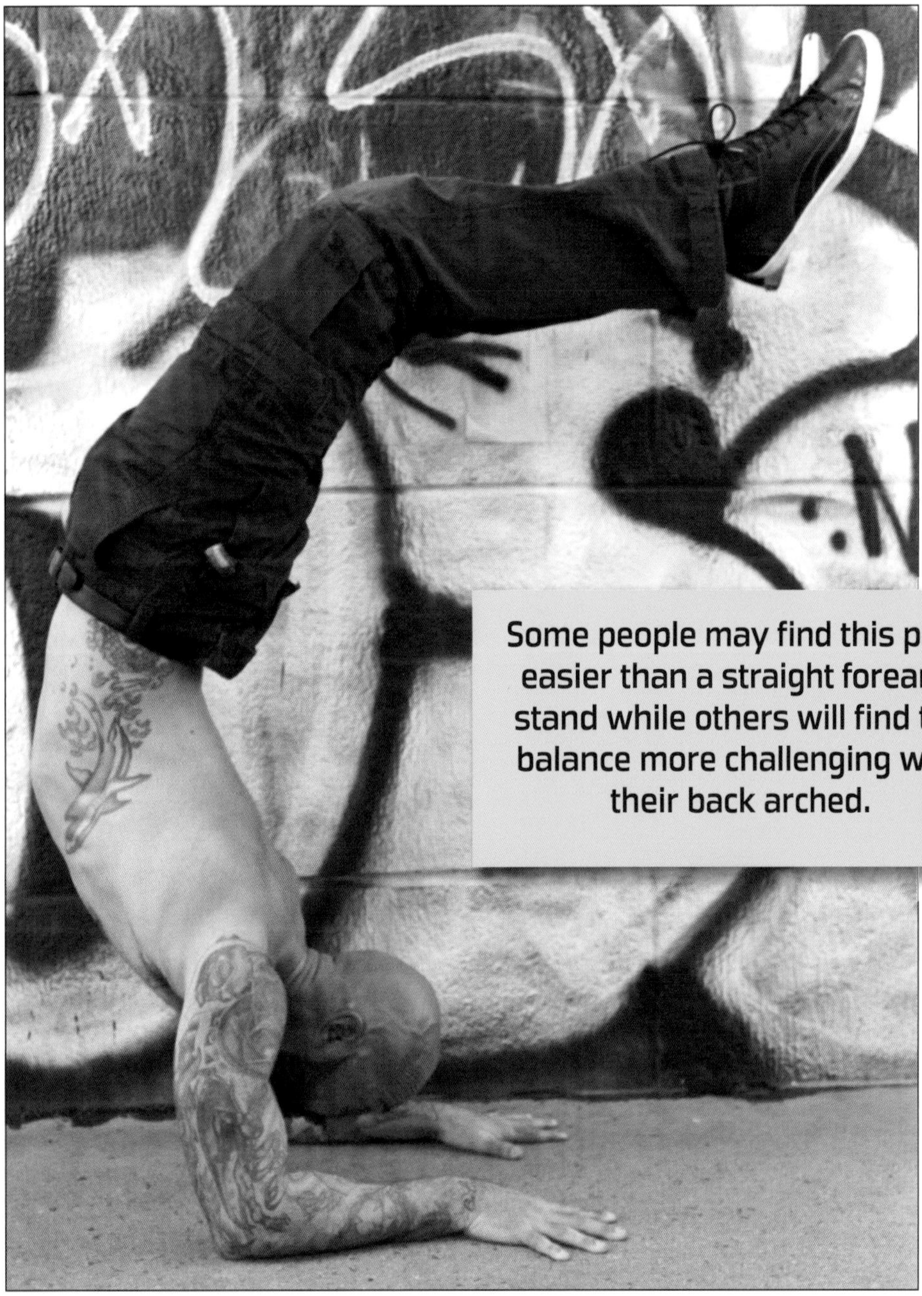

Some people may find this pose easier than a straight forearm stand while others will find the balance more challenging with their back arched.

Frog Stand

The two main factors that influence the difficulty of the various headstands, forearm stands and hand balances are the number of contact points and the position of your body. Also known as the crow pose, the frog stand limits you to just two relatively small points of contact — your hands. However, the tucked body position is much easier to control than the headstand or forearm stand. For this reason, the frog stand is generally easier to learn than a forearm stand or scorpion, even though those poses allow for more contact with the ground.

To practice the frog stand, you'll need to get into a deep squat and place your hands on the floor under your shoulders. Bend your elbows, get up on your toes and bring your knees to rest on the backs of your arms. It's almost like you are making a little shelf with your triceps on which to rest your legs. Keep your abs engaged and squeeze your hands and fingers like you are trying to grip the ground. Look out in front of your body as you lift up into position, not down at the floor.

When learning the frog stand, it is okay to begin with a deep elbow bend. With practice you can work towards straightening your arms and bringing your hips up higher. This will help you prepare to eventually transition to a handstand.

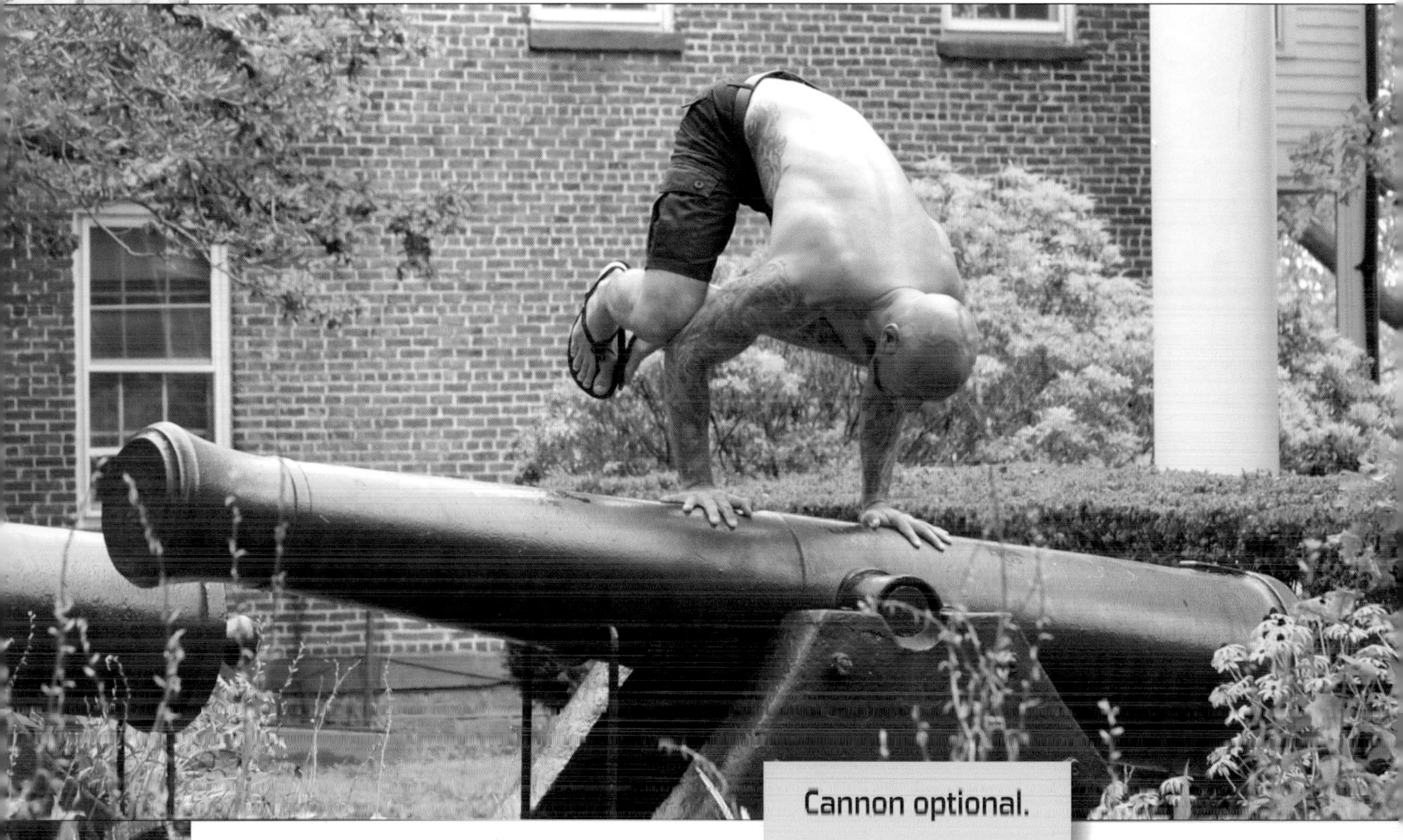

Cannon optional.

Handstand

Handstands are the ultimate inversion. They require precision, grace and total body strength in a way that few other exercises do. Like the other inversions, practicing against a wall is a nice way to learn, but the freestanding handstand is the real deal. If you aim to truly master your bodyweight, it is an essential skill.

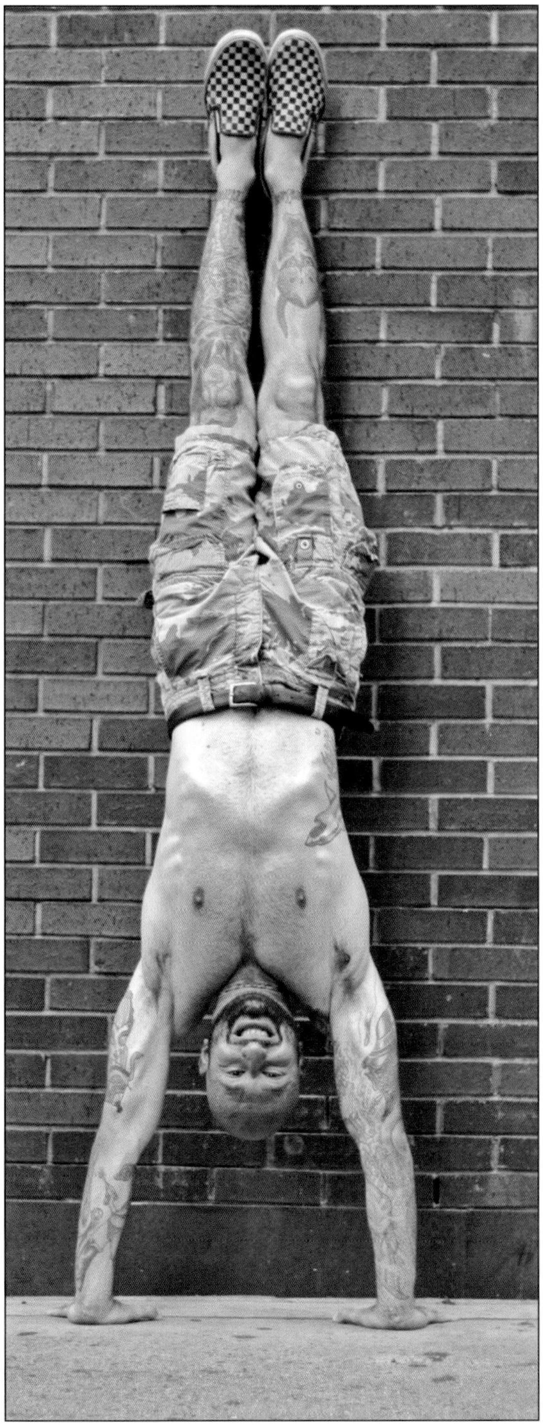

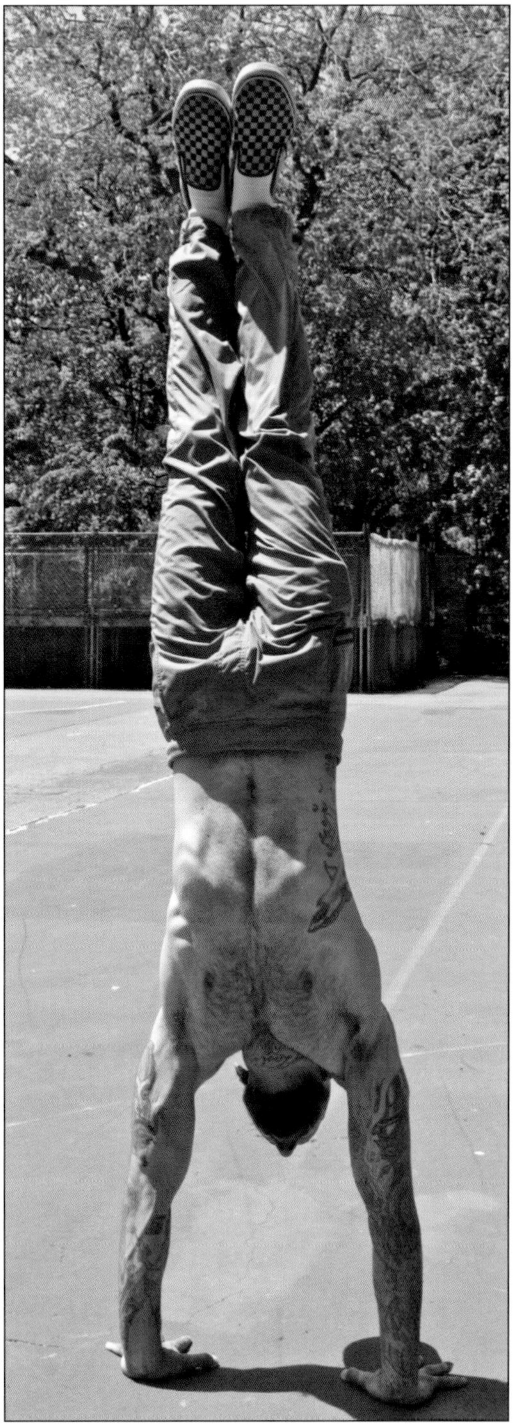

Kicking Up

If you're going to kick-up into a handstand, make sure you keep your elbows locked the whole time. I've seen quite a few beginners fall on their head during their first kick-up attempt because they let their arms bend just a little bit. Your arms tend to be stronger when they are locked out than they are with a bend in them and that's especially true in this case.

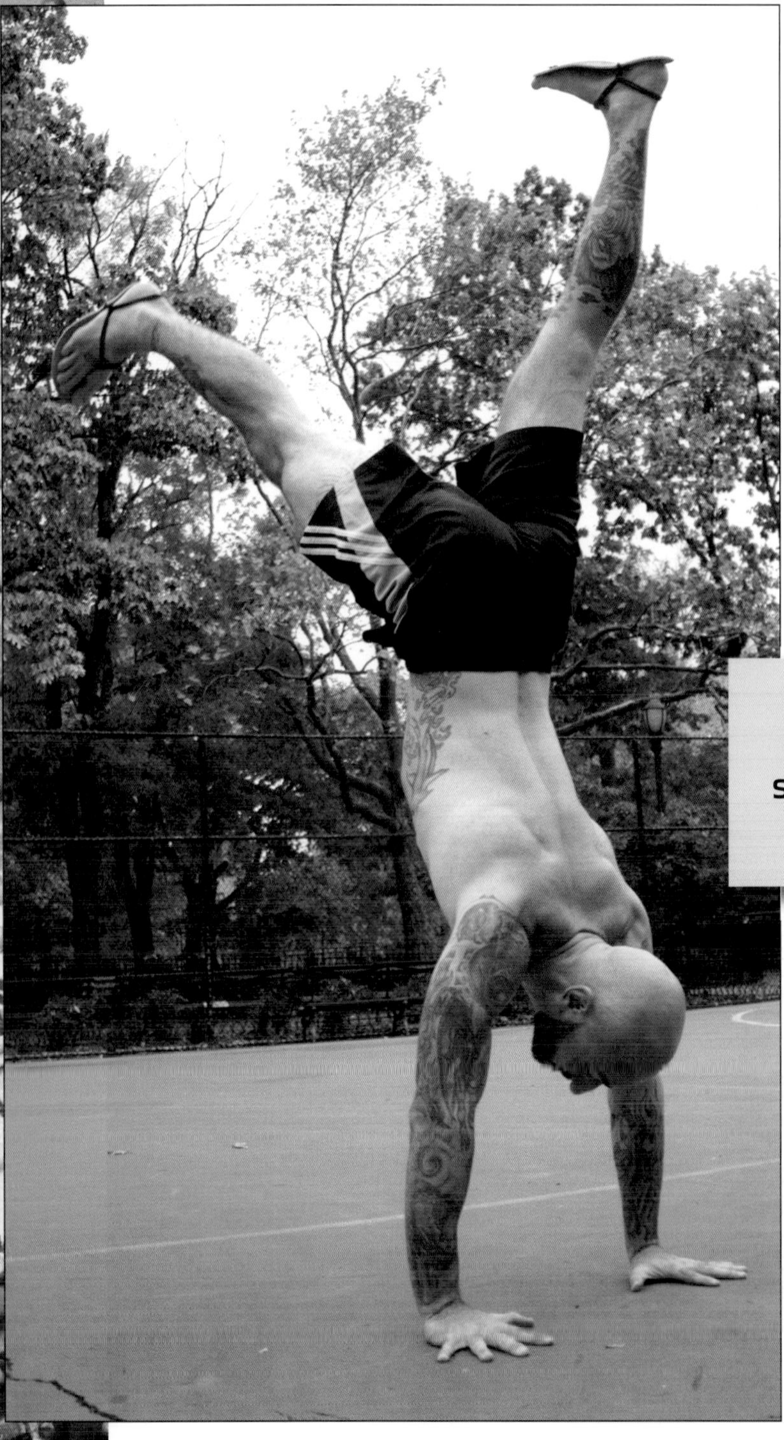

Start out practicing your handstand kick-up against a wall, leaving a little room for your back to arch. It will likely be easier for you to hold your handstand this way at first. In time you'll work towards getting your back straighter. With practice you can work up to gradually taking your feet off the wall. This will take different amounts of time for different people. If you are diligent in your training you will get there eventually, but don't expect it to happen overnight.

If you're going to kick-up into a handstand, make sure you keep your elbows locked the whole time.

Donkey Kick

Another way to kick into a handstand is to start in a position similar to the top of a divebomber push-up. From here, bend your legs and jump both feet right up to hip level with your knees tucked in by your trunk. Then it's just a matter of extending your legs into the air. Remember to keep your hips right over your hands. The hips tend to lead the rest of the body wherever they go.

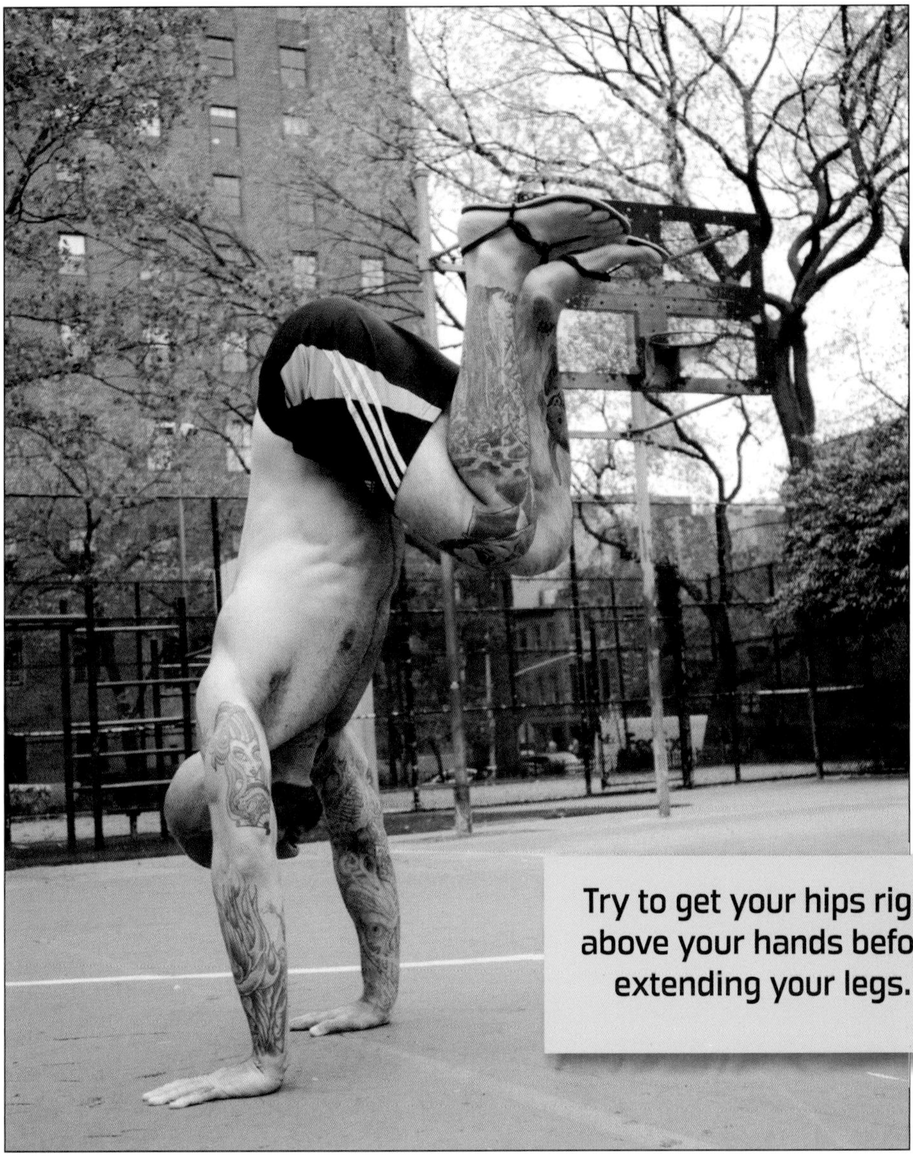

Try to get your hips right above your hands before extending your legs.

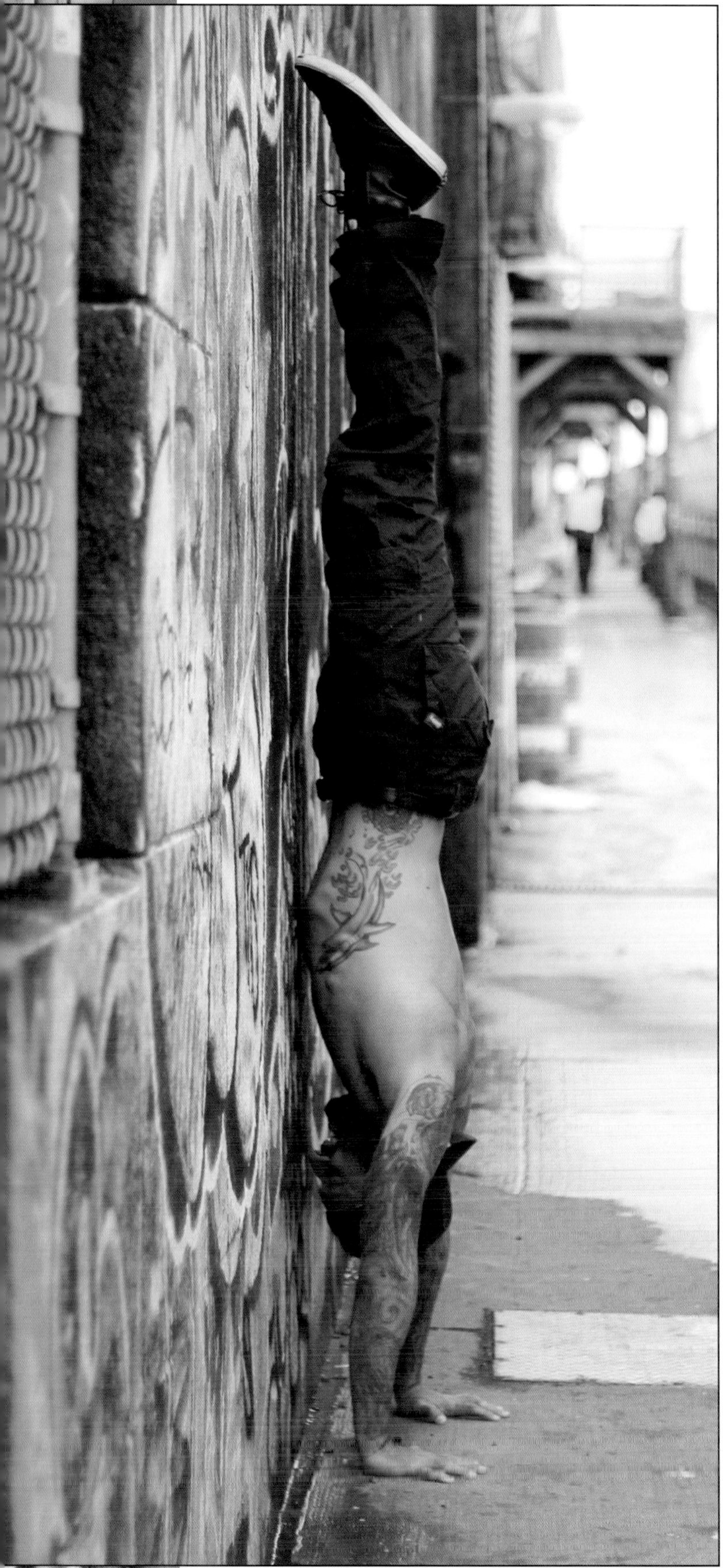

Facing The Wall

Though I recommend people who are new to handstands start out by practicing while facing *away* from a wall, doing the opposite is worthwhile to practice once you get the feel of being upside down on your hands. Getting into a handstand this way requires more strength than kicking up, but it can be very helpful with finding the alignment.

Get into a push-up position with your feet against a wall, then start gradually walking your way up the wall until you're upside down. Try to get your hands as close to the wall as you can and press your chest all the way out. Beginners may start five or six inches from the wall, but you should aim to eventually get within an inch or two. Think about lengthening your spine to make your body as straight as possible; you'll likely feel a stretch in your shoulders and upper back. Squeeze your legs and glutes to get your whole body straight. While I don't want you to shrug your shoulders during handstand push-ups, when holding the top position of a handstand, shrugging can help you lengthen your body and get your arms all the way under your shoulders. This can be a really helpful stretch if you're tight in your upper body.

Don't let your elbows flare out to the sides when practicing your handstand. Instead focus on keeping them in and back. This will help you fully lock out your arms and take advantage of your skeletal alignment. Just like when you stand on your legs, you want your bones to do some of the work when holding a handstand. Think about actively pressing the ground away from you as you lengthen your entire body.

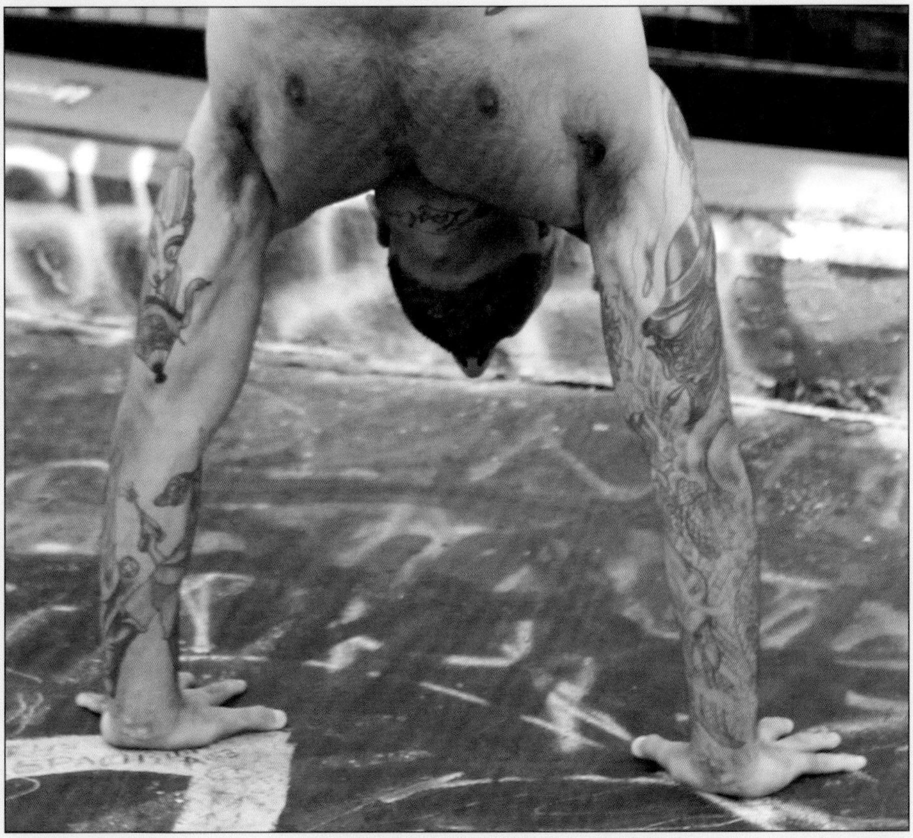

Press To Handstand

Pressing to a handstand is a much more challenging way to get into position. There are a few different ways to approach it. The simplest variation is to begin in a frog stand and try to lift yourself up by extending your legs as you press with your shoulders and arms. You can kick a bit with your legs to get some momentum if you don't have the strength to initiate this move with your arms alone. Be careful not to kick too hard though or you'll topple over.

You can also press to a handstand from your feet by bending over, placing your hands on the ground and shifting your weight forward onto your palms. Some people will find this easier than pressing from a frog stand, while others will find it more challenging, depending on individual factors. Feel free to practice from a shoulder-width standing position or with your legs in a straddle. The closer your feet are to each other, the more flexibility it requires. You can also bend your elbows a bit if you need to. Though starting with bent arms will require a bit more upper body strength, it can be helpful for those who lack the hip and/or shoulder mobility to begin with arms straight.

With either method, you'll need to grip the ground and engage your core as you raise your hips and legs up over your hands. Just like the donkey kick, get your hips all the way over your shoulders in order to find the proper alignment.

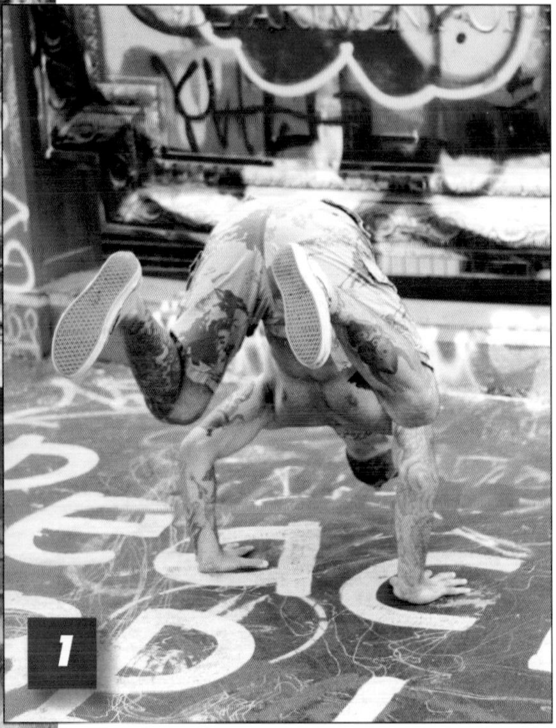
1

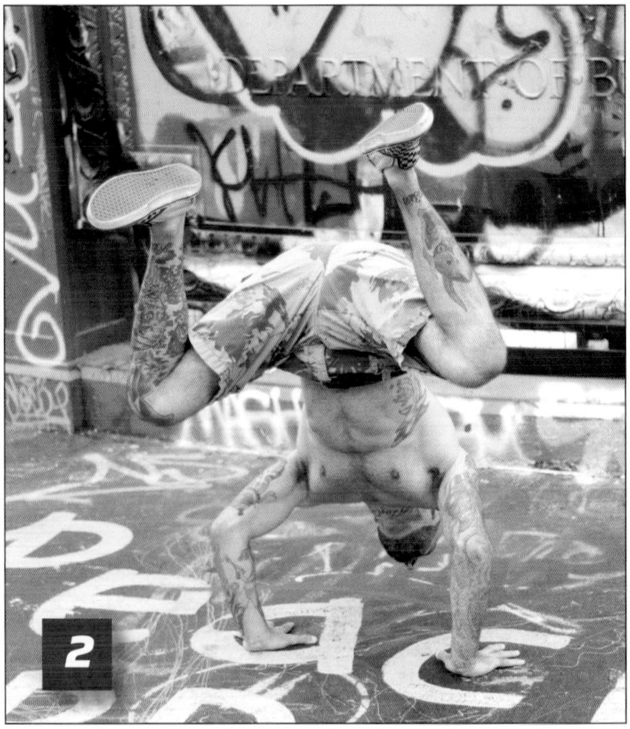
2

4

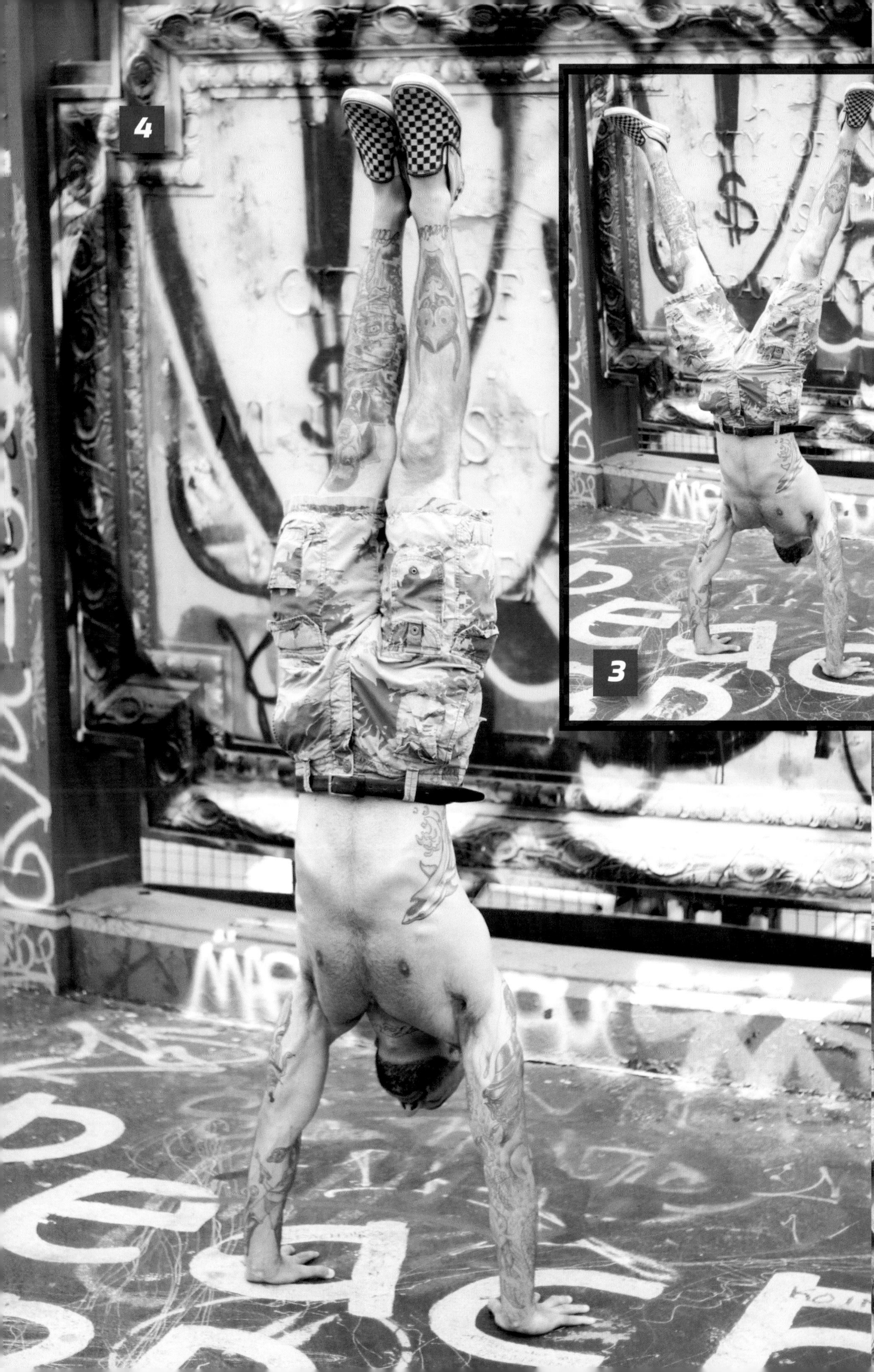

3

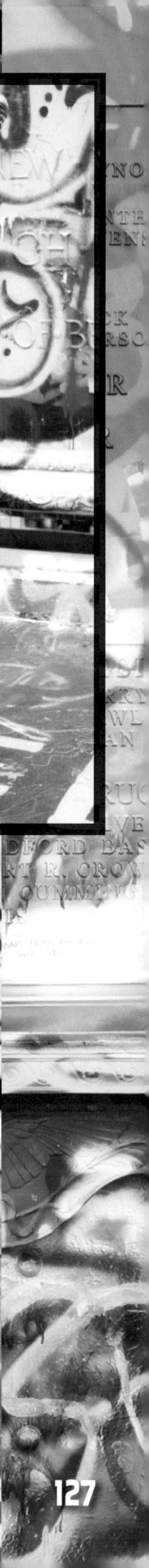

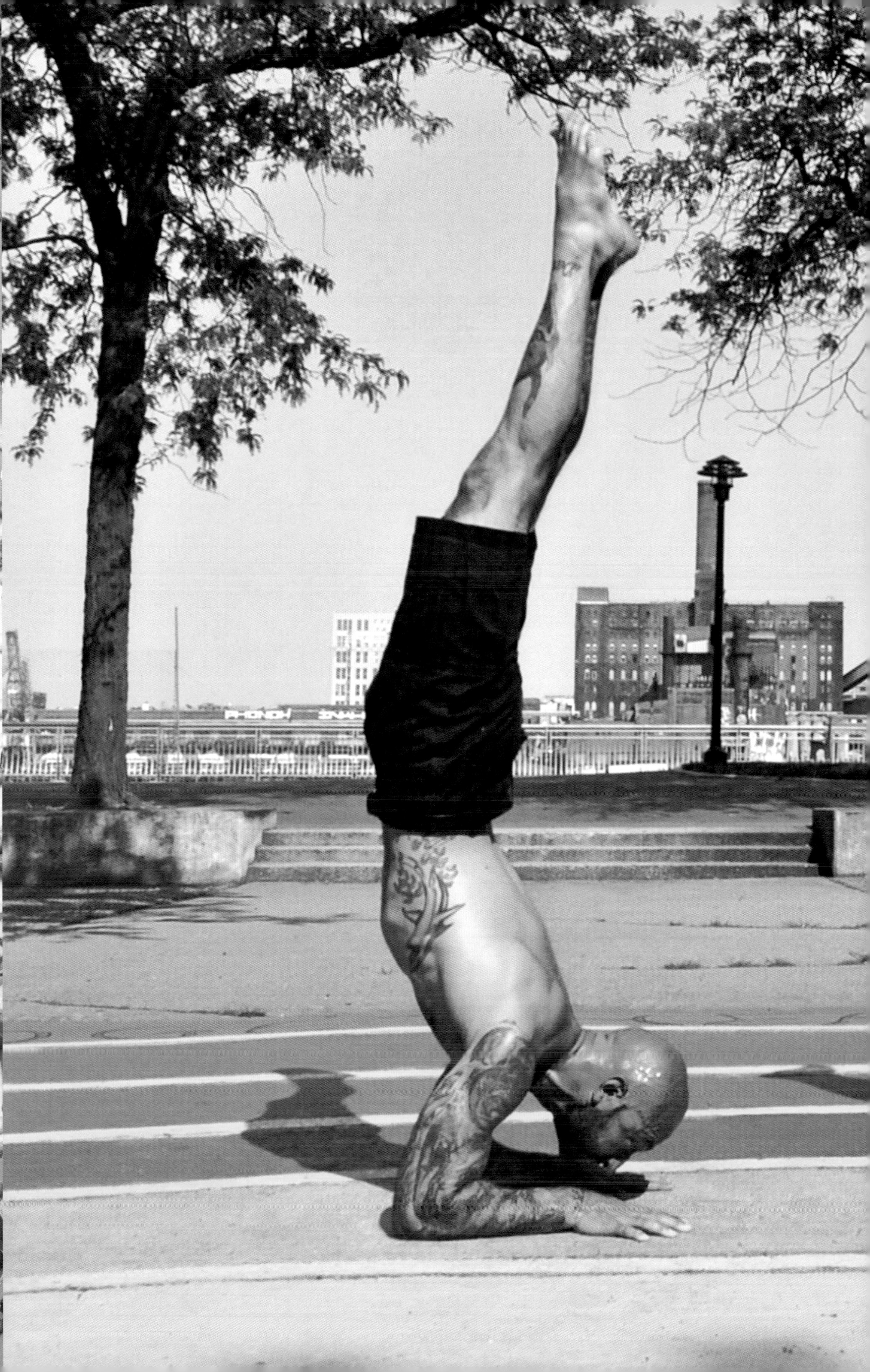

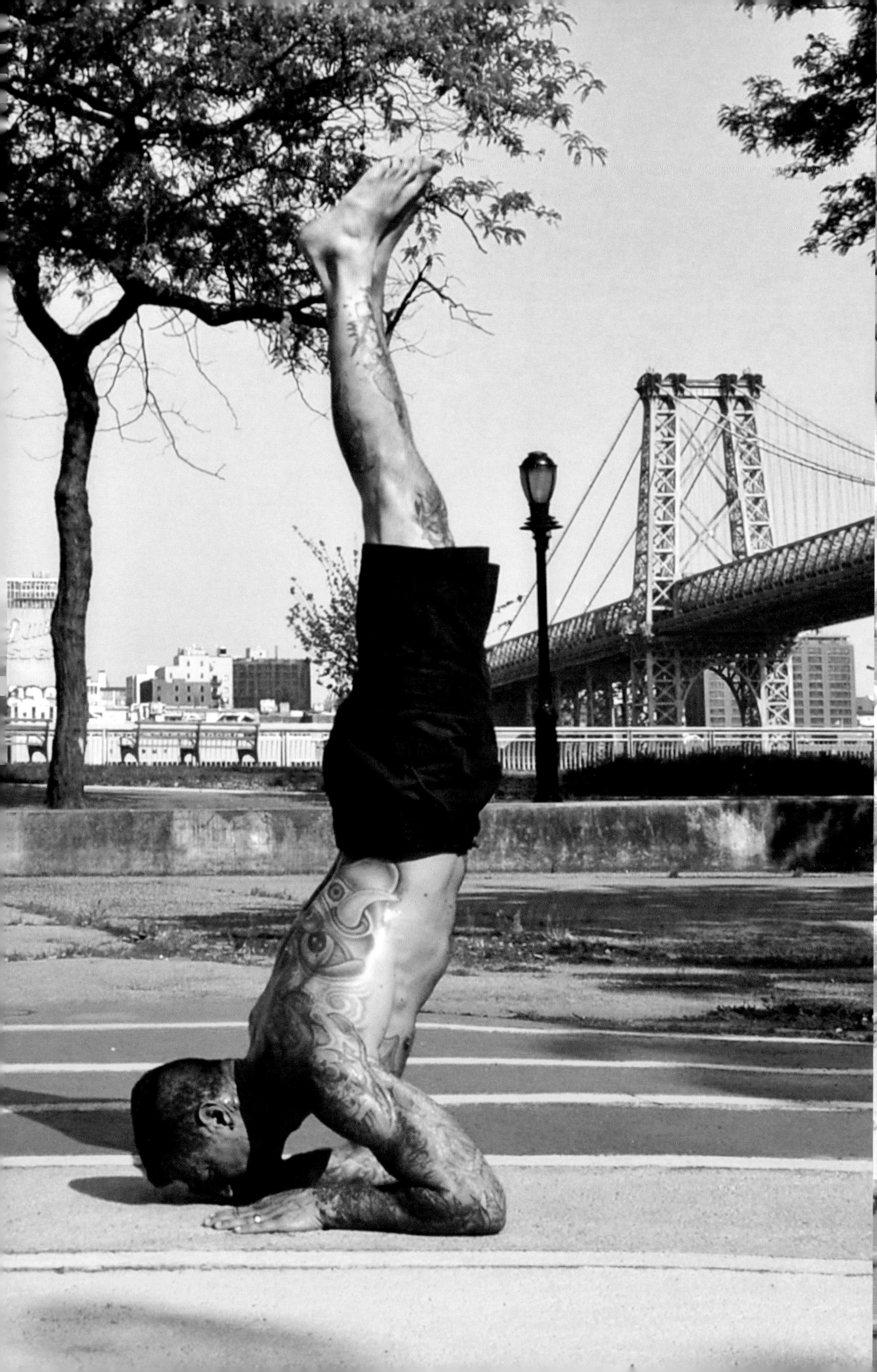

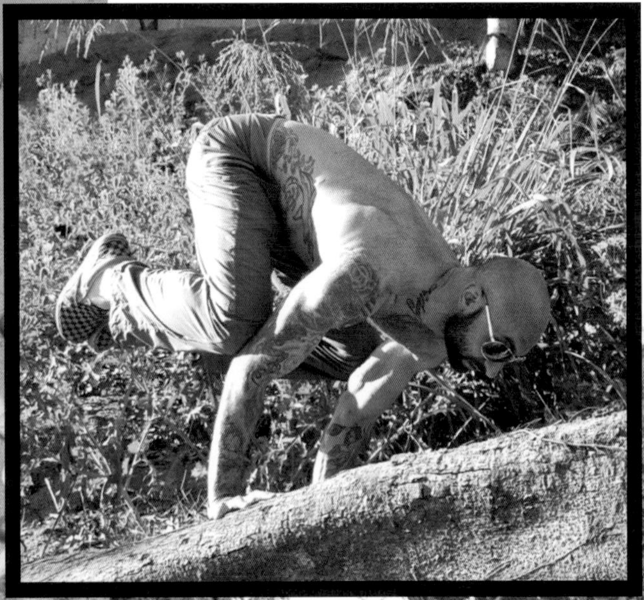

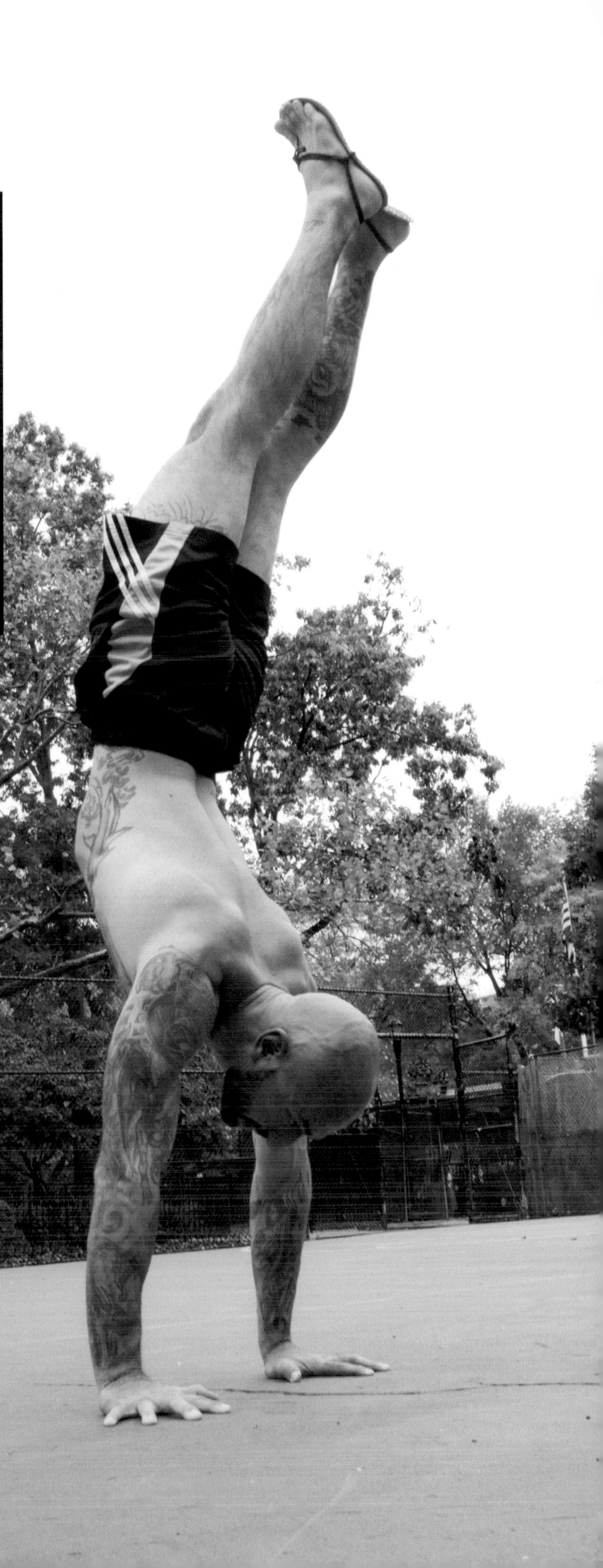

Beginners may find it easier to hold the handstand with an arched back.

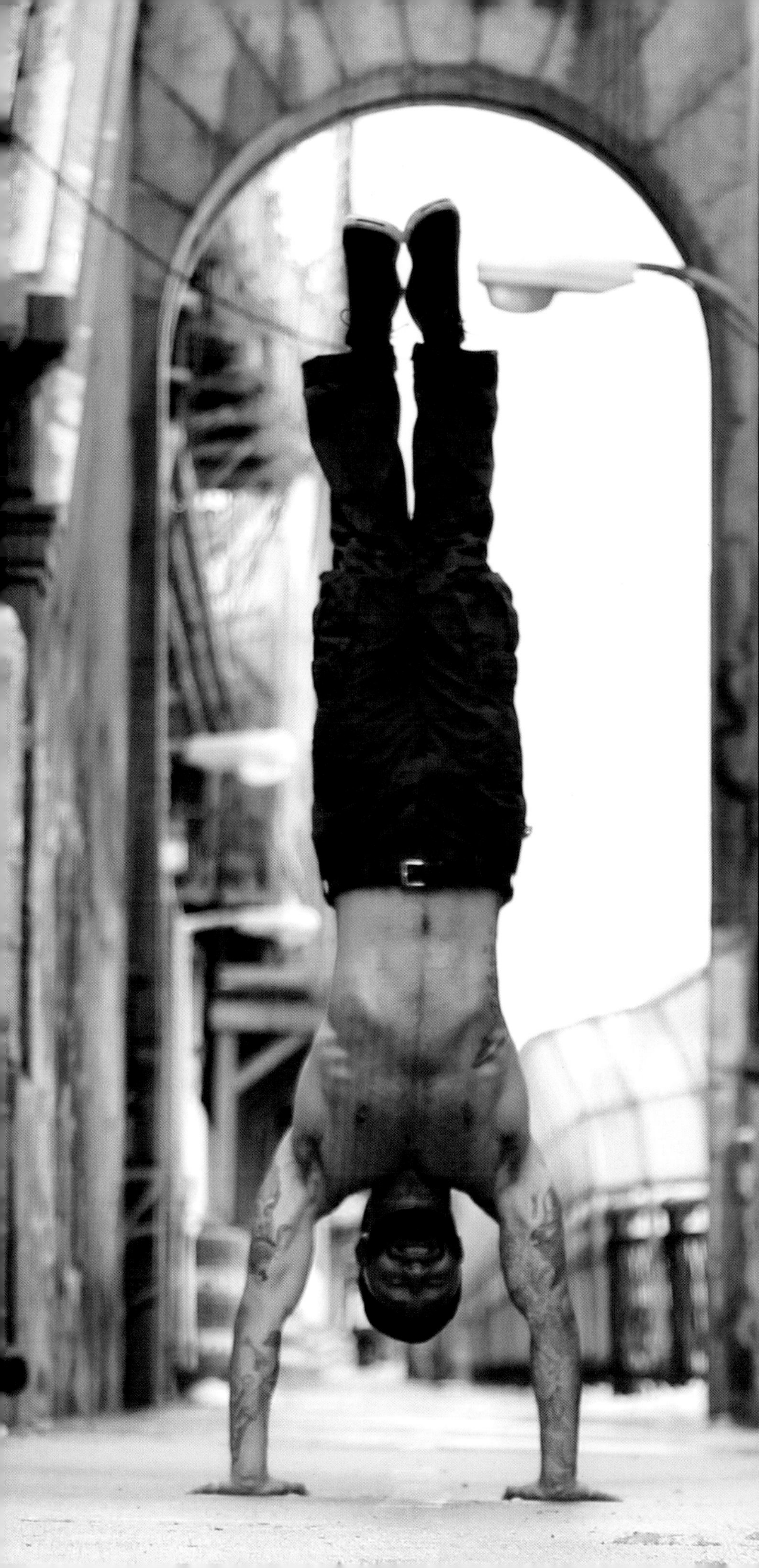

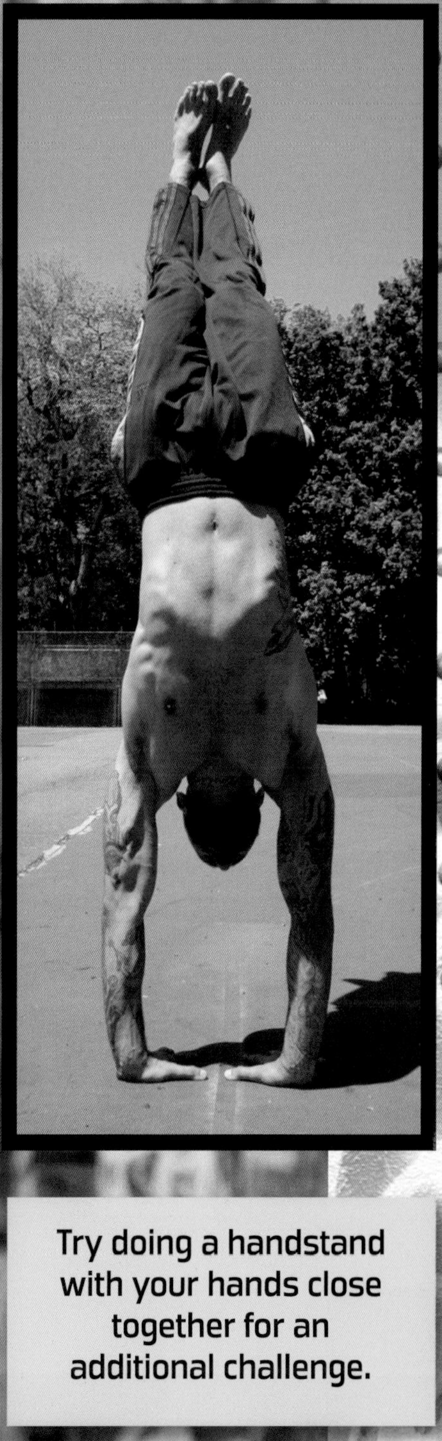

Try doing a handstand with your hands close together for an additional challenge.

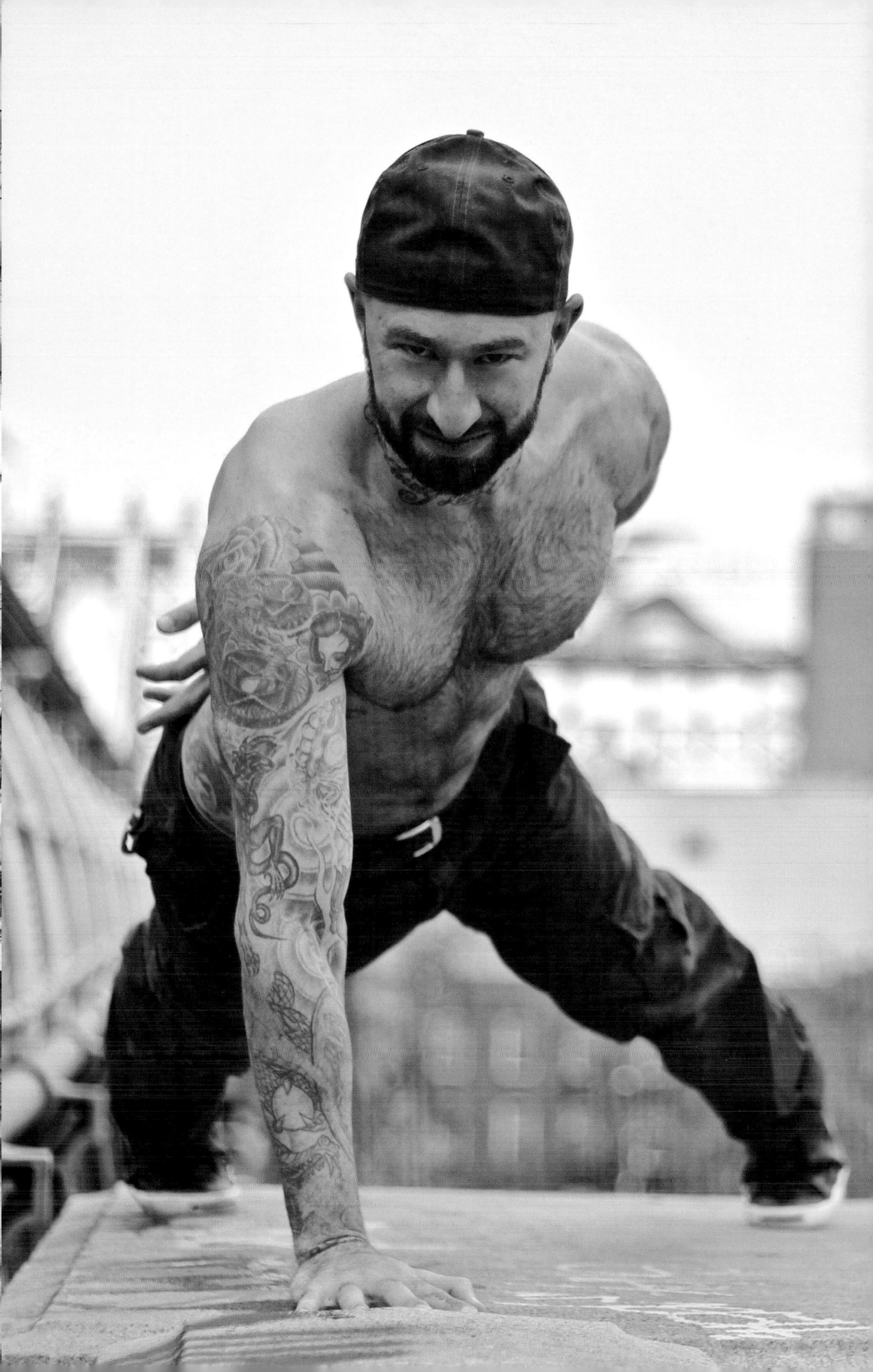

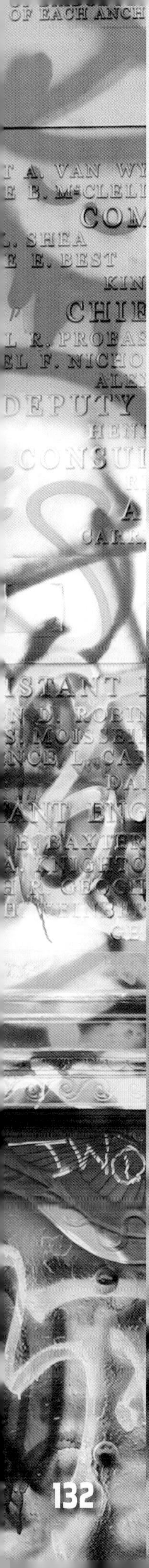

Chapter Seven:

Owning The One Arm Push-up

The one arm push-up is one of the most badass exercises on the planet. It demonstrates total body strength and control, and can do wonders for your pushing output. It's also an extremely versatile and adaptable exercise. Even within the world of one arm push-ups there are still many different variations and ways to progress things.

Only once you've gotten very comfortable with standard push-ups (and worked through the variations in Chapter Four) should you proceed with this move. You must also master the close push-up as a precursor to the one arm push-up. I recommend getting to the point where you can do at least 30 consecutive diamond (or arrowhead) push-ups before beginning one arm push-up training.

It should be noted that the form of a one arm push-up is a bit different from the standard two arm version. Your legs will need to be farther apart than in a regular push-up and your hand should be pretty much right beneath your body, rather than off to the side. The three points of contact (foot, hand, foot) will make a triangular formation. As a general guideline, the closer your feet are positioned to each other, the harder the exercise becomes. Begin with your feet nice and wide to help get the feel for the movement pattern. Eventually you may try working toward narrowing your stance.

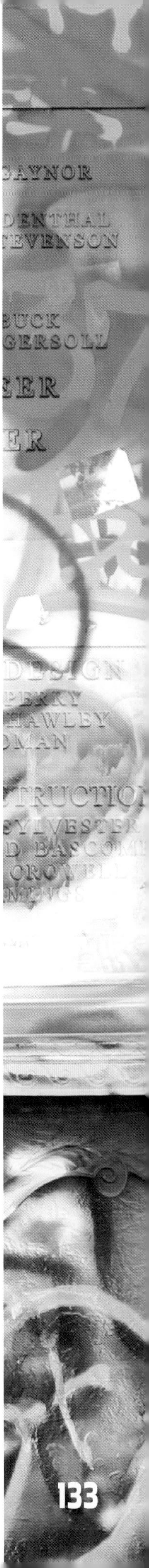

Incline One Arm Push-up

A lot of the techniques I recommend for learning the one arm push-up are the same as what I suggest for beginners who are learning to do push-ups with both arms. My favorite way to introduce the movement to someone new is to have them begin on an incline. You can best learn to get a feel for the movement and condition your joints by practicing one arm push-ups at an angle where you will have increased leverage.

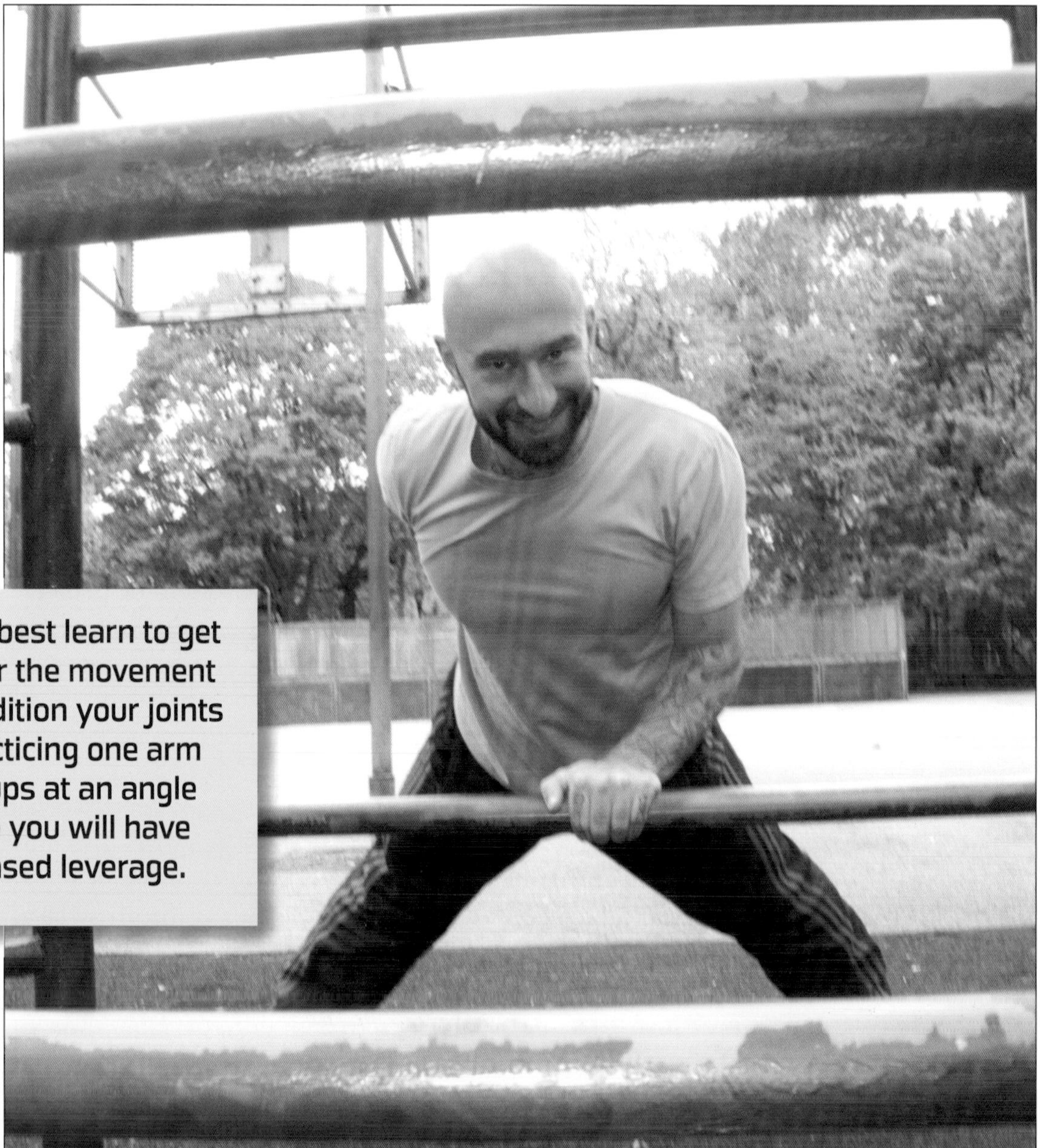

You can best learn to get a feel for the movement and condition your joints by practicing one arm push-ups at an angle where you will have increased leverage.

L7 Push-up

Not only is this variation a nice segue toward a one arm push-up, it's also a helpful approach toward a close grip wrist push-up. An L7 is to a diamond what the one and one push-up is to a normal push-up. One arm will rest on the back of the hand instead of the palm. When done with the right hand turned over, your fingers will look like the letter "L" and the number "7." Since having a lot of weight on the backs of the hands can be uncomfortable, this variation encourages you to push more with the opposite side. Focus on pushing primarily with your palm-down hand, relying on your opposite wrist primarily for stability.

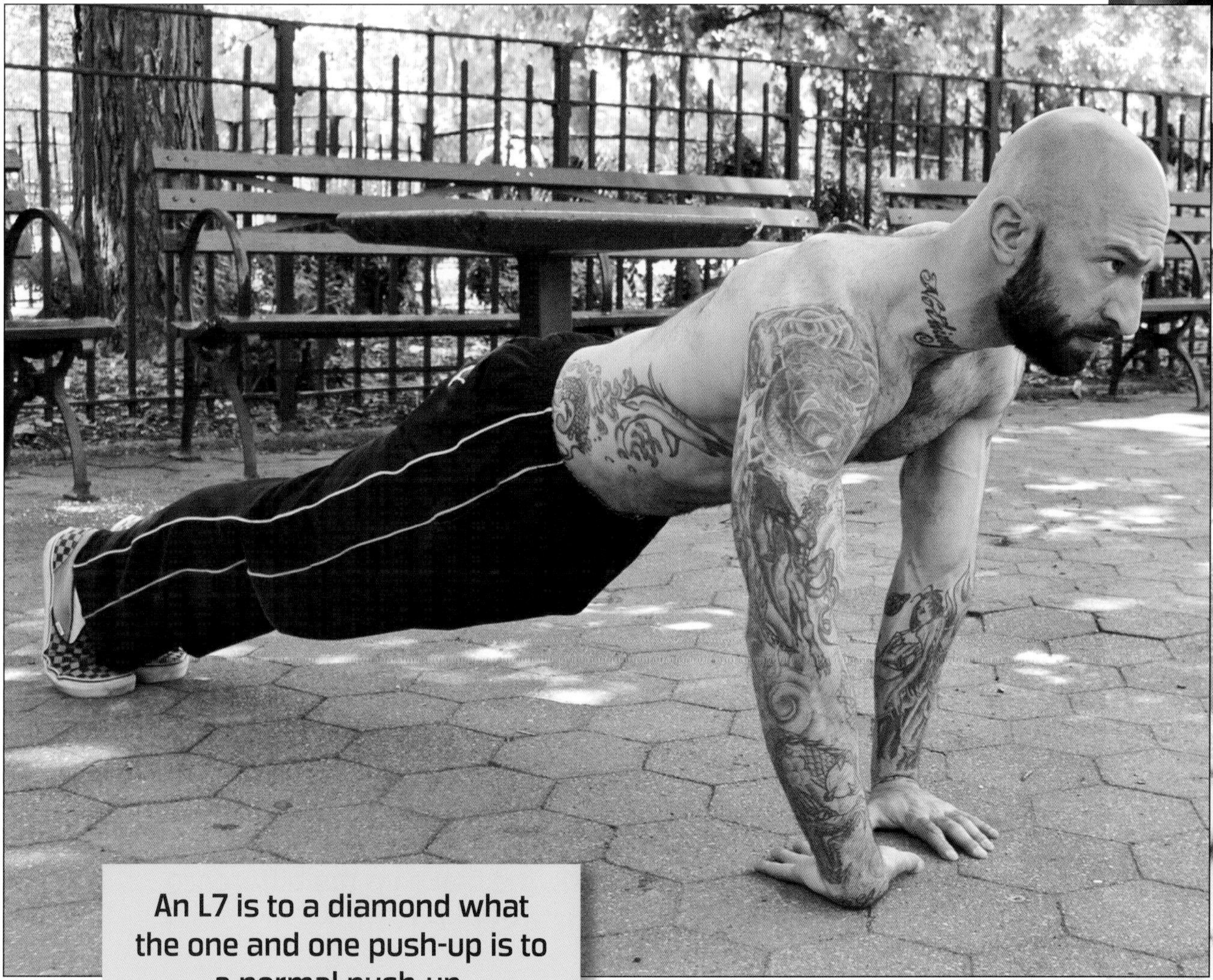

An L7 is to a diamond what the one and one push-up is to a normal push-up.

Self Assisted One Arm Push-up

A self assisted one arm push-up involves reaching your secondary arm out to the side and resting it on a raised object like a ledge, brick or medicine ball. Again, the idea is to use your primary arm to do the majority of the work and make up the difference with the extended arm. This technique is also helpful due to the fact that it teaches you the proper position for the torso during a full one arm push-up. Though a small degree of rotation may be unavoidable, aim to keep your upper-body as close to parallel with the ground as you can.

Though similar to an archer push-up, this variation should be performed one arm at a time, due to the nature of the opposite hand being elevated. Also keep your movement as vertical as possible to simulate a one arm push-up, as opposed to moving side to side as you would in an archer.

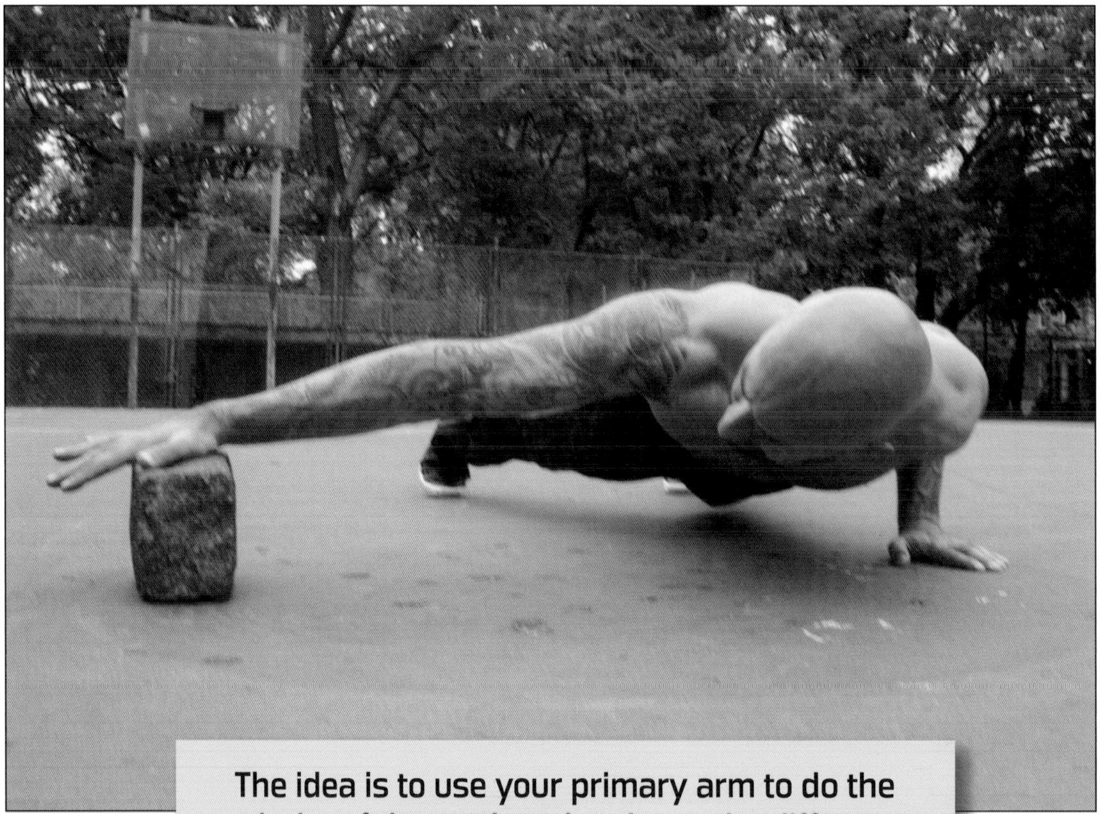

The idea is to use your primary arm to do the majority of the work and make up the difference with the extended arm.

Negatives

Performing the lowering phase of a one arm push-up can be a gateway to the full exercise as it helps you learn the movement pattern in a *neurological* sense. The brain has an amazing way of learning! Strength isn't all about muscles — it's about knowing how to use your muscles.

Get into the top position of a one arm push-up and squeeze your whole body tight as you slowly lower yourself down with control. Remember to keep your elbow in by your side. When you get to the bottom, push yourself back up with both arms, then take one away and do it again. You may wind up dropping quickly at first, but in time you will develop better control.

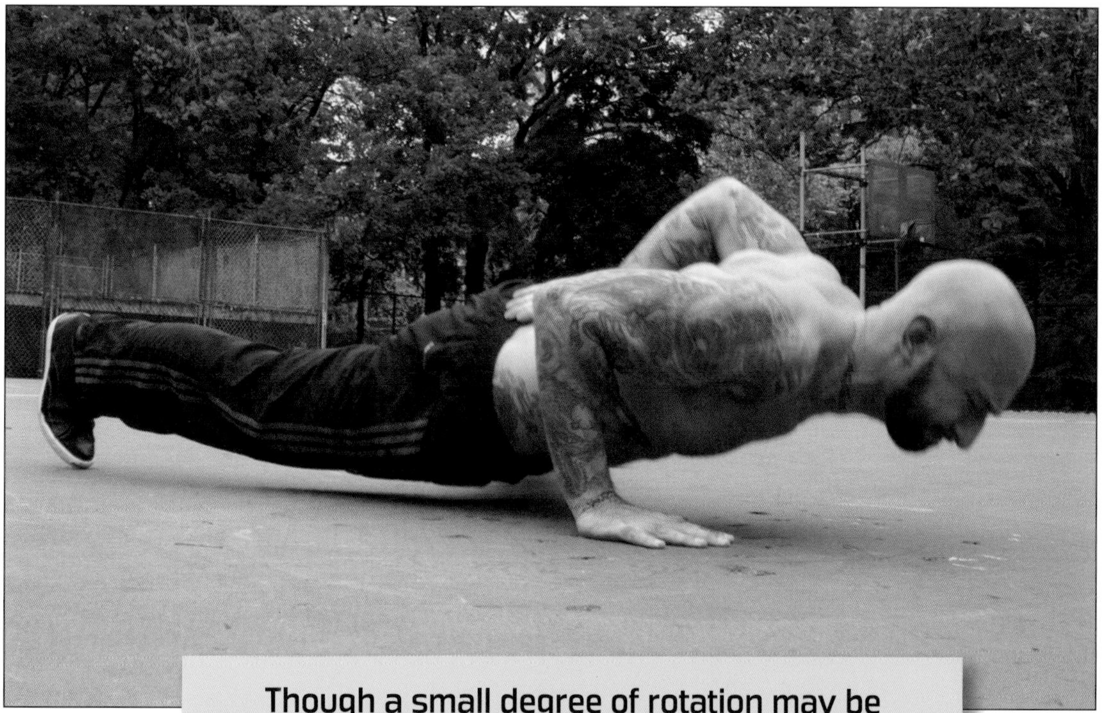

Though a small degree of rotation may be unavoidable, aim to keep your upper-body as close to parallel with the ground as you can.

One Arm Push-up

The phrase "one arm push-up" is a little misleading. It's impossible to do any type of push-up without using your entire body! If you don't contract your hips, legs, abs and glutes there's absolutely no way you can do a proper one arm push-up.

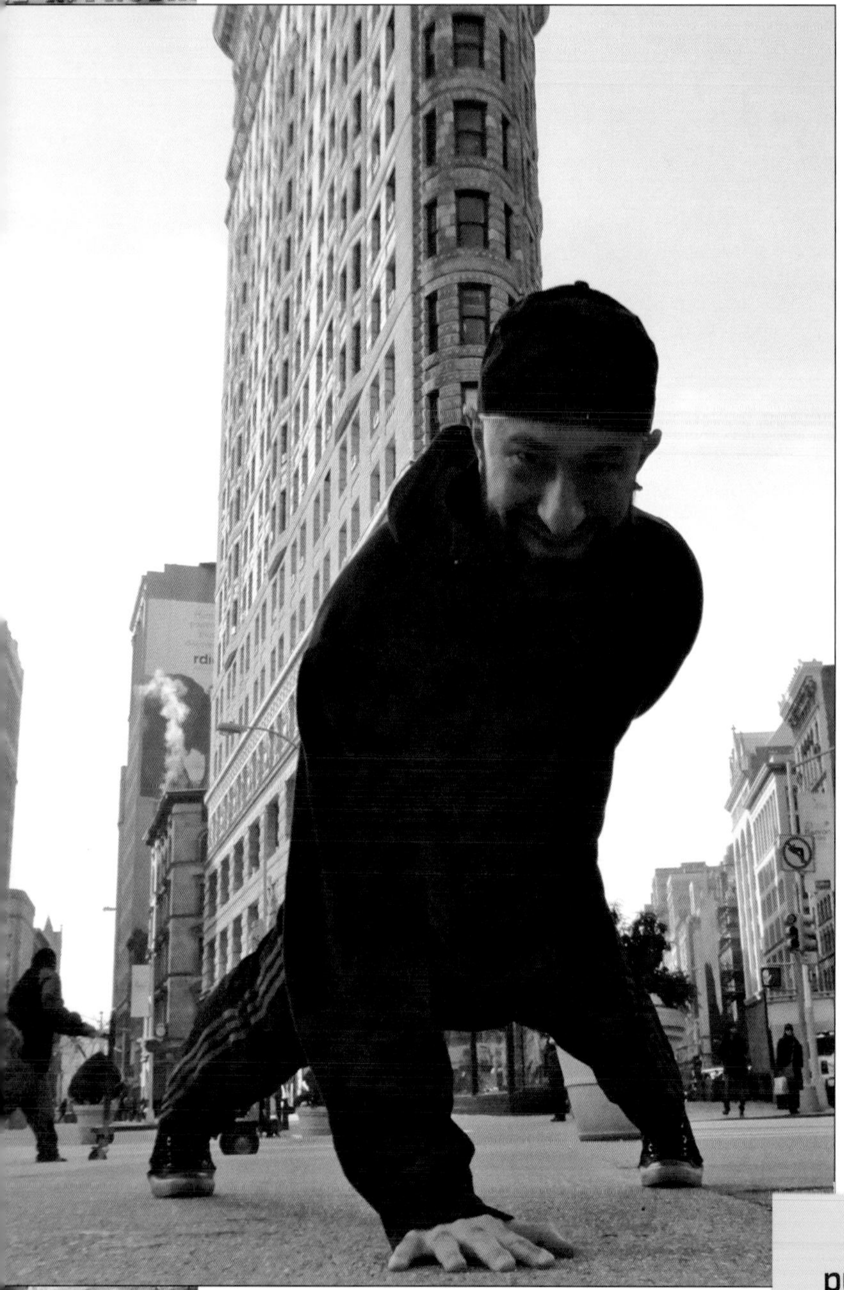

Make sure you keep your pressing arm close to your body. Just like a diamond or close grip push-up, your arm should gently graze your ribs on the way down as well as the way up. Your other arm can be held against your body or placed behind the back.

Remember that the standard one arm push-up involves the legs being in a straddle position. Though some people will tell you that this isn't a true one arm push-up, feet wide is most certainly the gold standard for the exercise. The torso remains mostly parallel to the ground, the elbow stays in and the hips move ever so slightly towards the pressing arm to maintain balance as the body lowers down.

A one arm push-up with the feet together is a more difficult move, but it's so much more difficult to pull off without significant bowing to the side that it isn't really practical to use as a training tool. If you're going to move your hips to the side, you might as well straddle your legs to minimize that movement.

The standard one arm push-up involves the legs being in a straddle position.

Fingertip, Knuckle And Back Of The Hand One Arm Push-ups

Obviously, the main thing that makes any of these one arm push-up variations harder than the standard type is supporting all your weight on the fingertips, knuckles or back of just one hand. Before attempting any of these variations, I suggest being able to perform at least 30 reps with the two arm equivalent. You also must be able to do several consecutive one arm push-ups on your palm. The surface you use can also affect the difficulty of the exercise. Doing any of these on pavement is not recommended until you've gotten the feel for practicing them on gentler surfaces.

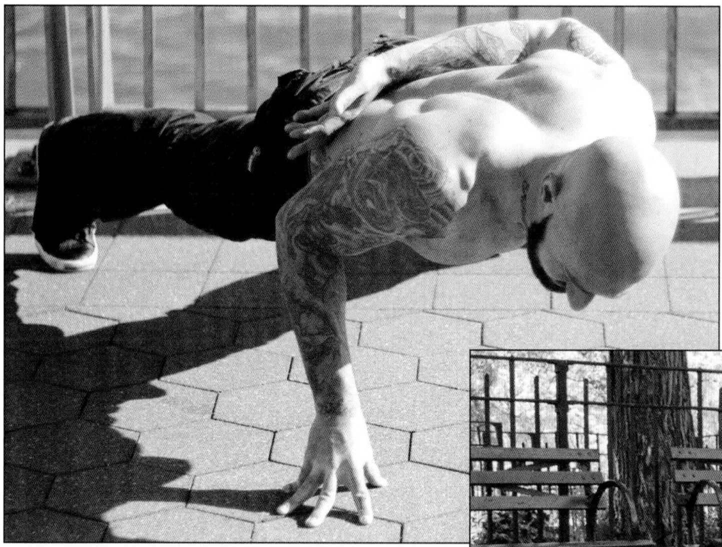

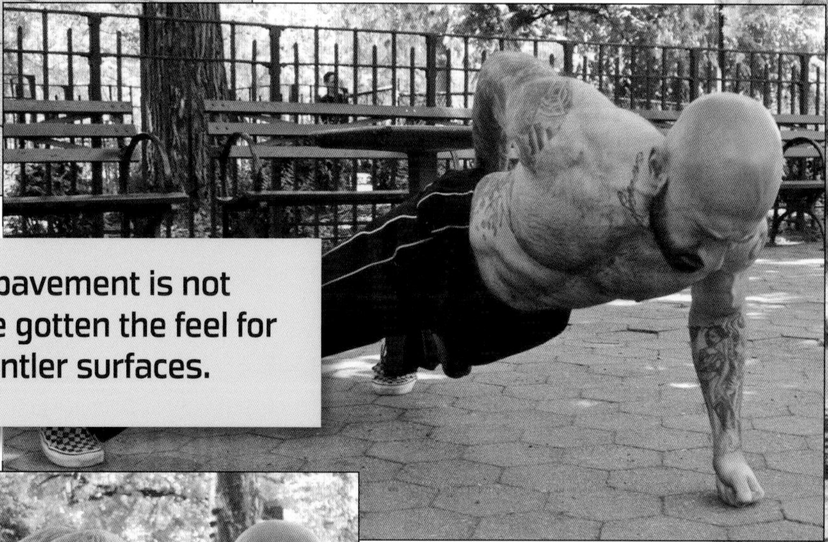

Doing any of these on pavement is not recommended until you've gotten the feel for practicing them on gentler surfaces.

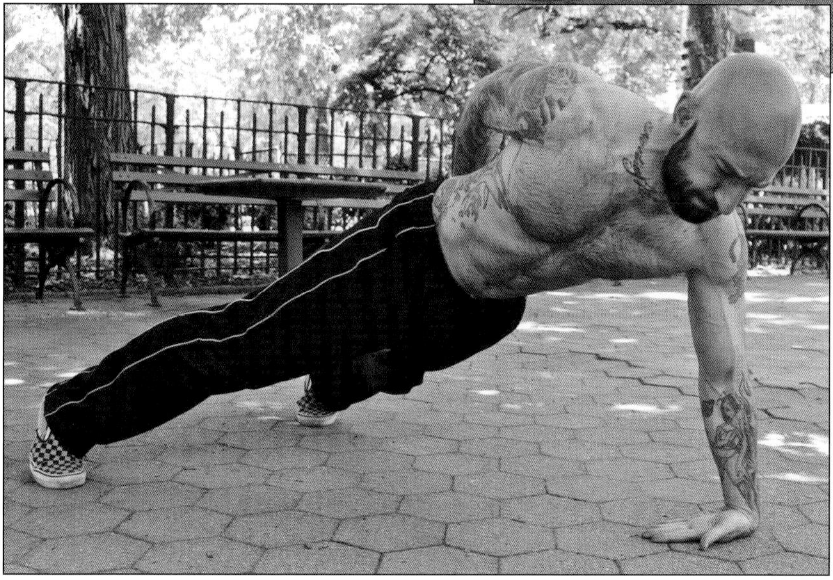

One Arm/One Leg Push-up

If you can do a few clean one arm push-ups, it shouldn't take too much practice to get the hang of lifting up the leg opposite from your pushing arm. Even though one foot is off the ground, you still want to keep your legs apart to maintain your balance. You might find it helpful to reach your free arm away from your body for balance as well.

The cross-stability required for this move is a bit more intense than a standard one armer, but if you take it slow and steady a little practice can go a long way. Make sure you use opposing limbs for this variant (right arm/left leg or vice versa).

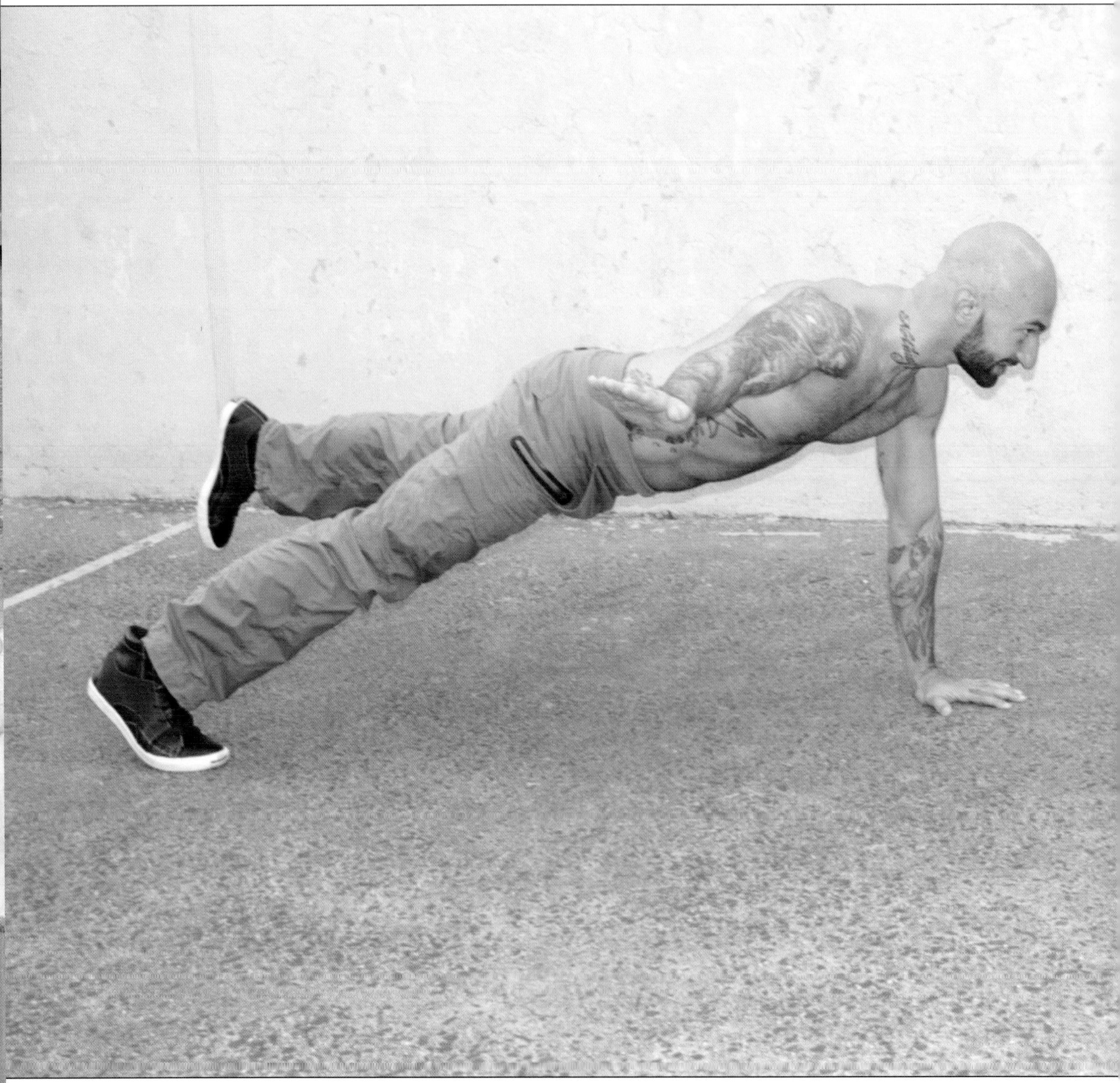

Make sure you use opposing limbs for this variant (right arm/left leg or vice versa).

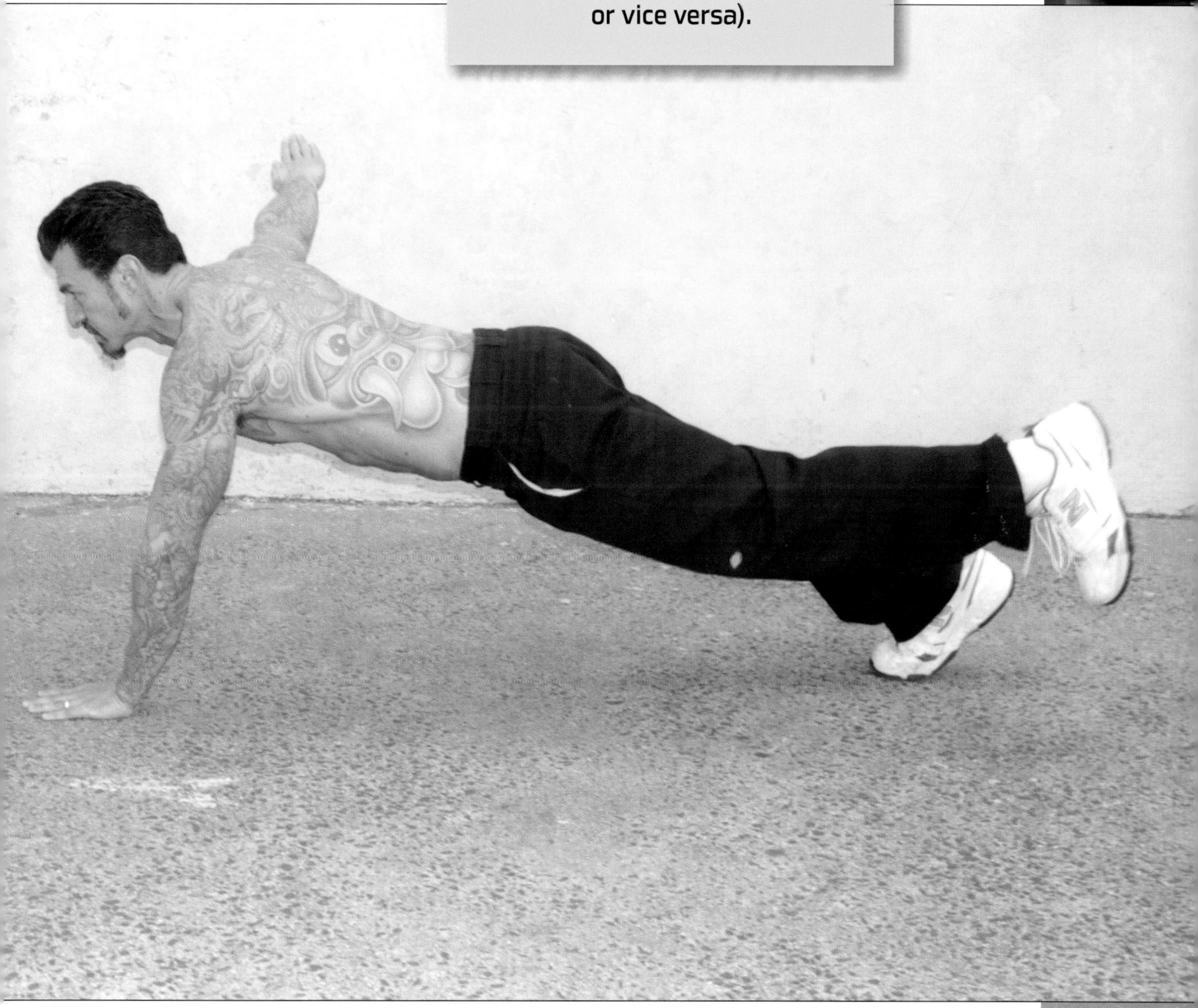

Plyo One Arm Push-up

If you practice enough one arm push-ups, you may eventually get strong enough to catch some air. Like any plyometric exercise, make sure you absorb the impact during the negative phase of the exercise. Avoid landing with your arm fully locked out on this type of move.

When you get a feel for the plyo one arm push-up, you might try clapping your hand to your chest, or waving it out in the air. I recommend getting to the point where you can perform at least five consecutive one arm push-ups before attempting plyos.

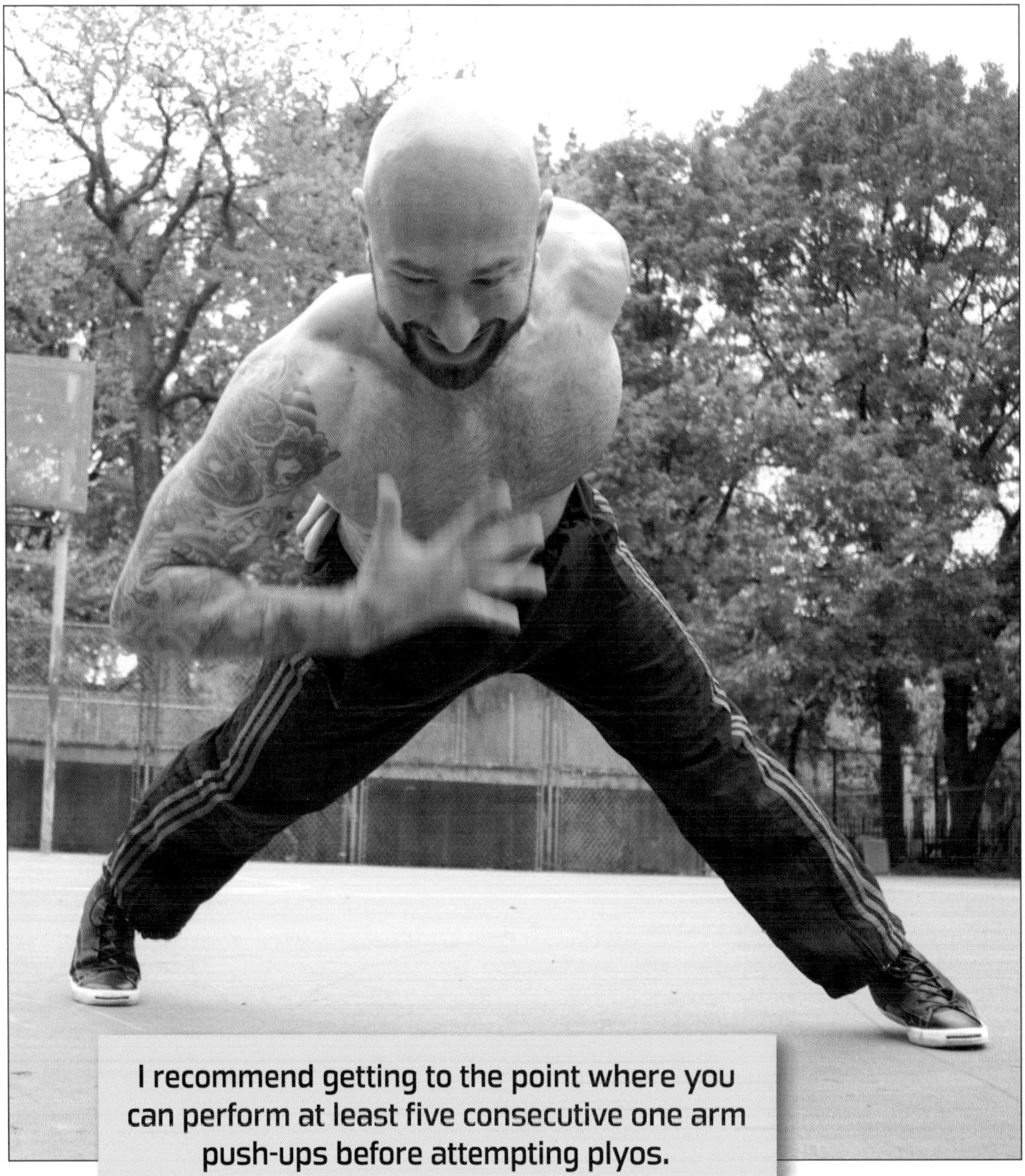

I recommend getting to the point where you can perform at least five consecutive one arm push-ups before attempting plyos.

Ultimate One Arm Push-up

In theory, performing a perfect one arm push-up with your feet touching each other and the body totally straight through the entire range of motion is the hardest push-up variation there could be. You'll only have two contact points instead of the three you'd have in a wide stance one arm push-up, and unlike the one arm/one leg push-up — which is surprisingly easy by comparison — you don't have a leg in the air to reach out and balance with.

The core strength and balance required to perform just one rep is only outdone by the amount of pressing power that your arm will need to generate in order to compensate for the change in hip position that placing the feet alongside each other entails. It's truly the ultimate one arm push-up!

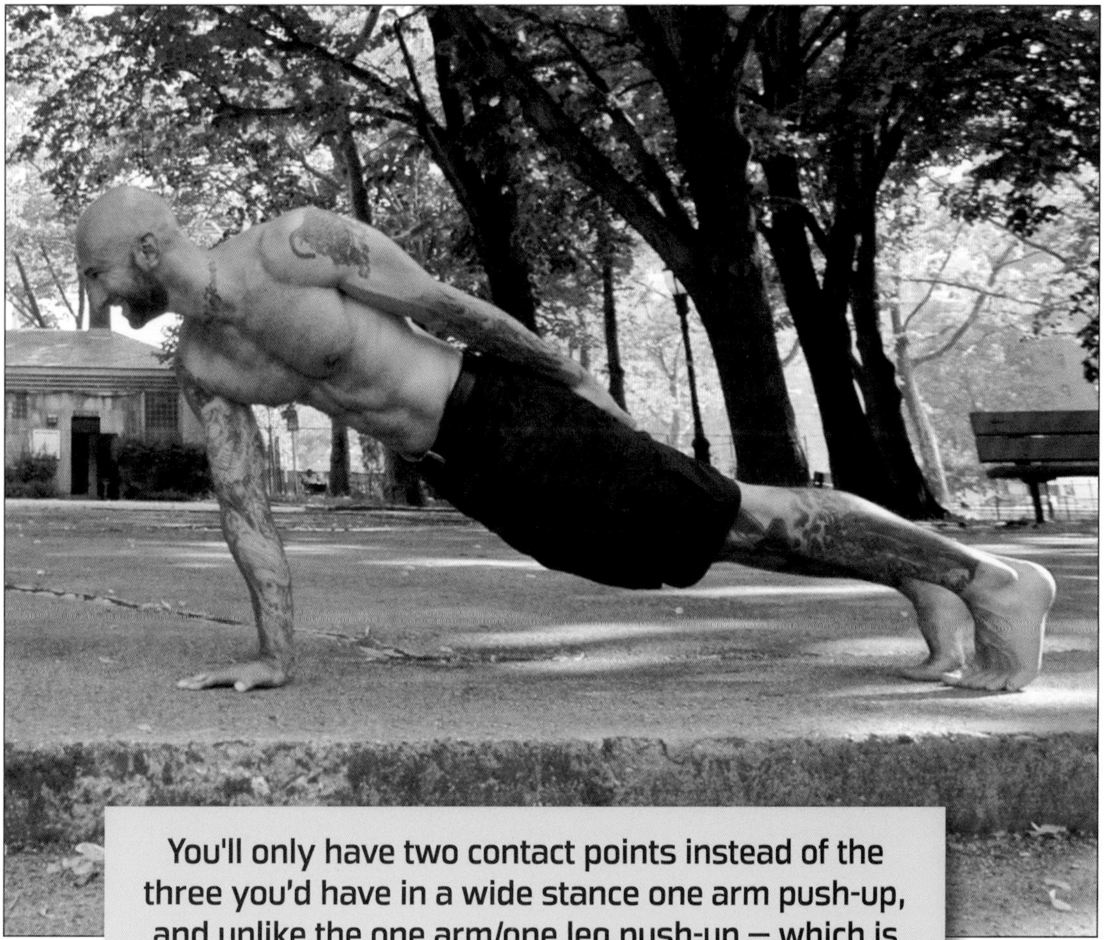

You'll only have two contact points instead of the three you'd have in a wide stance one arm push-up, and unlike the one arm/one leg push-up – which is surprisingly easy by comparison – you don't have a leg in the air to reach out and balance with.

Nobody's Perfect

The truth is, this variation is an ideal that will always stay just out of reach. Nobody has ever documented a perfectly straight feet-together one arm push-up and I'm not holding my breath for it to happen any time soon. Perfection is an illusion. There can never be a truly perfect one arm push-up, but sometimes it's good to have these ideals in our training. They motivate and inspire us to push ourselves. However, they can also be troublesome when they give us false expectations. Know that a truly perfect one arm push-up is a very subjective thing. Working out and being fit is about more than any one single skill and obsessing over perfection can actually impede growth. It's more practical to get your reps up with your feet apart than struggle for one rep of an exercise that is purely theoretical. Besides, a clean one arm push-up with the legs spread can be plenty challenging on its own!

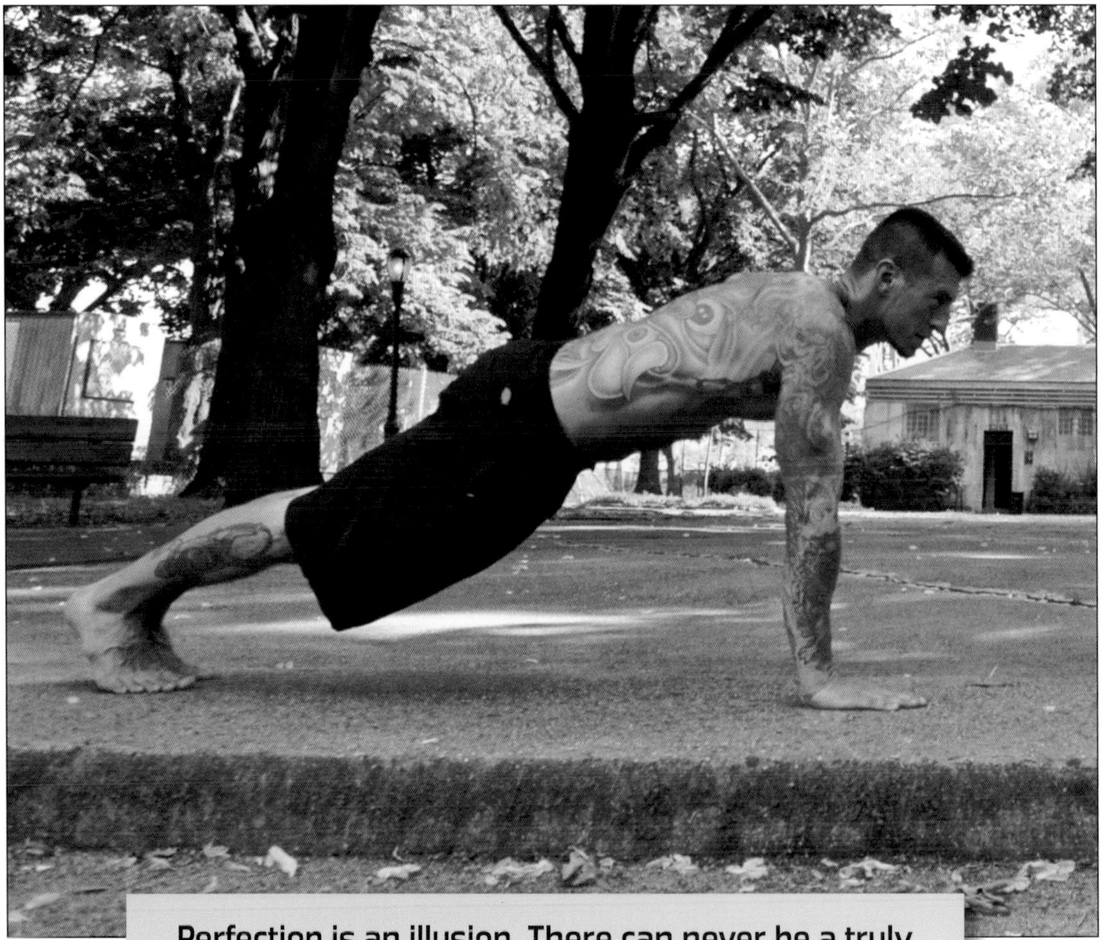

Perfection is an illusion. There can never be a truly perfect one arm push-up, but sometimes it's good to have these ideals in our training.

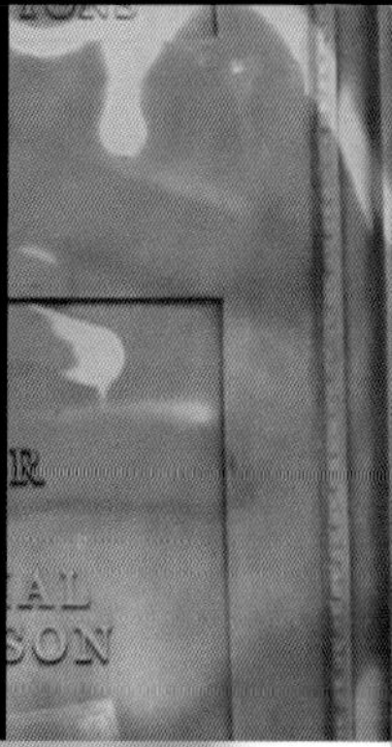

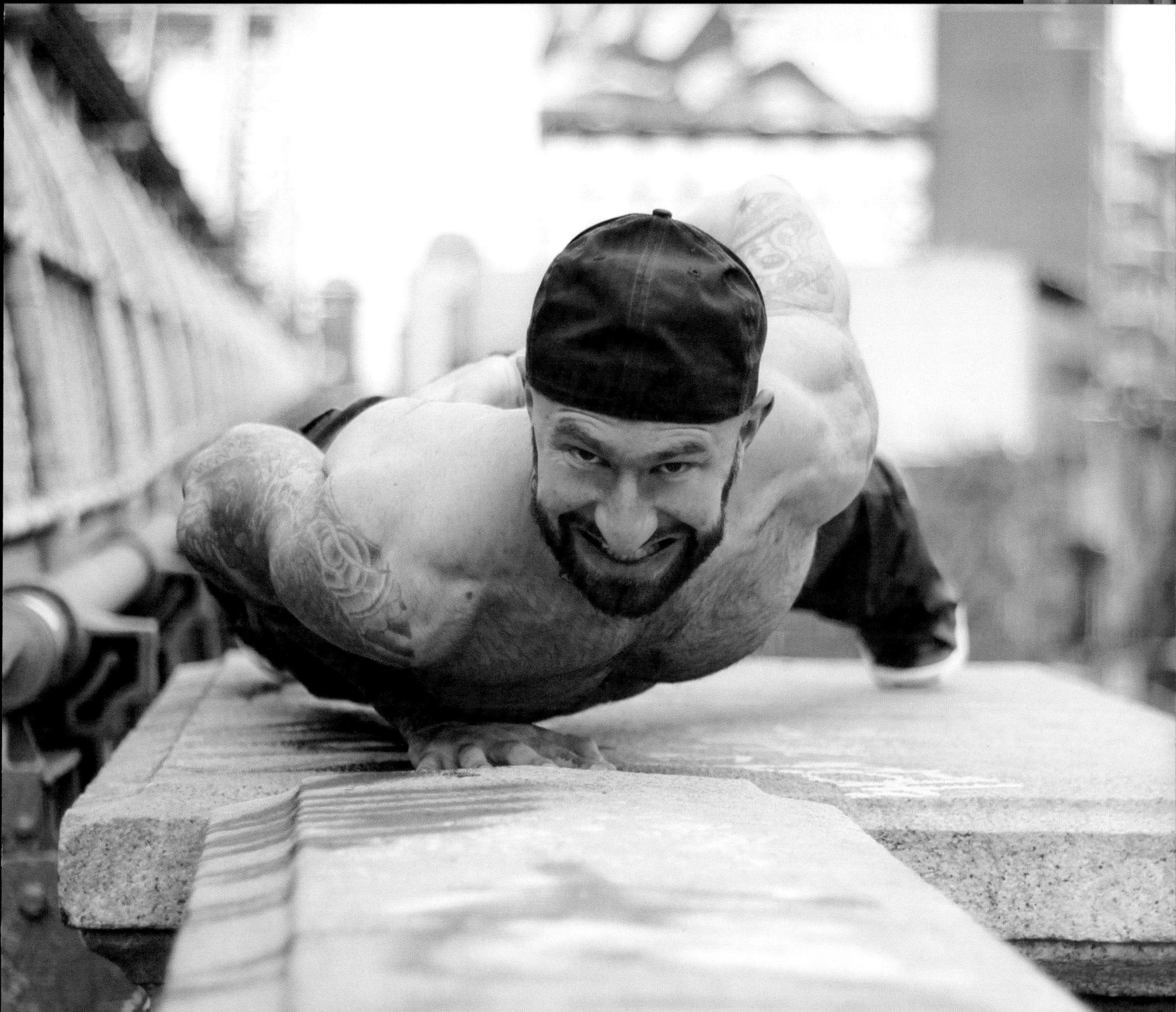

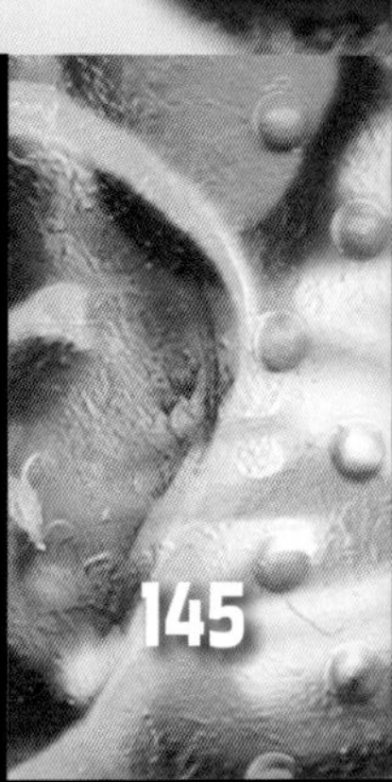

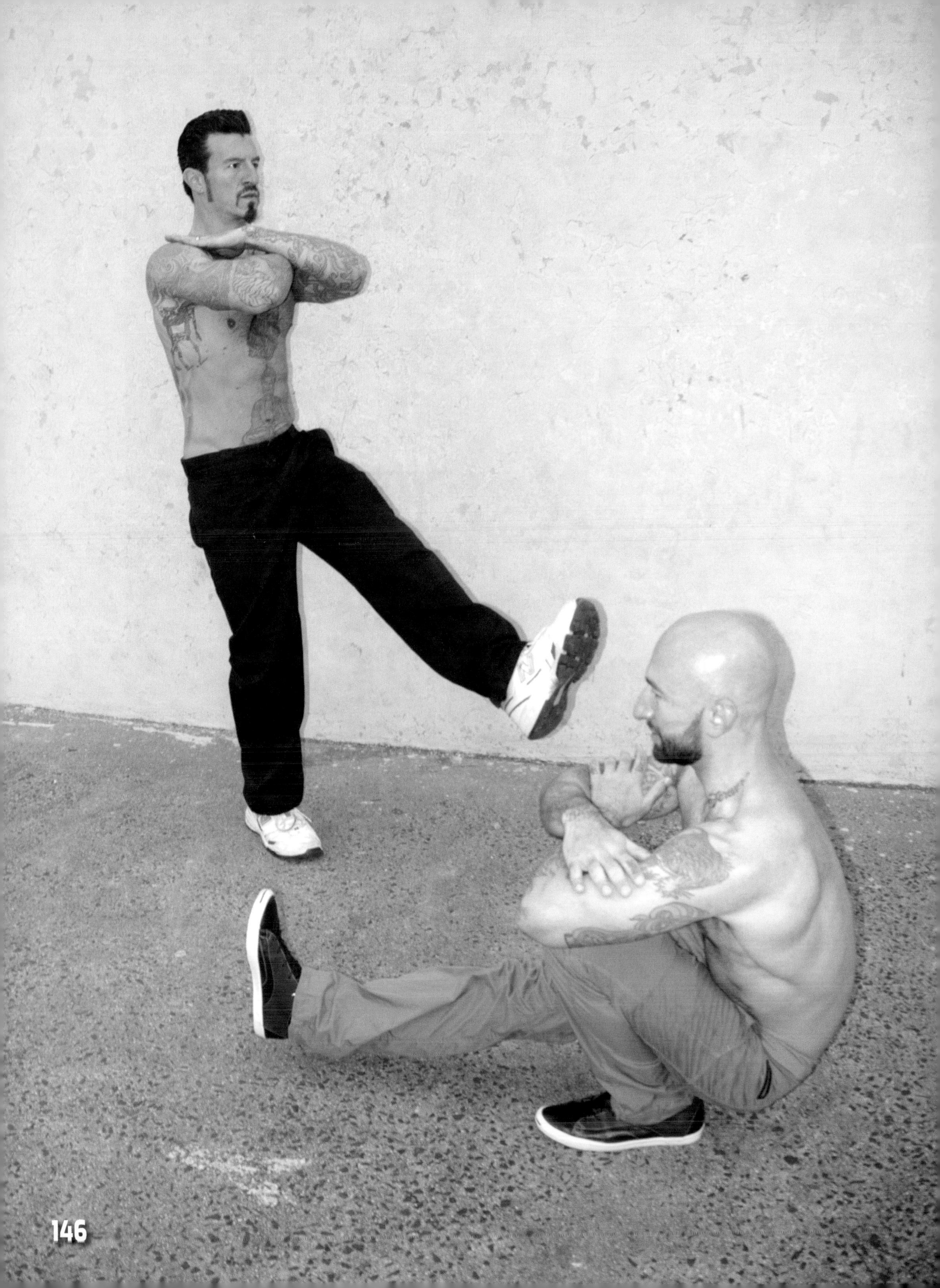

Chapter Eight:

Troubleshooting The Pistol Squat

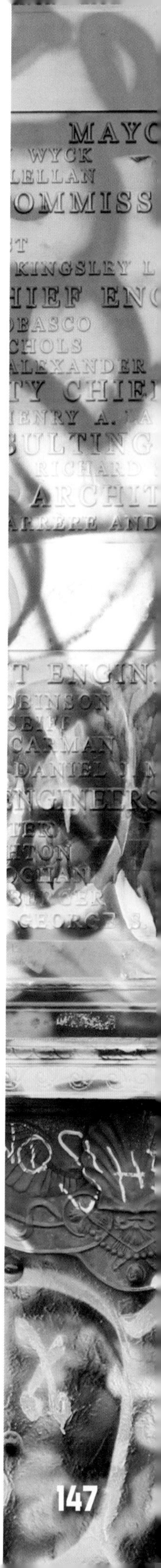

If you do squats for long enough, even advanced variations can eventually become fairly easy. While you can still get strong by doing high reps of an exercise, when you've made it into triple digit numbers in one set, it's probably better to just find a harder exercise and do fewer reps. At that point, one legged squats are the best way to progress your lower body strength without the need for weights or other extraneous equipment.

The pistol squat is the gold standard of single leg squats. It's one of those rare exercises that will challenge your strength, flexibility, balance and coordination. It's an elusive skill that demands practice, patience and perseverance to master. As a prerequisite, it's good to be able to do lots of close stance squats with a full range of motion. Once you've mastered those, there are a few easier variations on the one legged squat that can help you on the road to the pistol. Start with these and take your time. A beginner should not expect to get a pistol without months or possibly years of dedicated training.

One Legged Bench Squat

Just like a novice starting out with two legged squats, using a bench to catch yourself will help you build the stability and balance to eventually perform a freestanding one legged squat. Reach your opposite leg into the air and sit back onto an object that will leave you with a 90 degree angle at your knee. You'll likely lose control at the bottom the first time — this is fine. Plop down on the bench if you have to, then squeeze your abs (and your whole body) as you reach your arms out in front and pitch yourself forward to get up.

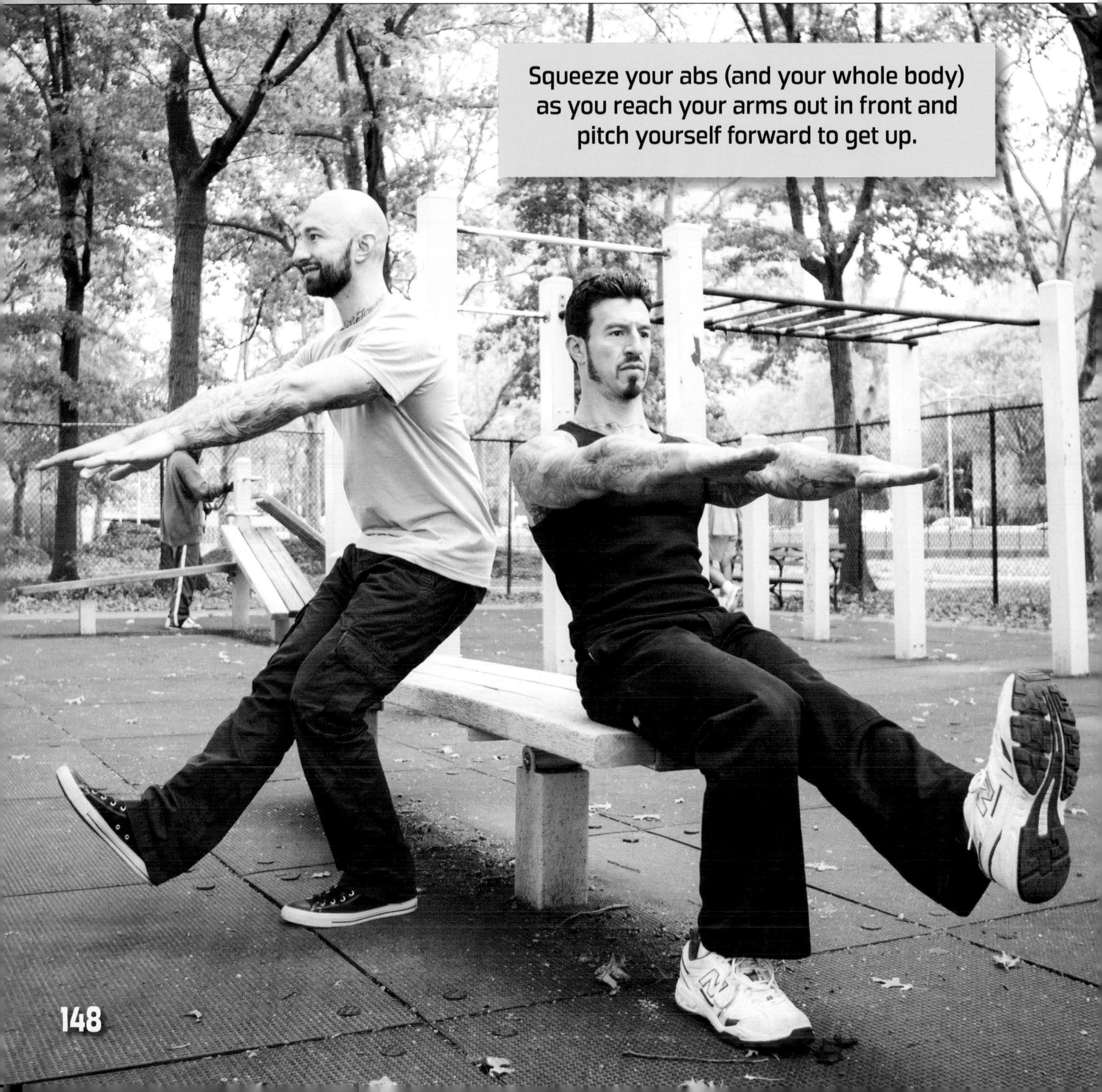

Squeeze your abs (and your whole body) as you reach your arms out in front and pitch yourself forward to get up.

Elevated One Leg Squat

Standing on top of an object while squatting on one leg will allow you to drop the opposite leg off the side of the object as you lower yourself down. This makes the exercise a bit easier as it lets you relax your free leg and focus all your attention on the squatting leg. It's also easier to balance this way as opposed to holding your free leg straight out in front or behind you. When you've built up to a few good reps, you should try moving to something lower down. Ideally, you'll be able to find an object just high enough to keep your outstretched foot from dragging on the ground.

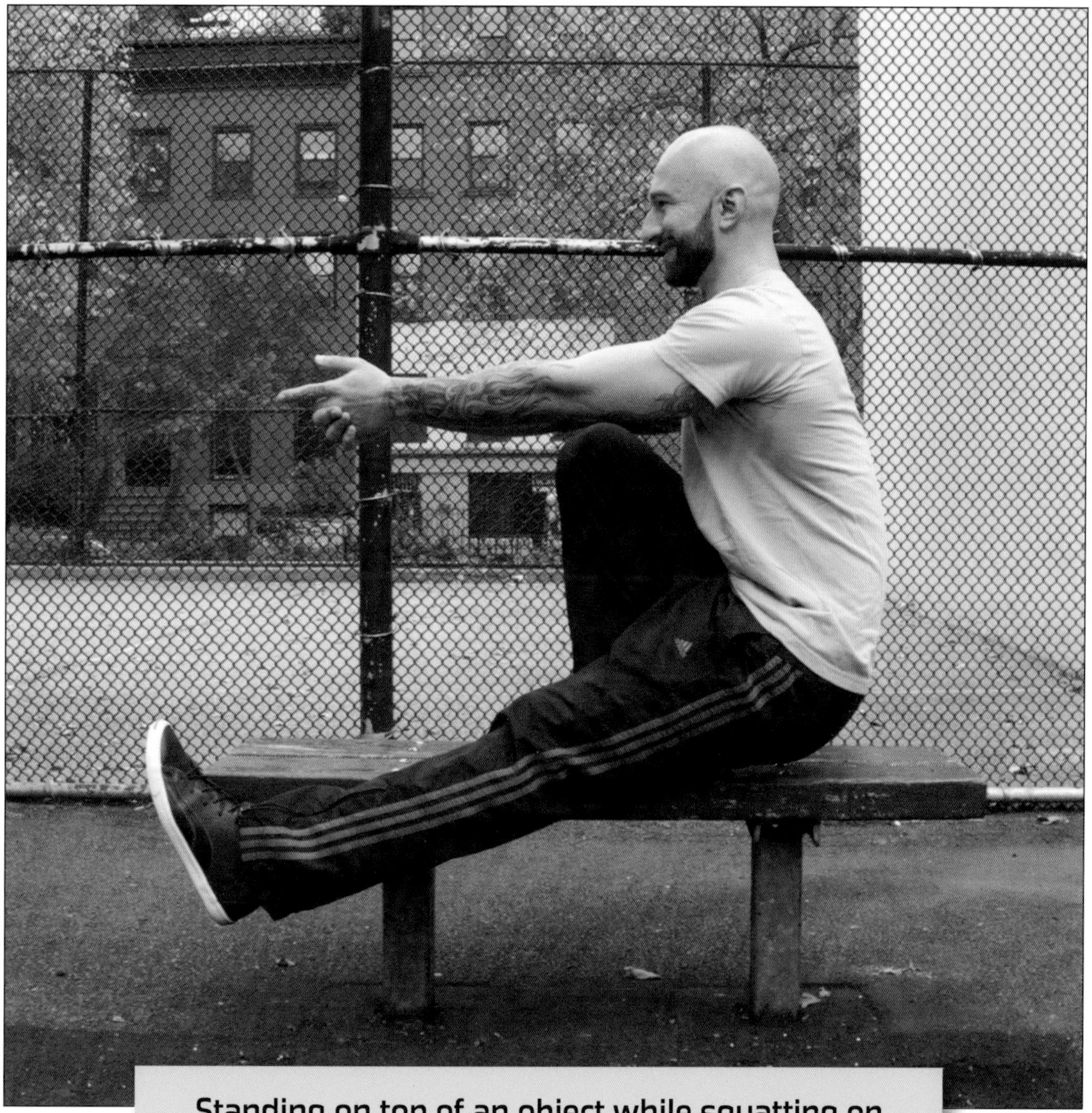

Standing on top of an object while squatting on one leg will allow you to drop the opposite leg off the side of the object as you lower yourself down.

Balance Of Power

While balance can be an issue with pistols, the two main things that hold people back from owning this move are a lack of strength and/or flexibility. Often it is a lack of both (though guys often mistakenly blame their flexibility when they simply lack the strength). One way to test to see if you have the requisite range of motion is to try an assisted pistol squat (aka an "assistol"). If you can lower yourself all the way to the proper bottom position while holding onto something in front of you (a pole, door frame, suspension trainer, etc.), then the issue is not as simple as being inflexible.

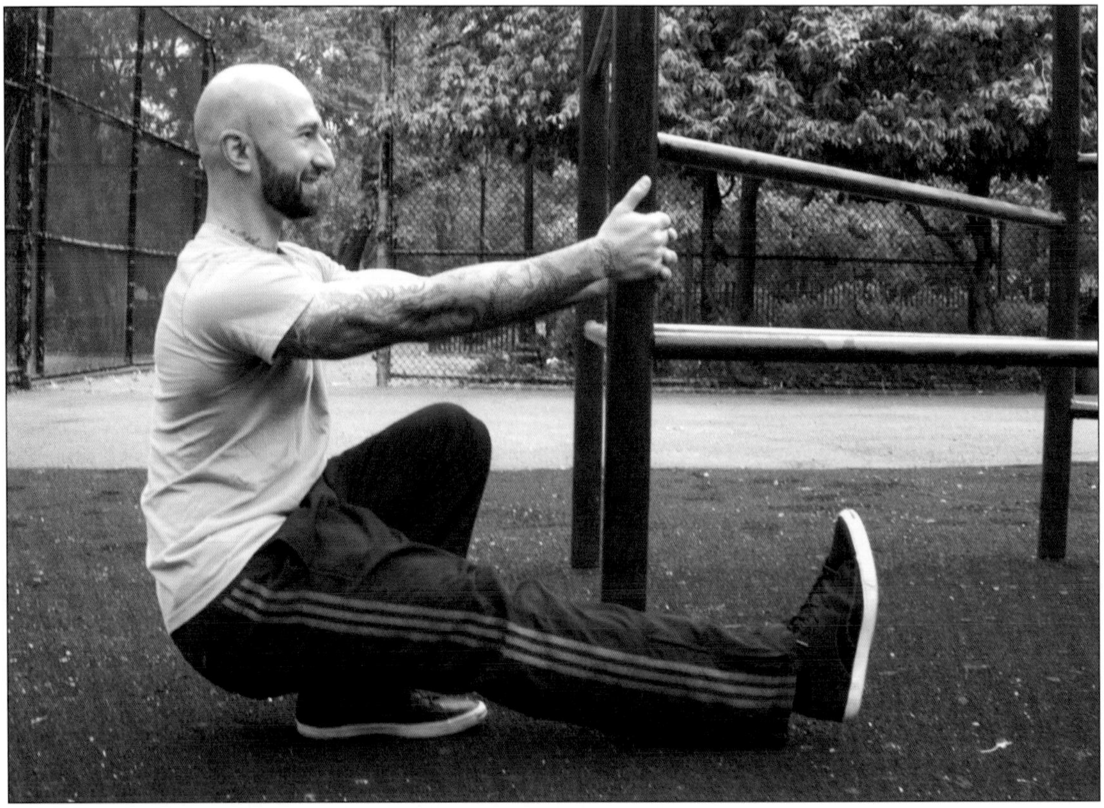

Part of what makes the pistol such a fantastic exercise is that it requires harmony between different areas of the body. The tighter you are in one spot, the stronger you're going to have to be in another. If there is tightness or weakness in any part of your legs or core, the pistol will continue to elude you. People who think a lack of flexibility is their most limiting factor are only seeing half of the picture. Like the back bridge, the problem that stops many folks from achieving the pistol is that they are tighter than they are strong. Your quads and hip flexors on your extended leg must be strong enough to overcome tightness in your hamstrings and lower back to keep it straight out in front. It need not stay totally parallel to the ground for the entire range of motion, but that heel definitely shouldn't touch the ground at any point during the exercise. For this to happen, you'll also need to be strong enough through your abdominals to stabilize your pelvis.

PUSHING THE LIMITS!

In theory, anyone who can do a full range-of-motion barbell back squat with their body weight on the bar should be able to do a pistol. In practice, this is rarely the case. The core strength and coordination needed to perform the pistol is very unique and requires skill specific work. Like anyone else, I had to put in my time and learn the mechanics of this move the old fashioned way — practice. If I make pistols look easy, it's only because I've been practicing them for over a decade.

In theory, anyone who can do a full range-of-motion barbell back squat with their body weight on the bar should be able to do a pistol.

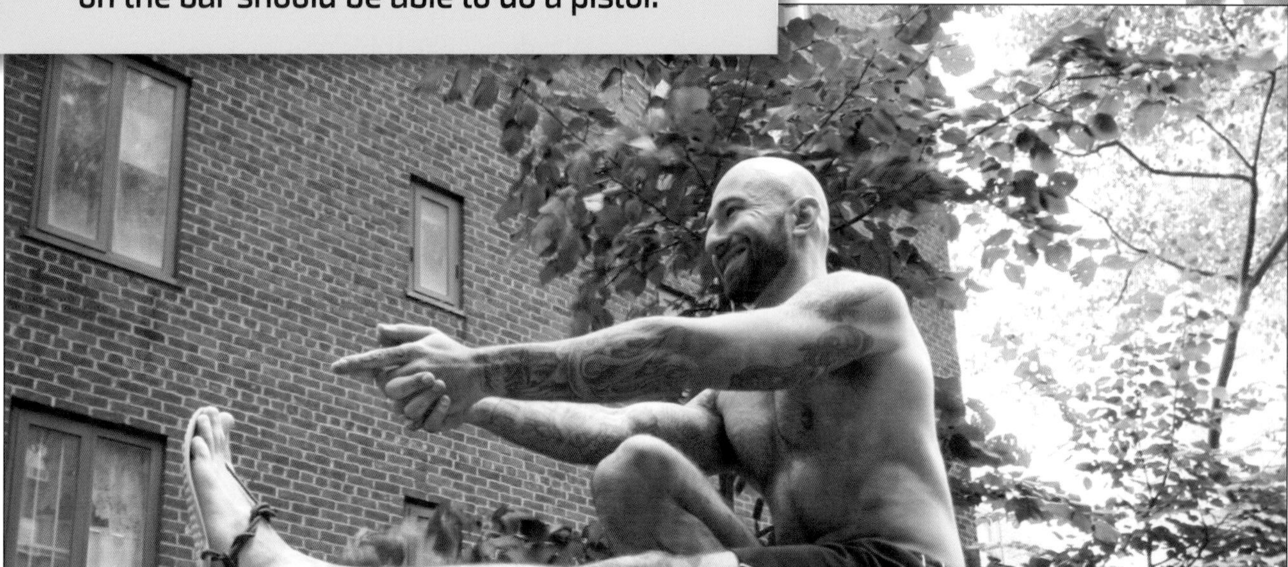

In practice, this is rarely the case.

Total Body Tension

If you still haven't figured it out, the key to bodyweight exercises is to use your whole body as one cohesive unit. This is especially true for the pistol — you need to squeeze everything you've got!

Beginners may find that their extended leg cramps up when attempting a pistol. This is quite common so make sure you brace your quads and keep your whole body engaged. You might try clasping your hands together with your arms straight in front of your chest to generate additional tension throughout your body. (Sticking your index finger out like a gun is optional.) Others will prefer to keep their hands apart. Either way, squeeze your abs tight like you're bracing for a punch in the stomach during the transition back to the top.

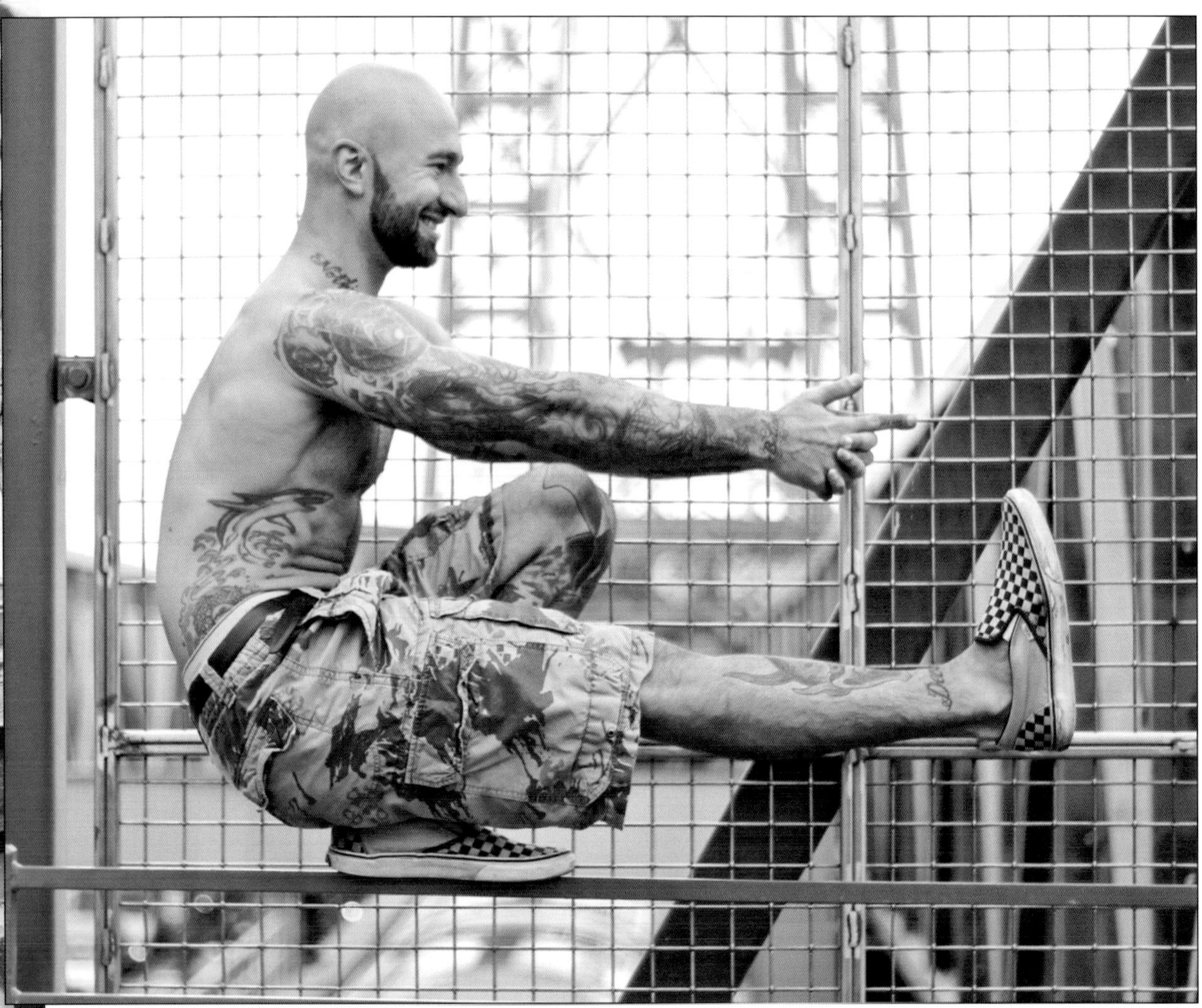

Partner Pistol

Having a training partner assist you through the sticking point of a pistol squat is another helpful technique when you're on the verge of your first official rep. Clasp hands with your partner and use them to provide stability through the transition (and pull you out of the hole if necessary). If your partner can do a pistol themselves, have them go up and down with you and do your reps as a team. Otherwise they can just pull you up from two legs.

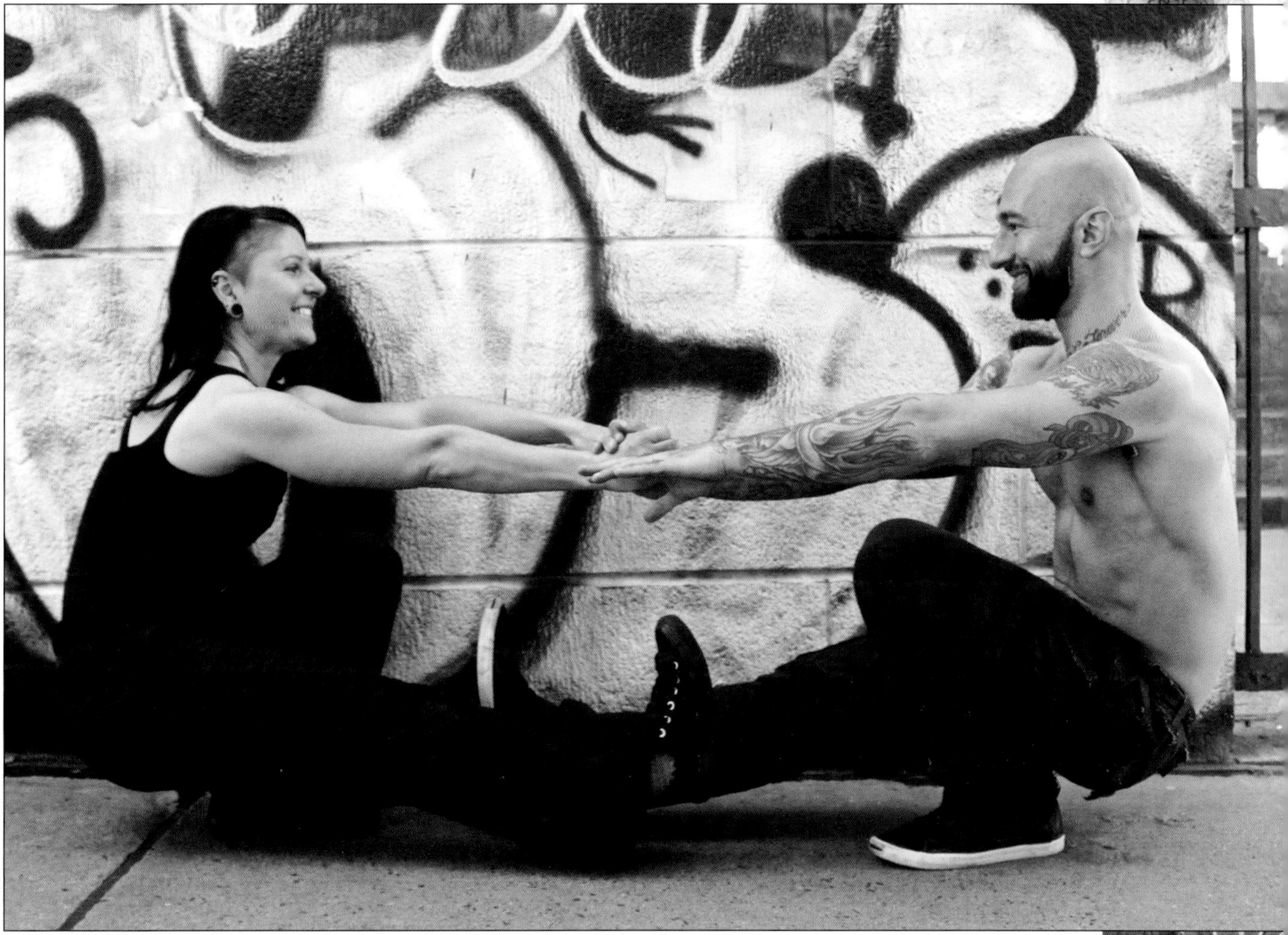

Counterweights

Pistols are one of those rare exercises that can actually be made easier for most people by *adding* weight. Holding a dumbbell or kettlebell in front of your chest can keep you balanced by pulling you forward, offsetting the weight of your hips moving back. It's almost like having a partner help you through the range of motion. Start with ten or fifteen pounds and work your way down to lighter weights. Eventually, you will get it free-standing.

Pistols are one of those rare exercises that can actually be made easier for most people by *adding* weight.

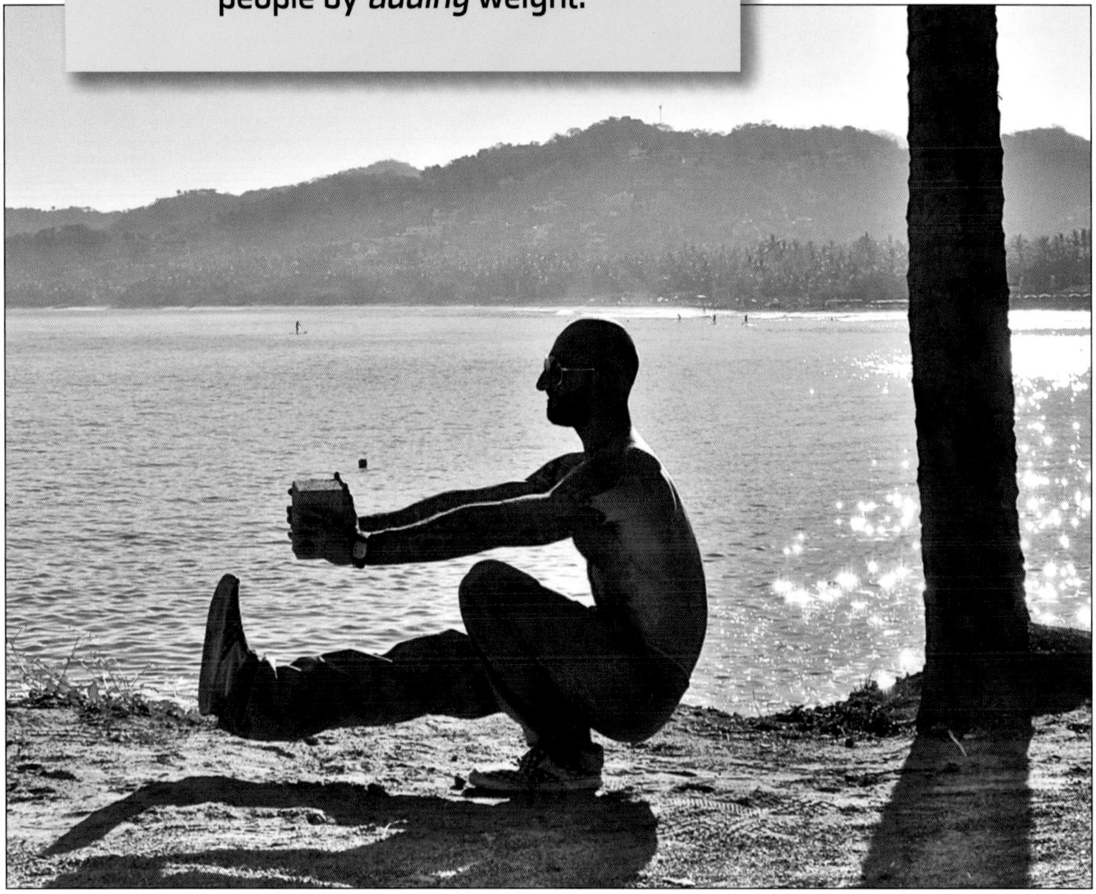

Raised Heels

Another way to make the pistol less difficult is to practice with the heel of your squatting leg on a slightly elevated surface (about an inch or so). Wearing a shoe with a raised heel is probably the easiest way to accomplish this, though you can also slide an object beneath your bare heel. This minor change in leverage can make the pistol significantly easier.

Though elevating your heel can be helpful for someone who is on the brink of a full-on pistol, I have mixed feelings about this technique, as it can put your knee into a compromised position if the heel is too high and/or too many reps are performed this way. Keep the elevation to an inch or less and keep your reps low. This technique should only be used for practice towards the real deal, not as an alternative to it. The eventual plan is to work up to flat-footed pistols on a level surface.

Just like the counterweight technique in which you begin with a heavier weight and work down to a lower one, you can gradually work away from relying on an elevated heel. Raising the heel of your squatting leg during a pistol is a bad habit, so don't use this technique too often or you could be preventing further progress.

Wearing a shoe with a raised heel can make the pistol less difficult.

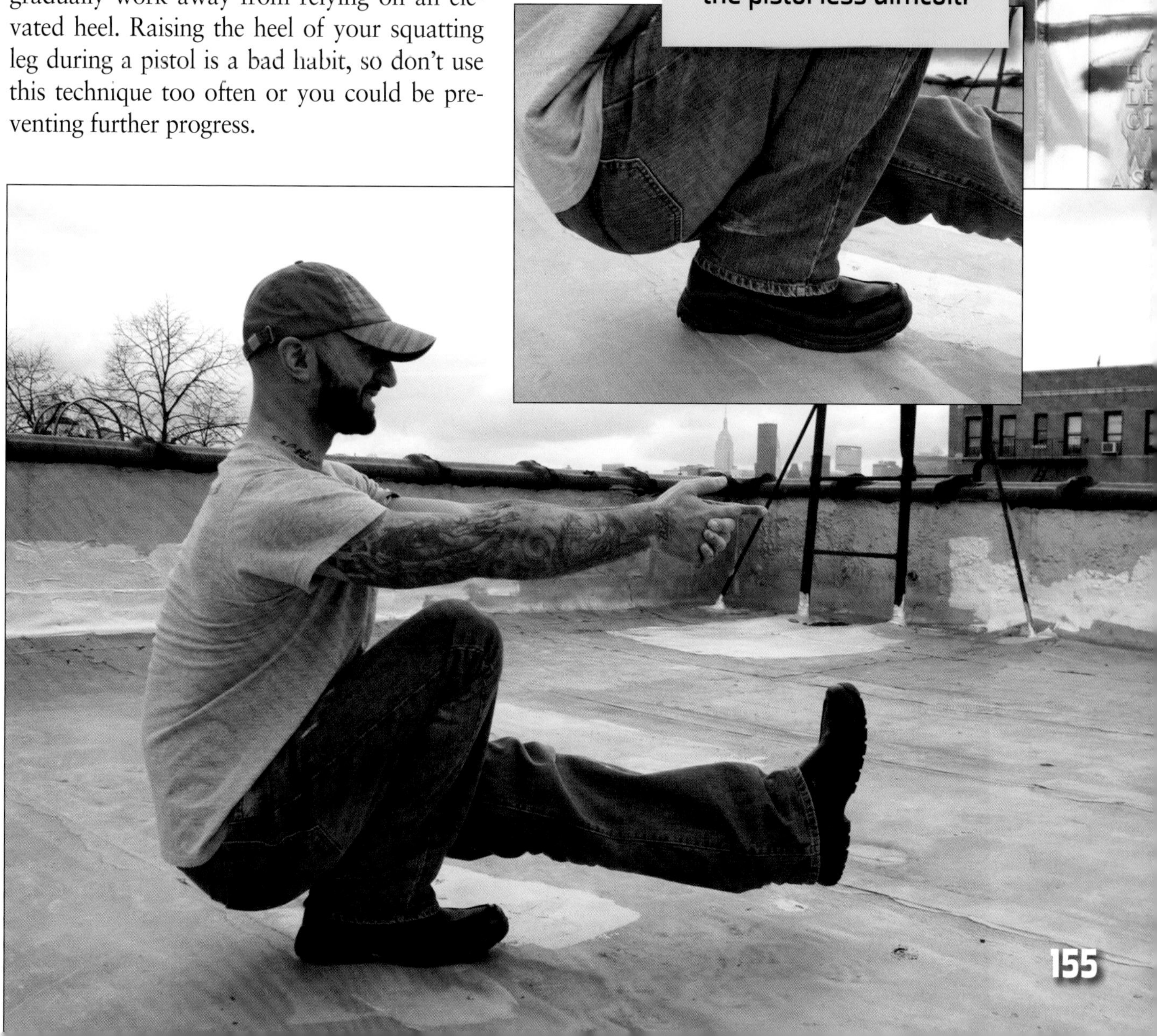

Pistol Switch

This drill is designed to help with the balance at the bottom of the pistol squat. If you are close to achieving a full pistol but struggle with this part of the exercise, practicing the pistol switch may help you get your first legit rep.

Begin in a deep squat position with your knees wide, then lift your right foot and quickly replace it with your right hand while reaching that leg toward your opposite hand. You'll

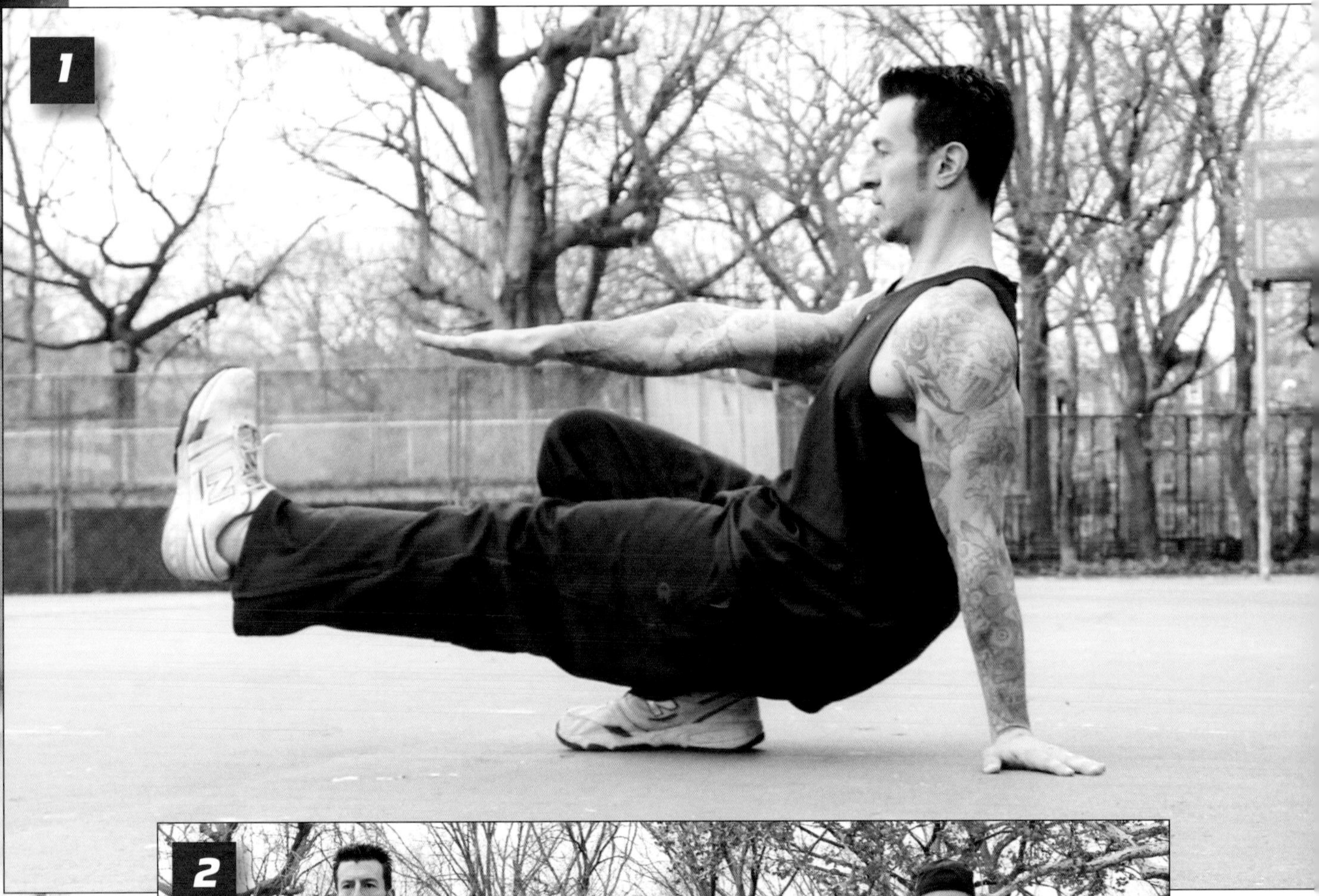

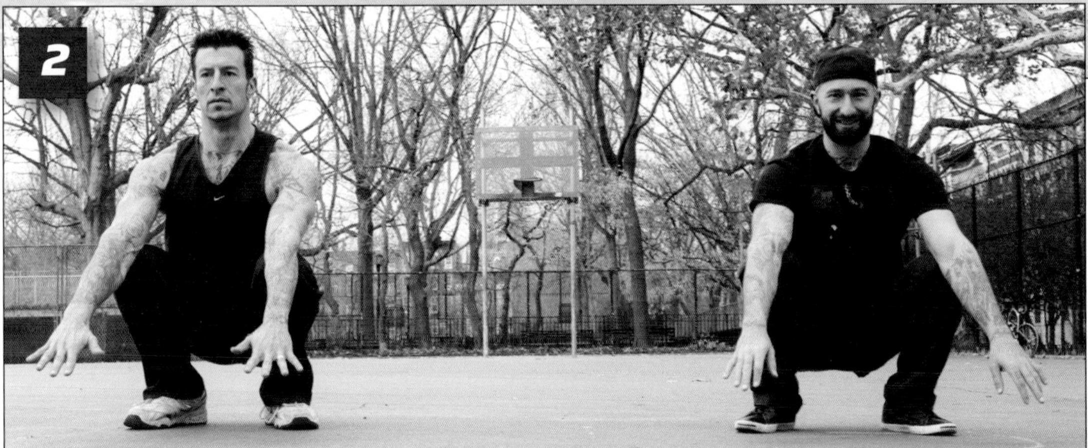

wind up at the bottom of the pistol position but with one hand supporting some of your weight. From here, reverse back to the initial position and attempt the switch on the left side.

With some practice, you can work on slowly taking the weight off your hand while you are on one foot in order to find the balance for the bottom of the pistol squat. Reach your arms all the way in front of you while you squeeze your abs tight and flex your extended leg. You'll likely need to round your back pretty deep at first to keep from falling on your butt. Also remember to flex as much as possible from the ankle of your squatting leg. Just don't forget that you want your heel to stay down.

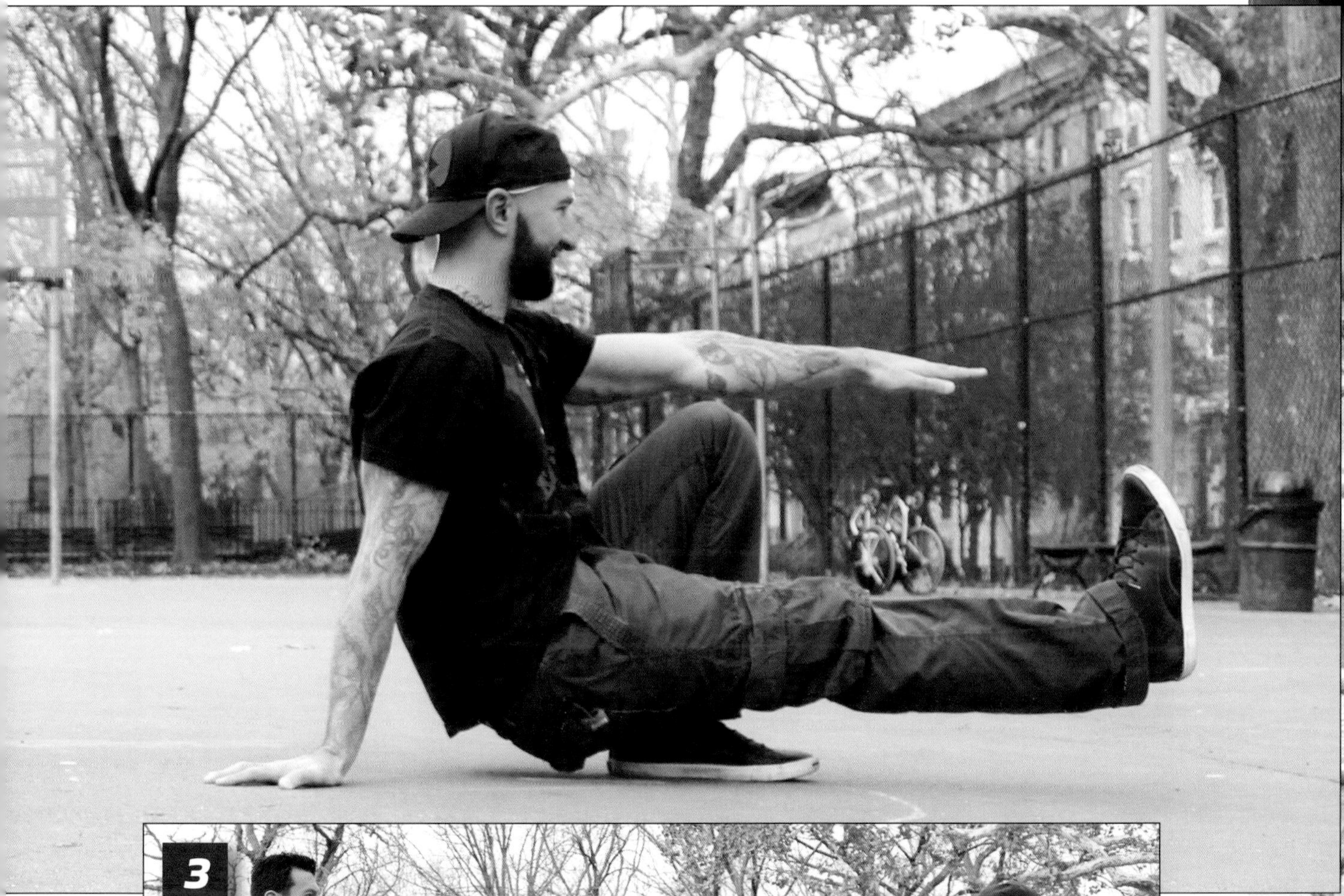

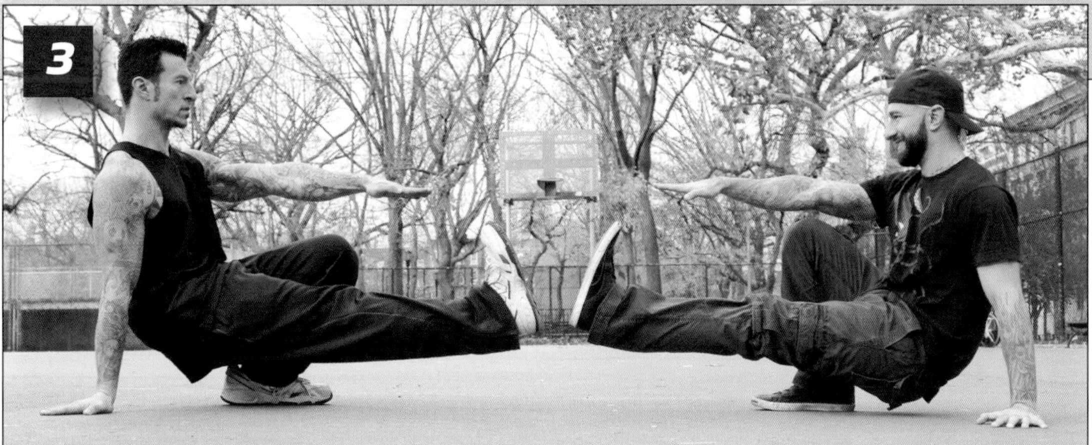

Hold It

Another helpful technique if you're on the brink of your first pistol is to practice slow negatives with brief isometric holds at the key transitional positions on the way down. Stop when you are a quarter of the way down and hold for a slow three count. Do the same at the half way and three quarter positions. Eventually make that three count into a five count. Once you can do that, you'll have your first pistol very soon.

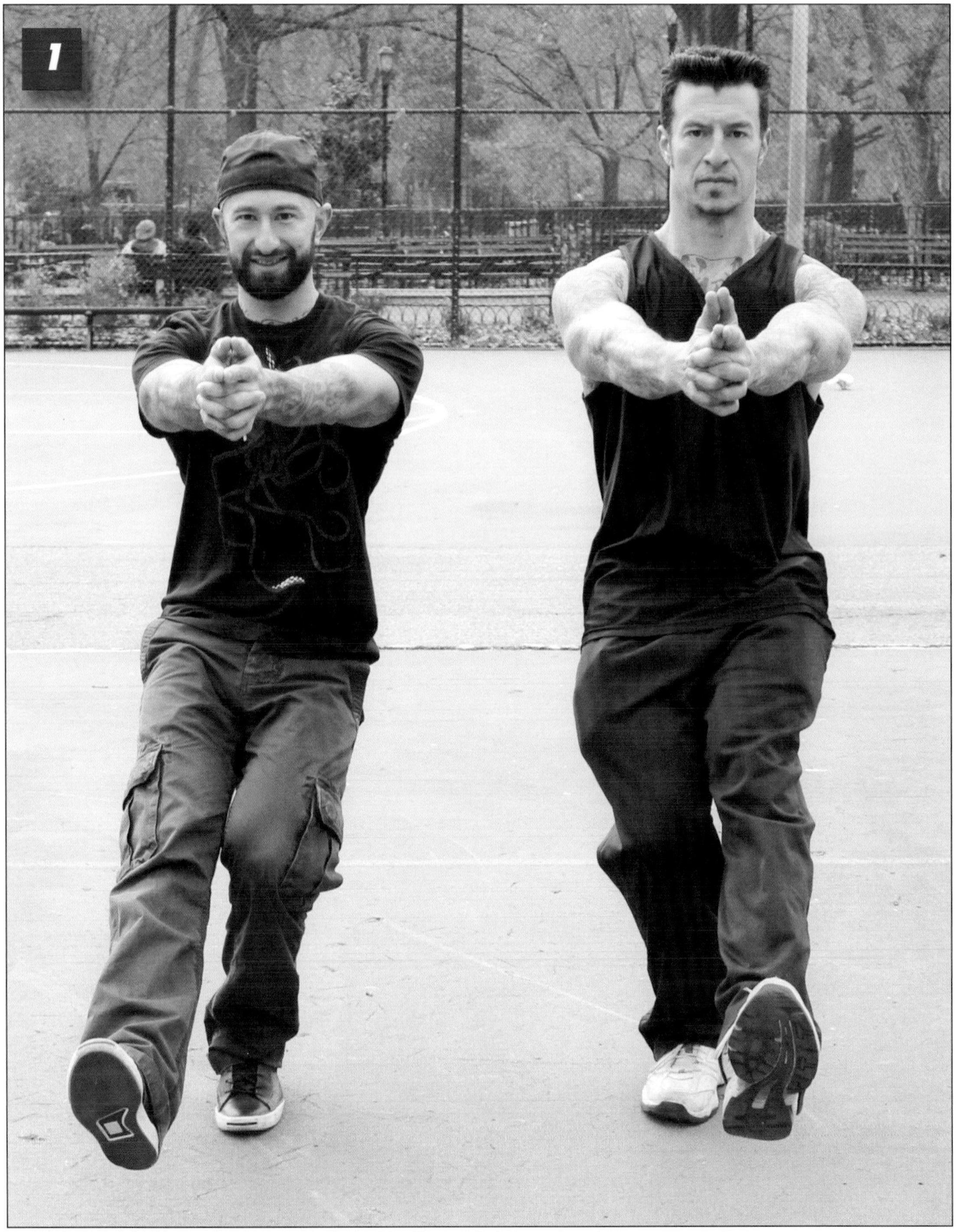

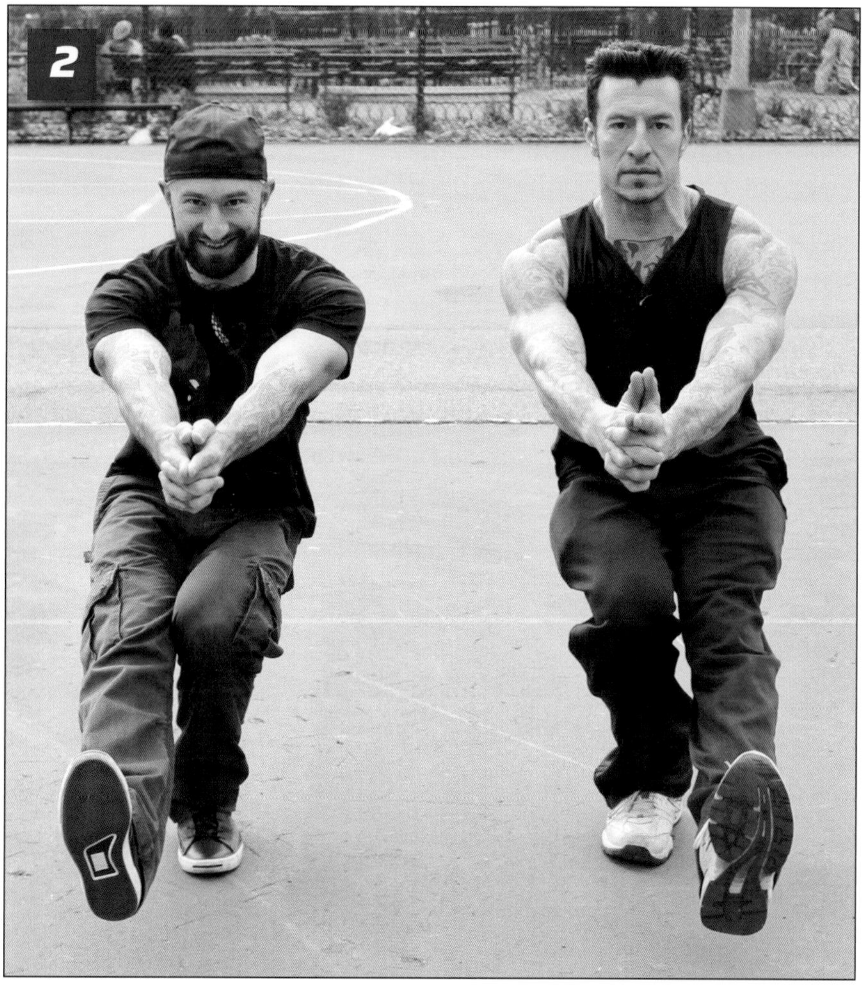
2

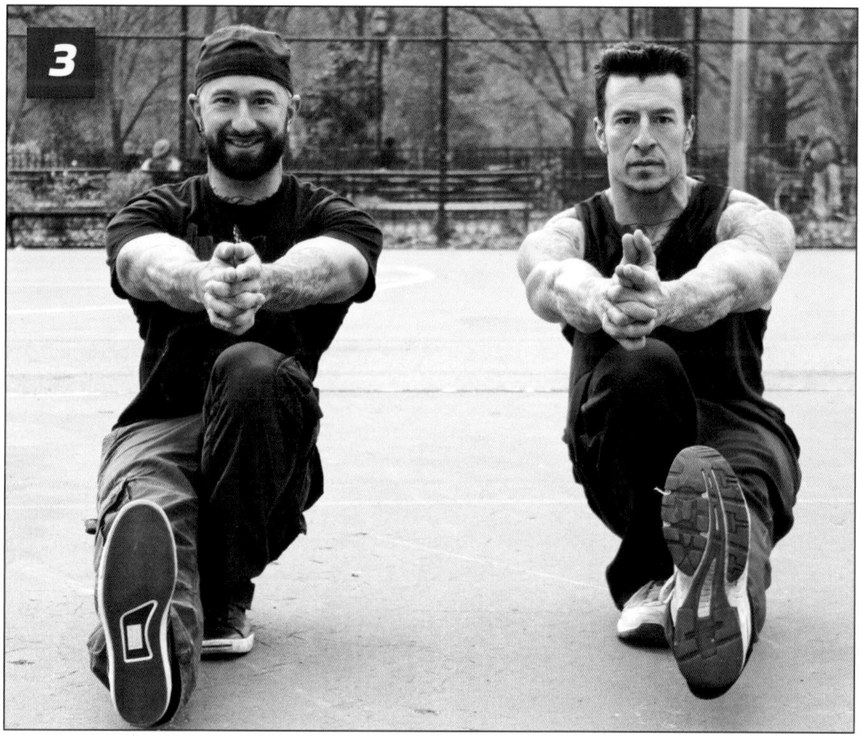
3

Round And Round

Some people have taken issue with the pistol squat due to the fact that it's virtually impossible to do one without sacrificing your neutral spine position to some extent. A lot of people are overly paranoid about their lower back, but as I've said, the spine is designed to flex and extend.

If you are doing squats with weight on your back, you need to maintain a neutral spine. However, since your spine isn't loaded during a bodyweight pistol, the lumbar curve shouldn't be an issue, though attempting to minimize that curve will make the exercise more challenging (which usually leads to increased strength). Additionally, tightening your stomach and creating abdominal pressure from the inside out further protects and stabilizes your spine during the pistol.

Like the "perfect" one arm push-up, a perfect pistol with a neutral spine is a nice vision to have in mind while you perform the exercise, but understand that it is an idealized view of reality. Just as your hips will inevitably move to the side during a feet-together one arm push-up, your lower back has to round a bit to perform a pistol.

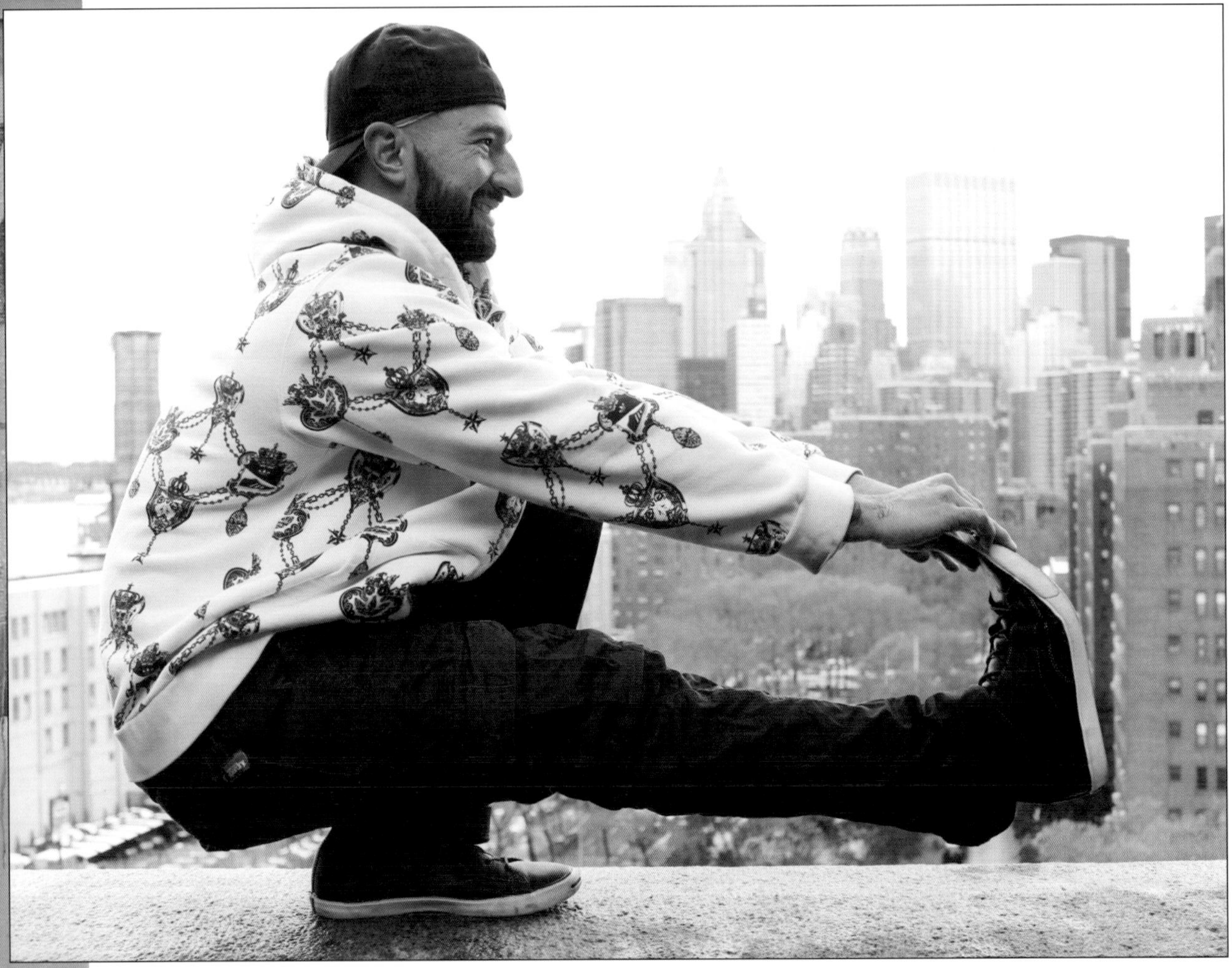

Knees And Toes

The other big concern I hear from people when I tell them to practice pistols is the safety of their knees. While there is potential for injury with advanced calisthenics, there is potential for injury with all types of physical pursuits. And the more advanced things become, the more that risk grows.

Regardless of whether you are lifting weights, doing calisthenics, or racing a triathlon (all things I've done), the keys to avoiding injury are the same: train consistently, progress slowly and respect your body.

As long as you practice proper form, avoid trying to move to harder variations before you are ready and keep your training volume appropriate, you should be able to progress to pistols and eventually practice them as a regular part of your training without any joint problems. In fact, your hips, knees and ankles should get *stronger* from doing them.

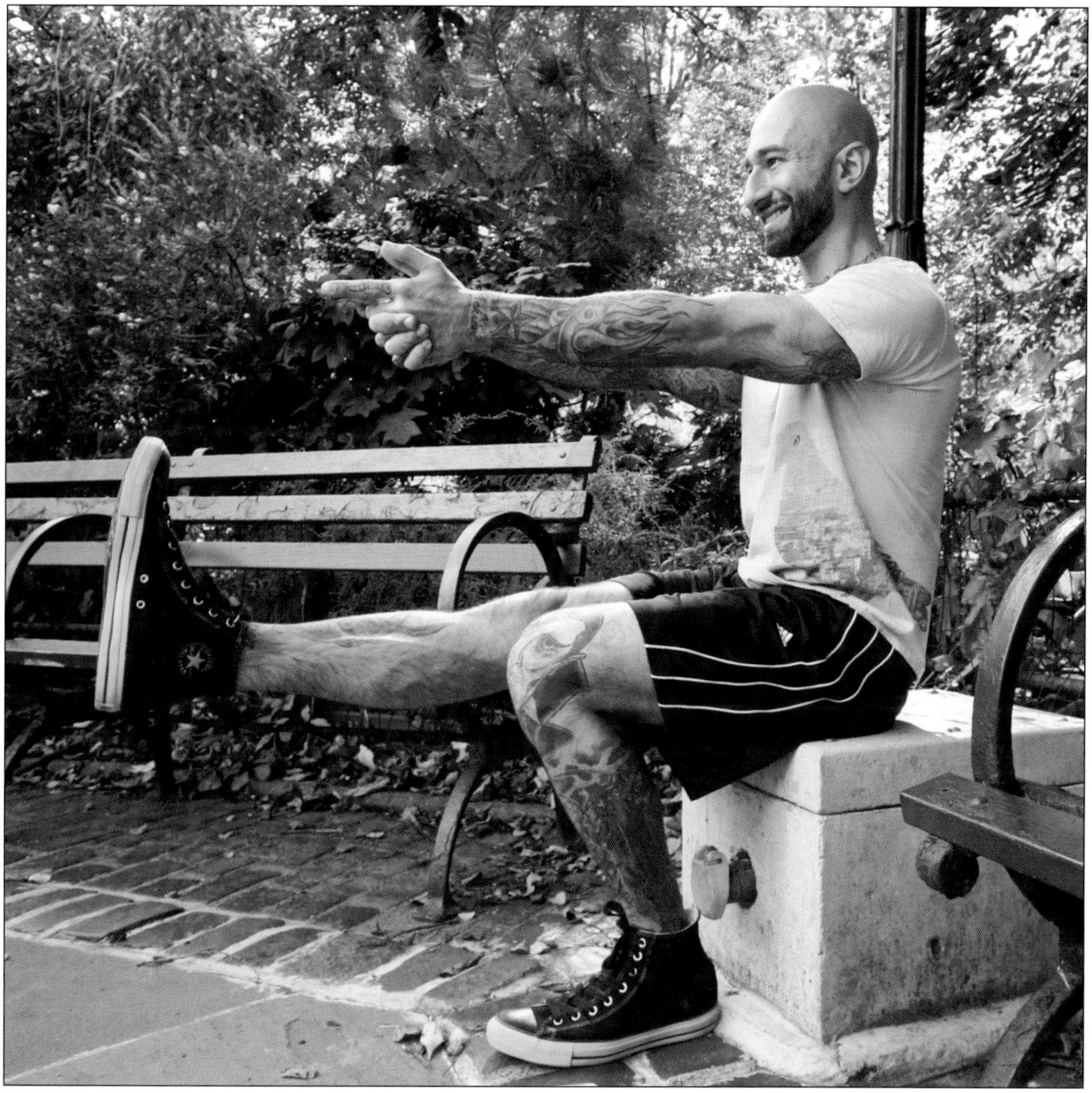

Remember that while strength training makes your connective tissue stronger, it can be slower to act on ligaments, tendons and cartilage as compared to muscle. You must build to harder exercises gradually over many months and years. You can push the limits but you must acknowledge them first. Don't try to get to the full pistol without putting in the necessary work.

Arm Position

As bodyweight training is all about manipulating leverage, there are always subtle ways to make an exercise easier or more difficult. In a one arm push-up, you can change the leverage by positioning your legs closer together or farther apart. To make a pistol squat harder, you can try gradually working your arms from in front of your body to behind your back.

When learning the pistol, it is best to reach your arms out in front. This will keep your weight more evenly distributed as you sit back into your squat, making it easier to balance and maintaining more favorable leverage for your muscles. You may even try holding onto your toes for balance (doing so will also increase the stretch, an added benefit for many of us).

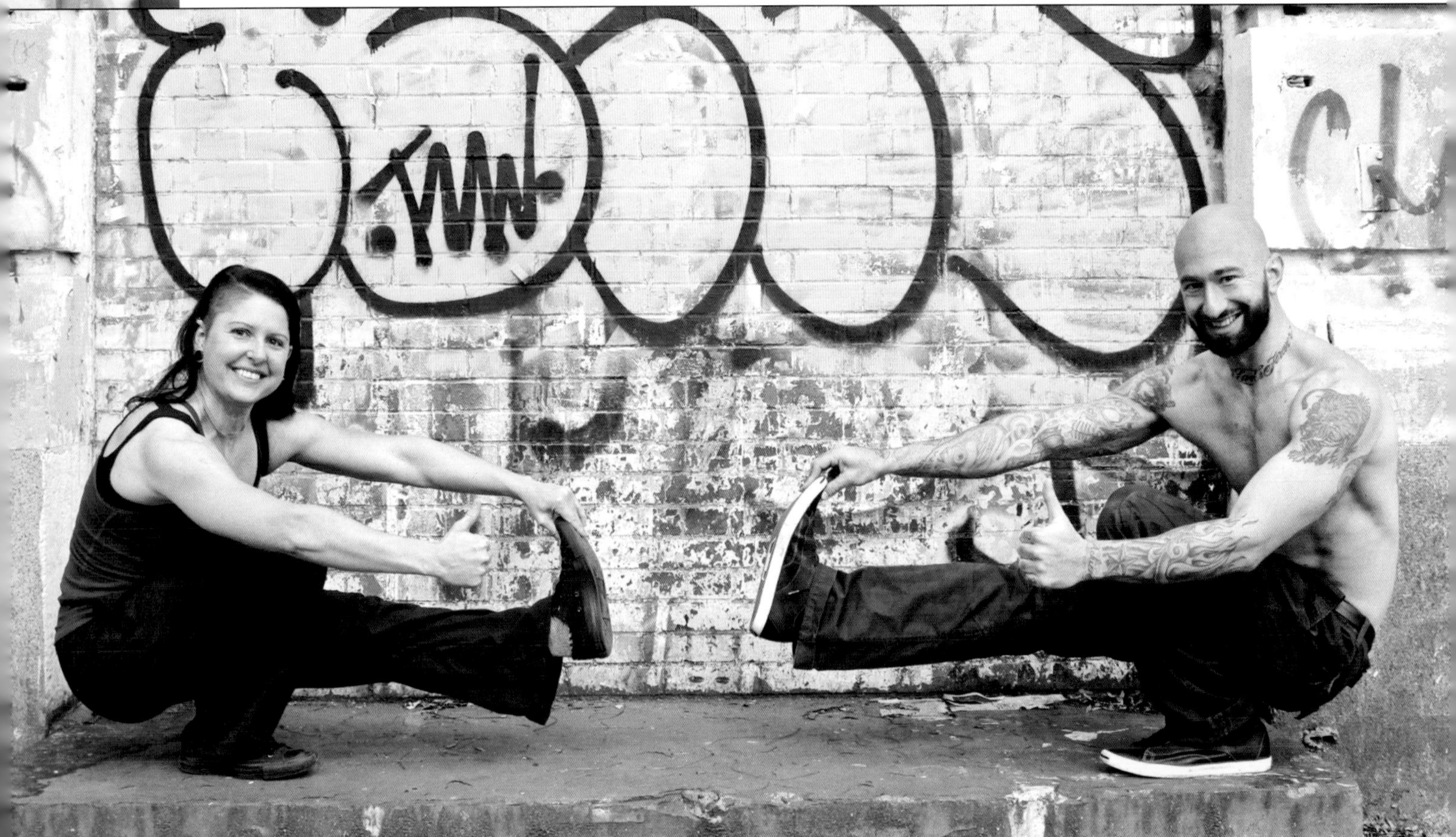

Pushing The Limits!

Once you can do several pistols with your hands in front however, try performing a pistol while crossing your arms at your shoulders, placing your hands behind your head, or harder still — clasping your hands behind your back.

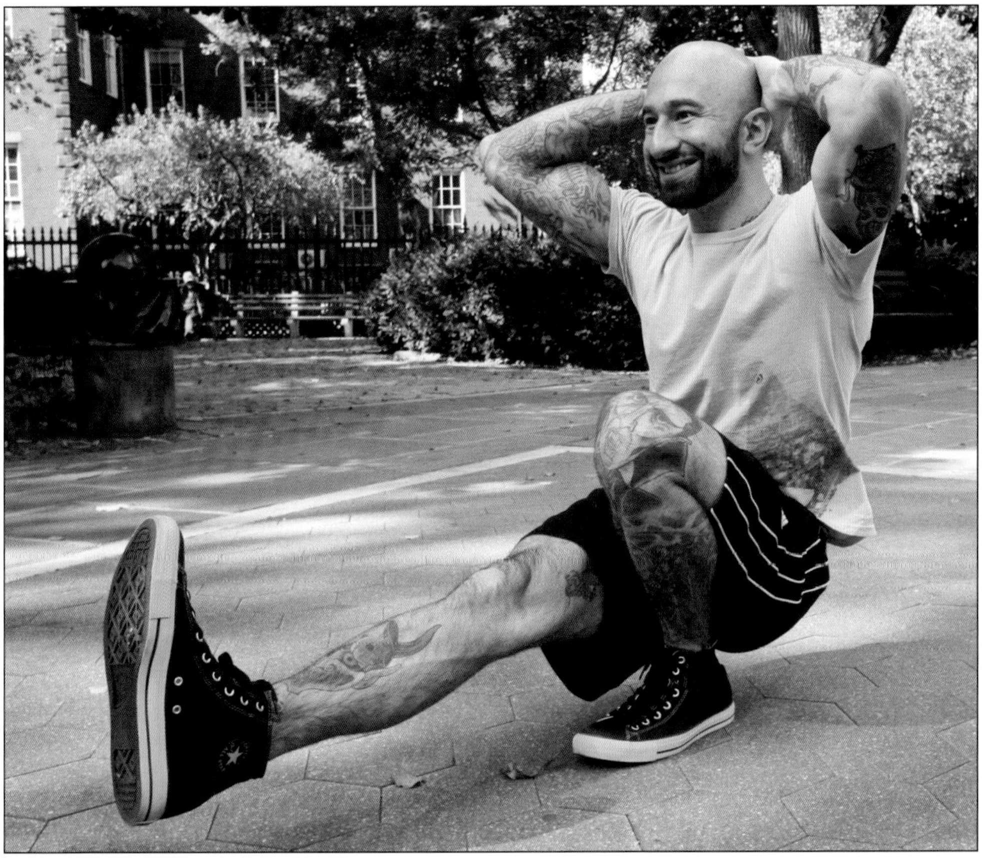

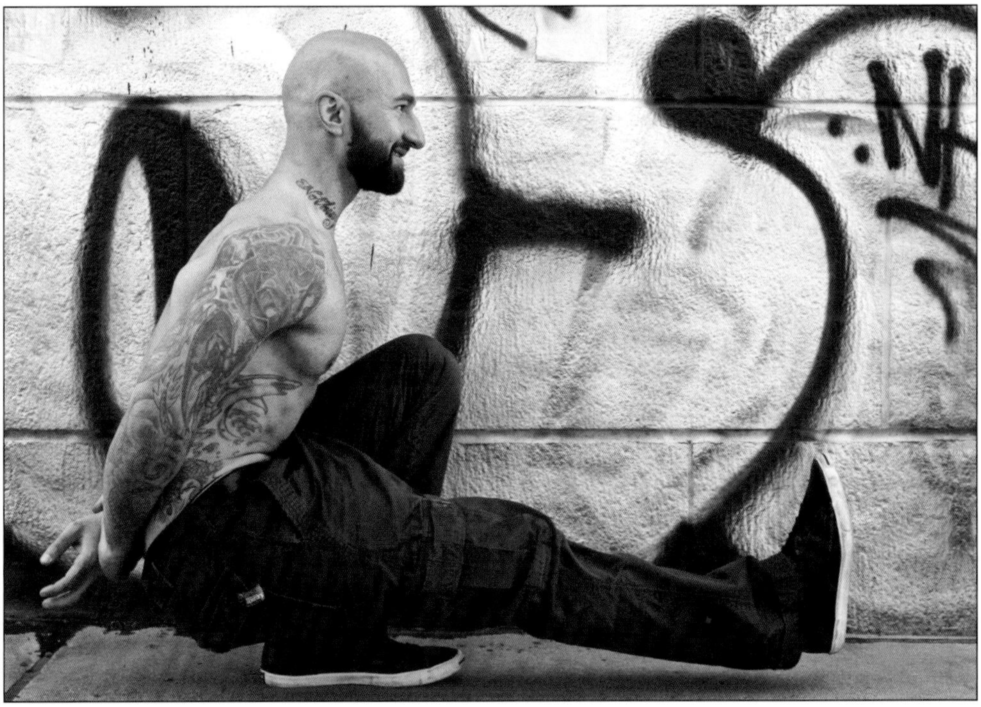

Walking Pistol

After you can do a few pistols on each leg, walking pistols are a fantastic way to increase your reps. The one legged equivalent of the walking lunge, alternating legs while moving forward will allow each leg a little extra rest between reps, giving you the opportunity to do more reps in a single set than going one leg at a time. These can become a serious cardio workout as well once you develop the ability to do lots of reps on each leg. Additionally, some people might find that the forward momentum of walking in and out of each rep makes the exercise a bit more manageable.

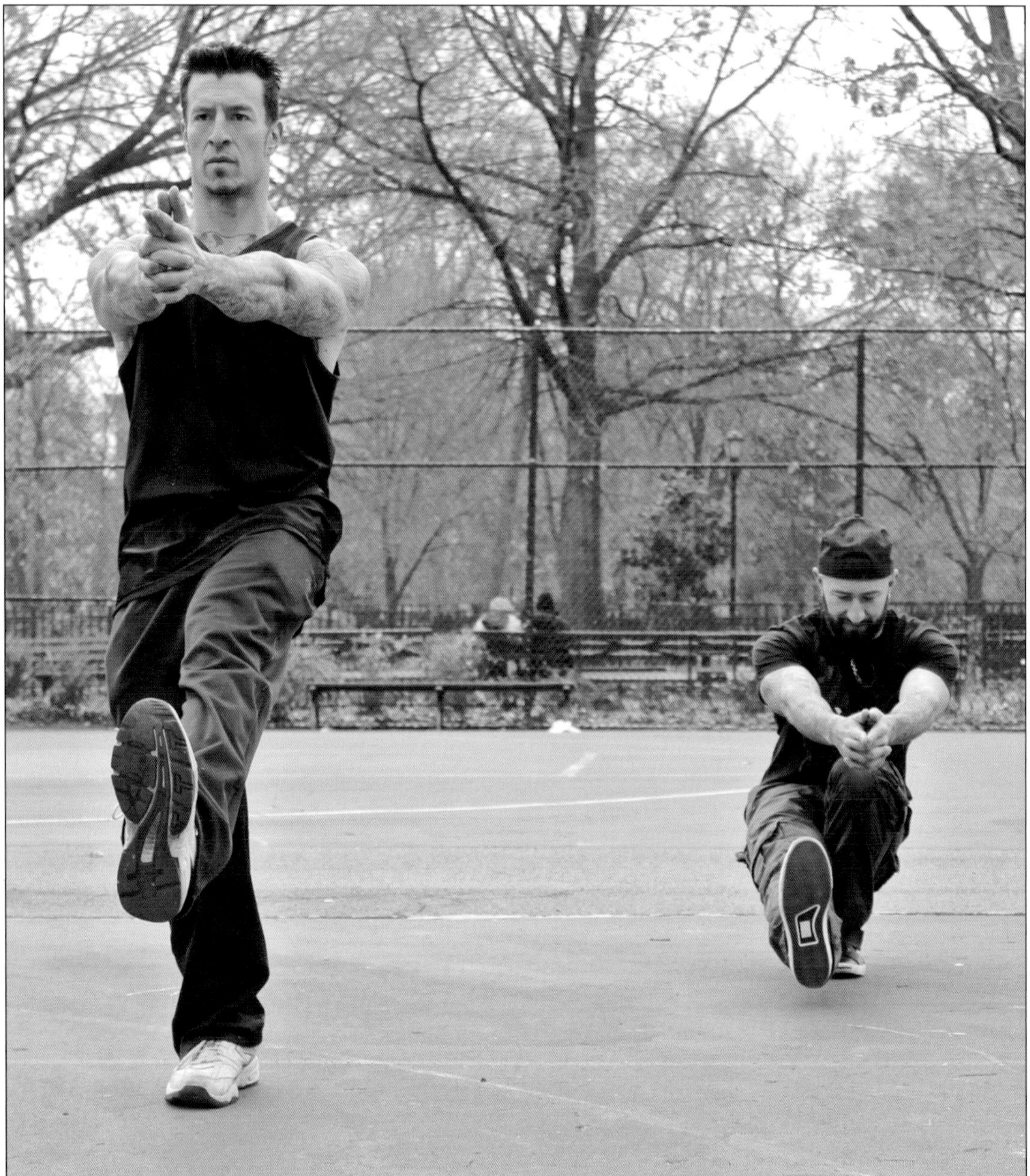

Plyo Pistol

Think you've got strong legs? Challenge yourself to jump at the top of your pistol squat. You may even try jumping onto an object such as a step or bench. Start with something nice and low — this is a very advanced move — try it at your own risk!

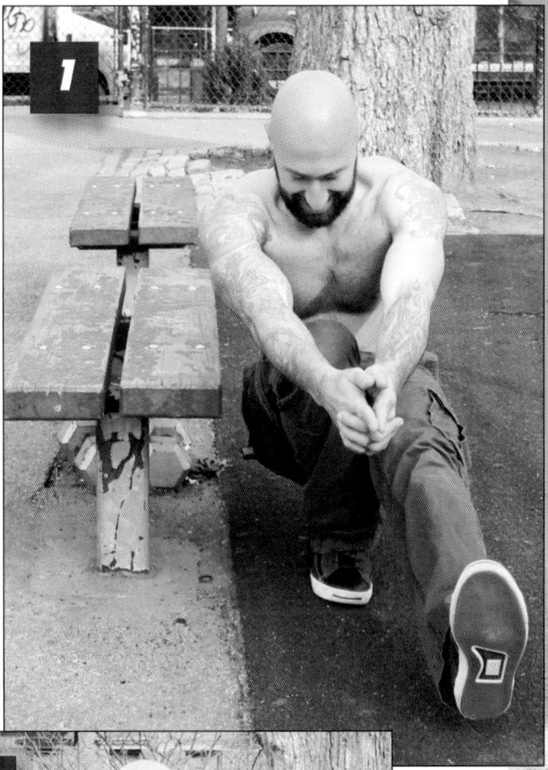

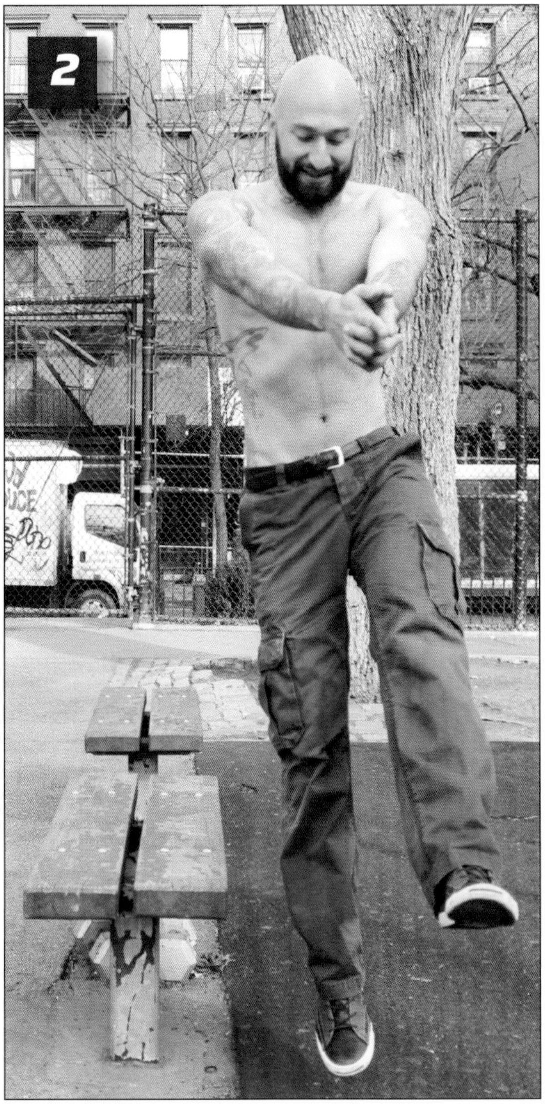

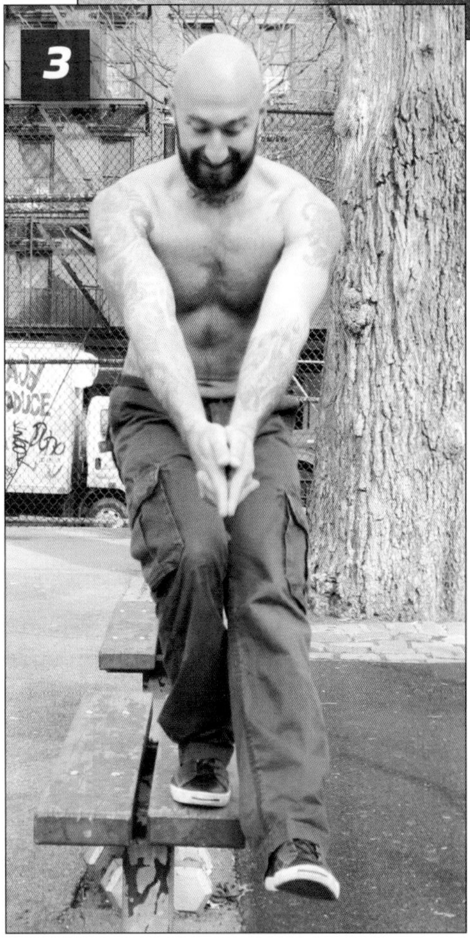

Shrimp Squat

If you think pistol squats are the be-all-and-end-all of bodyweight leg exercises, think again. The shrimp squat is a challenging single-leg bodyweight movement that can humble any sharpshooting pistol squatter.

To perform a shrimp squat, begin in an upright position then bend one knee so you can grab your ankle behind your back (just like you would if you were stretching your quads). From here, slowly lower yourself down until your back knee touches the ground behind the heel of the squatting leg. Try to go down as controlled as possible, though most first timers will find themselves dropping through the last few inches of the range of motion (you might want to try this exercise on a soft surface when starting out). If you are having a hard time, you may choose to begin from the ground up instead. Once you can do a few reps this way, you should be able to gradually work on getting down with more control.

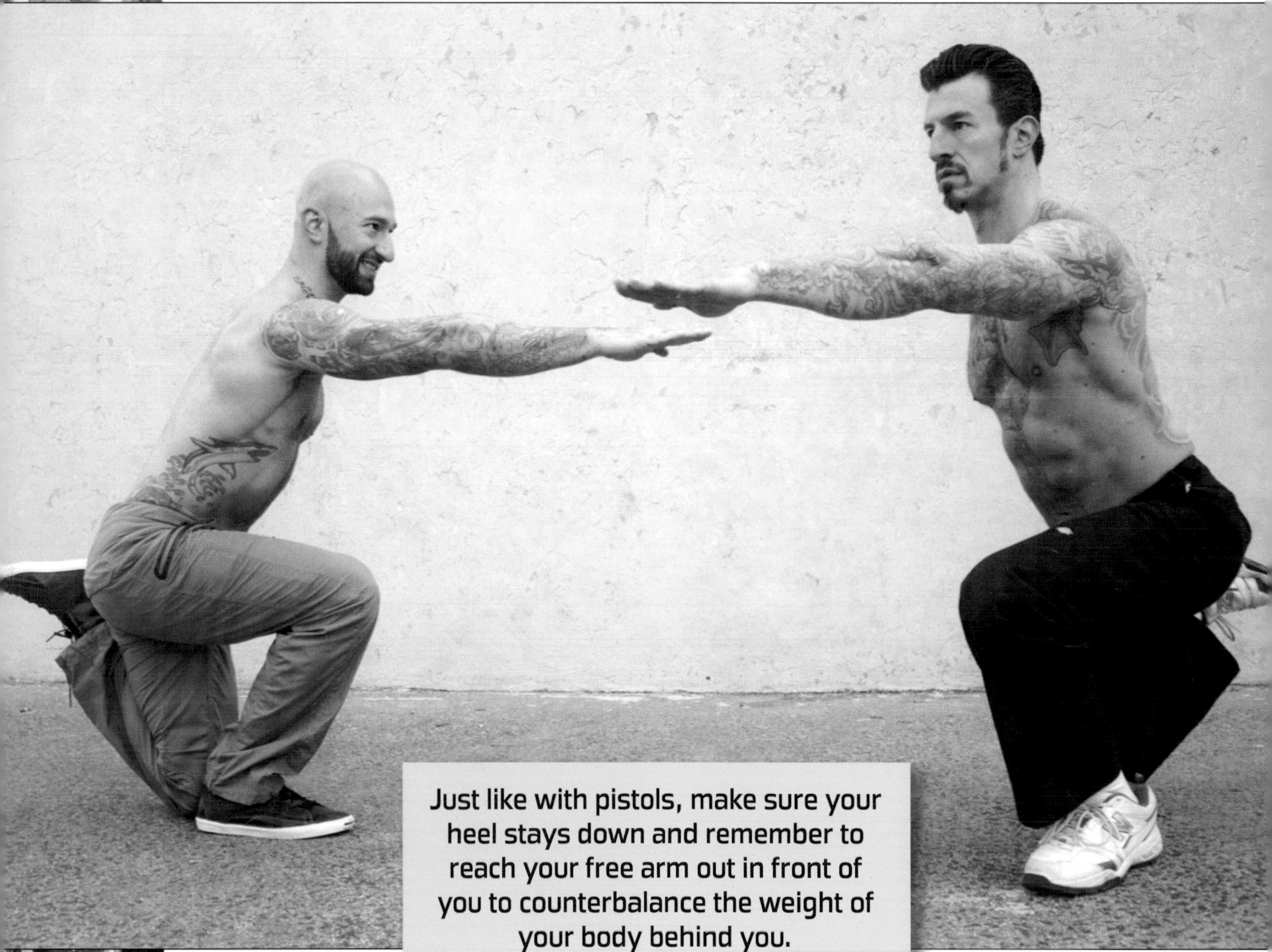

Just like with pistols, make sure your heel stays down and remember to reach your free arm out in front of you to counterbalance the weight of your body behind you.

Just like with pistols, make sure your heel stays down and remember to reach your free arm out in front of you to counterbalance the weight of your body behind you. You'll also need to pitch your chest forward on the way up to keep from falling backward.

Once you get the hang of the standard version, you can attempt an advanced shrimp squat by holding your ankle with both hands. This will put you at a serious mechanical disadvantage, plus you'll no longer be able to use your free arm for balance. It takes a lot of leg strength to do an advanced shrimp squat, but of course it also takes core strength.

Pitch your chest forward on the way up to keep from falling backward.

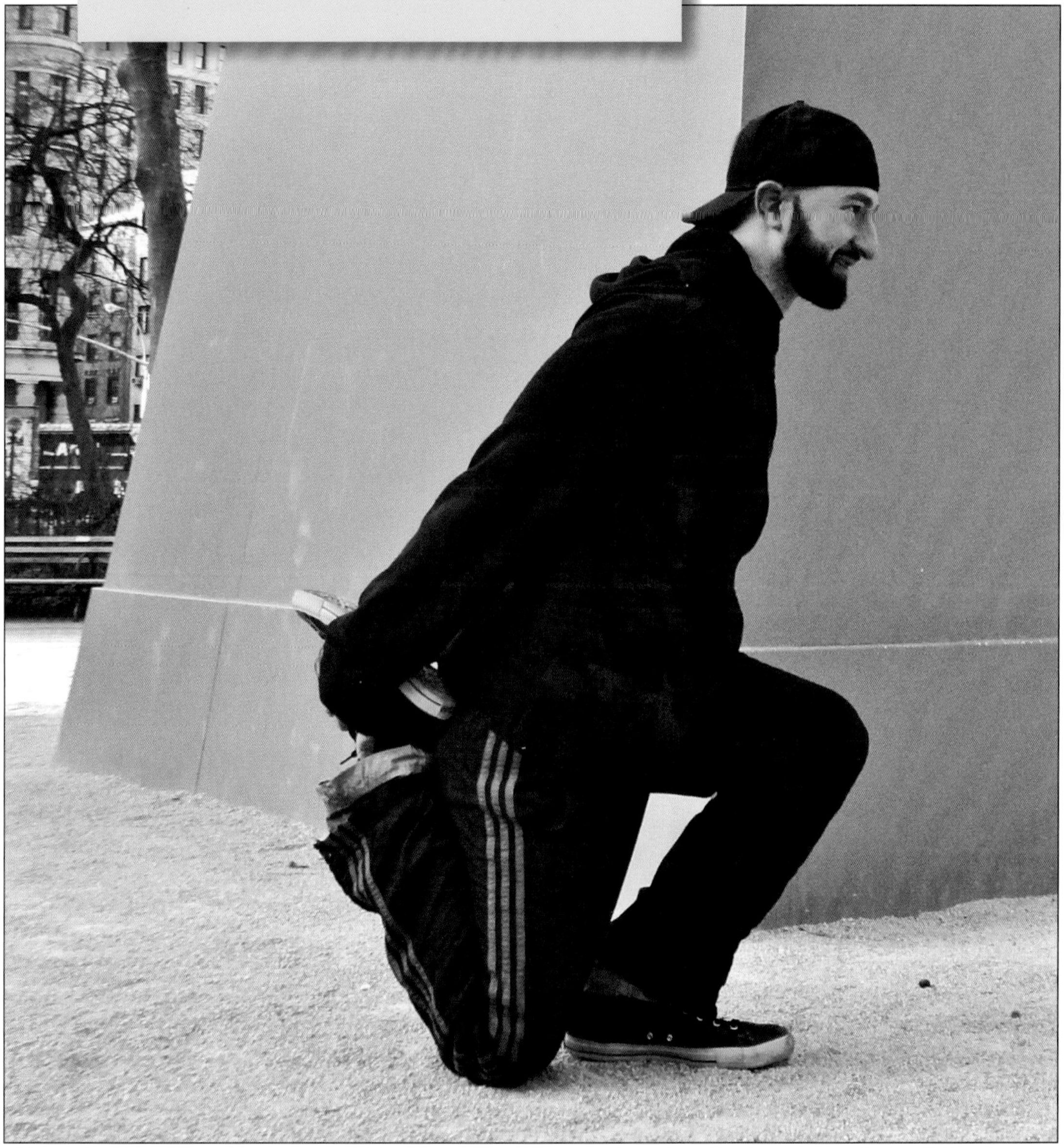

Jumbo Shrimp Squat

You can also add difficulty to the shrimp by doing it while standing on a platform. Unlike the pistol, which is easier when elevated, performing a shrimp this way allows for a bigger range of motion, as your knee can go deeper than the level of your foot.

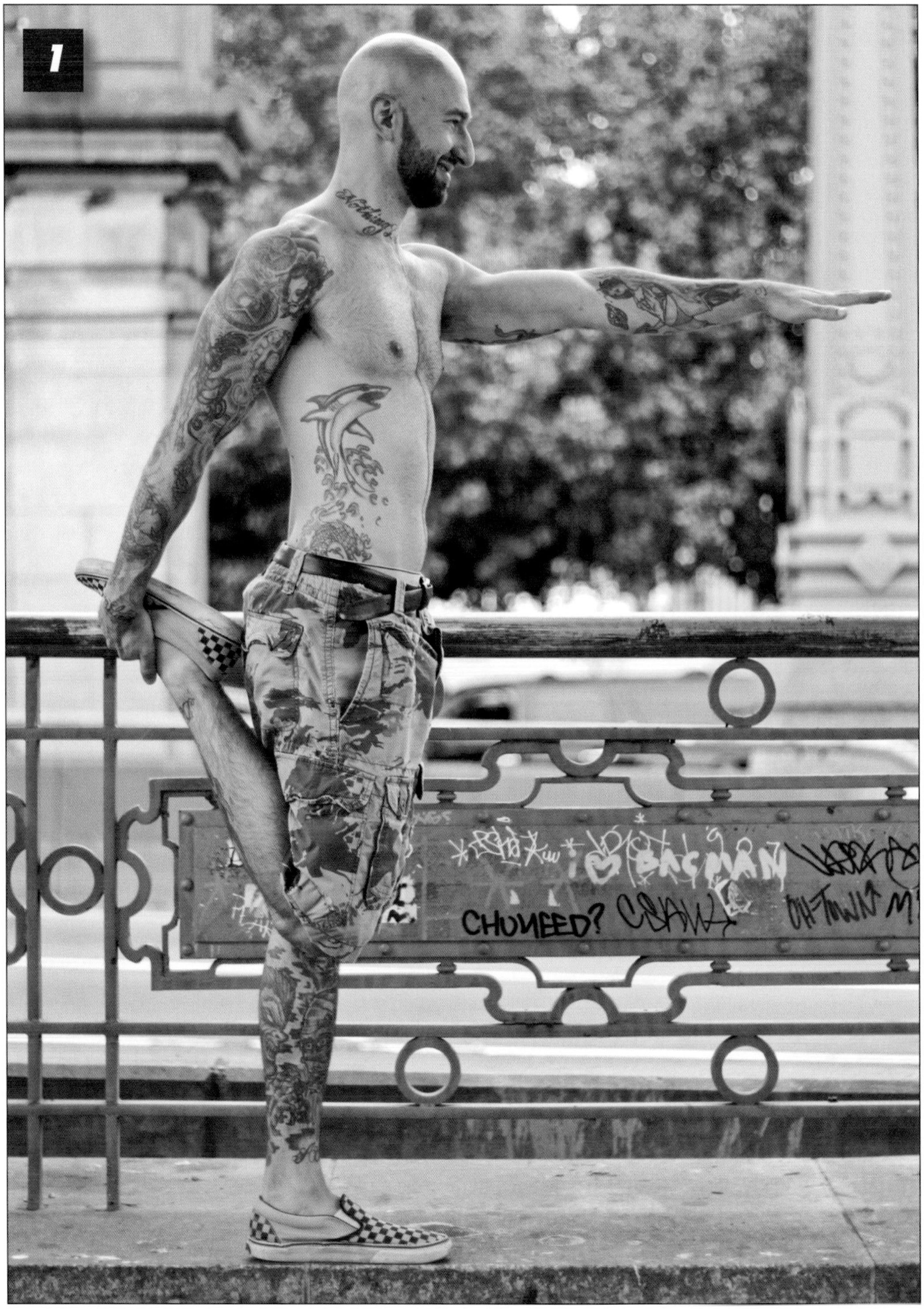

The flexibility can also become a greater challenge with this variant. You'll likely need to allow your bottom knee to come forward as you pass below the depth of the elevated object on which you're positioned.

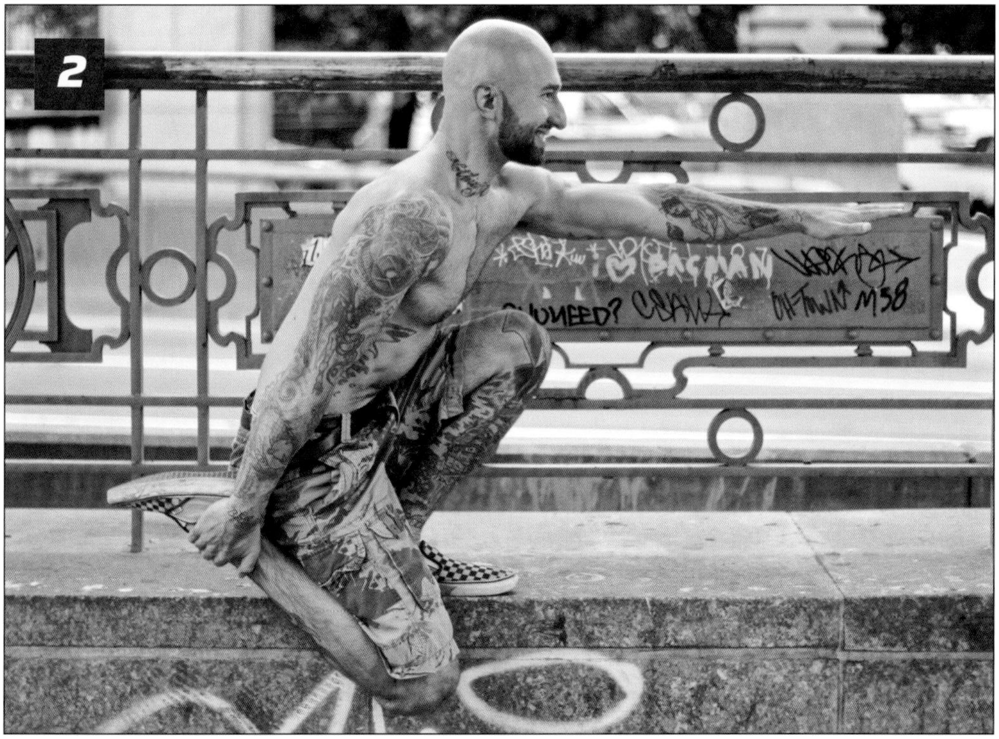

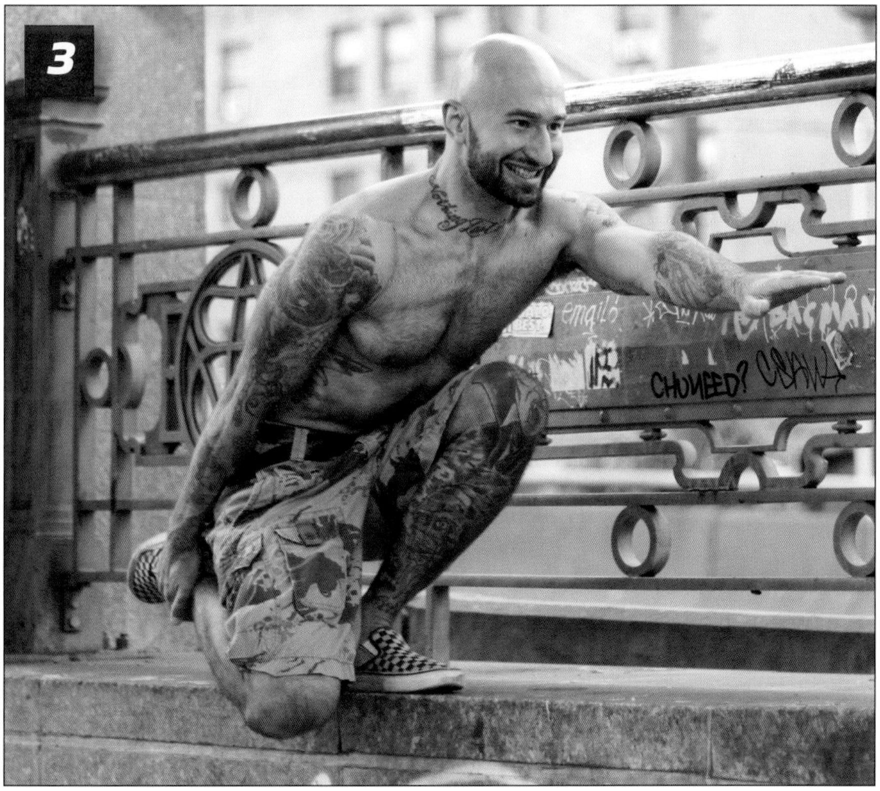

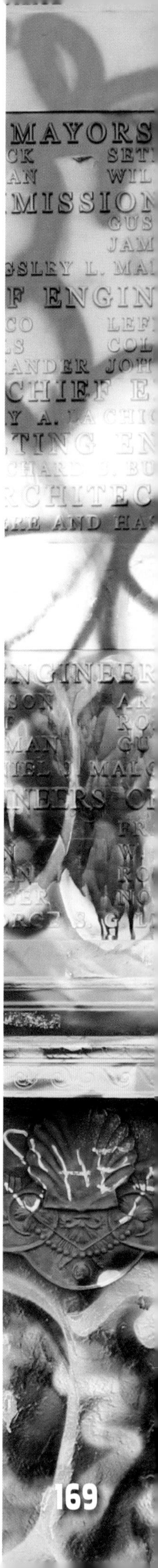

Hover Lunge

Another challenging aspect of the shrimp is the flexibility — your quads and hip flexors will need to be quite mobile to achieve this move (especially in the no-handed version). If you're struggling with this aspect of the exercise, you could try an easier variation where the back leg simply hovers behind you. It's looks sort of like a back lunge but your rear foot never touches the ground.

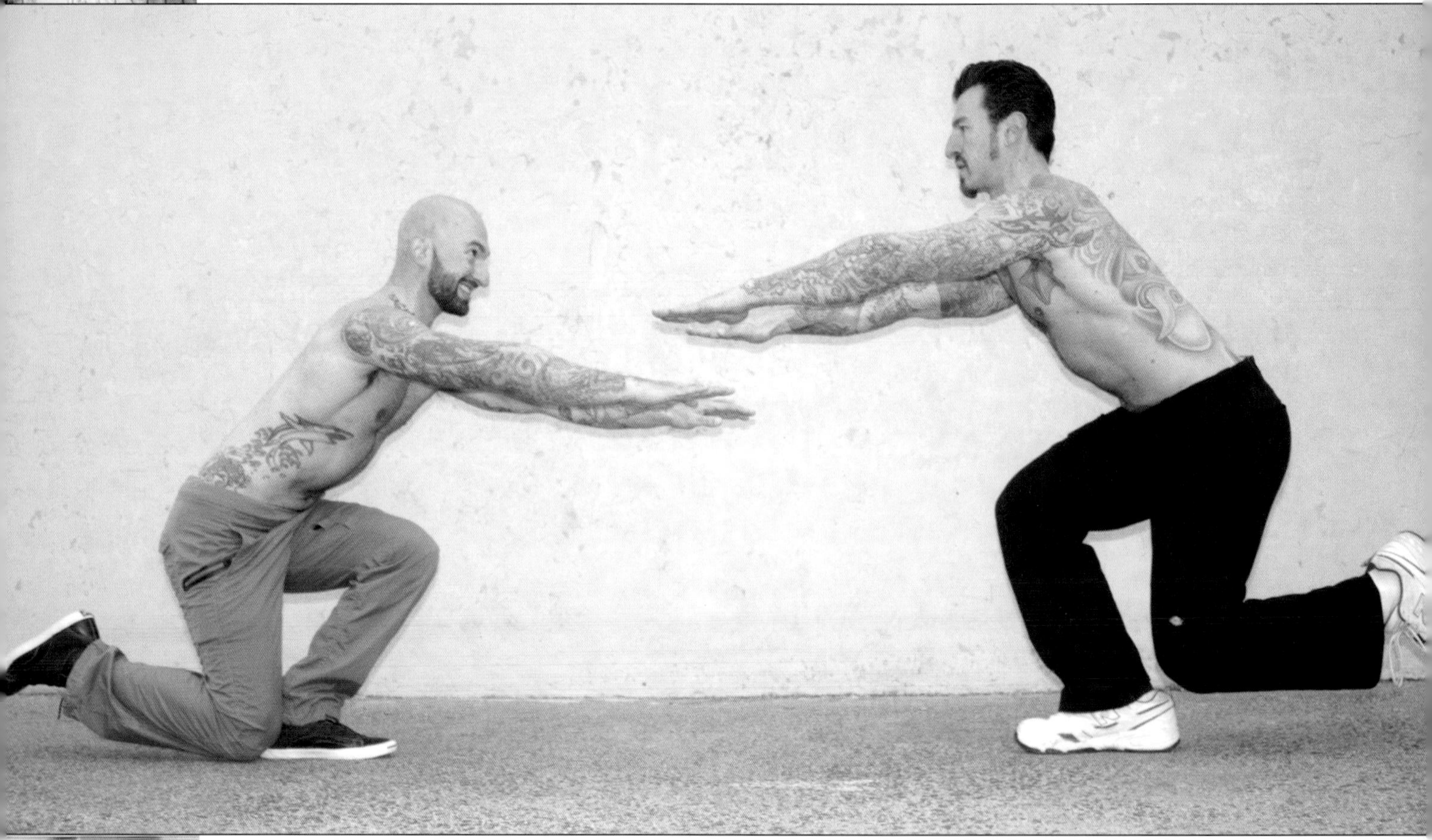

If your legs are strong, yet you lack the ability to do a pistol, the issue may be core strength. As anyone who's attempted a pistol knows, part of the challenge is keeping the non-squatting leg straight out in front. The L-sit is an excellent move to help you get a feel for using your core to assist your quads and hip flexors in keeping the legs extended. (More on L-sits in Appendix A.)

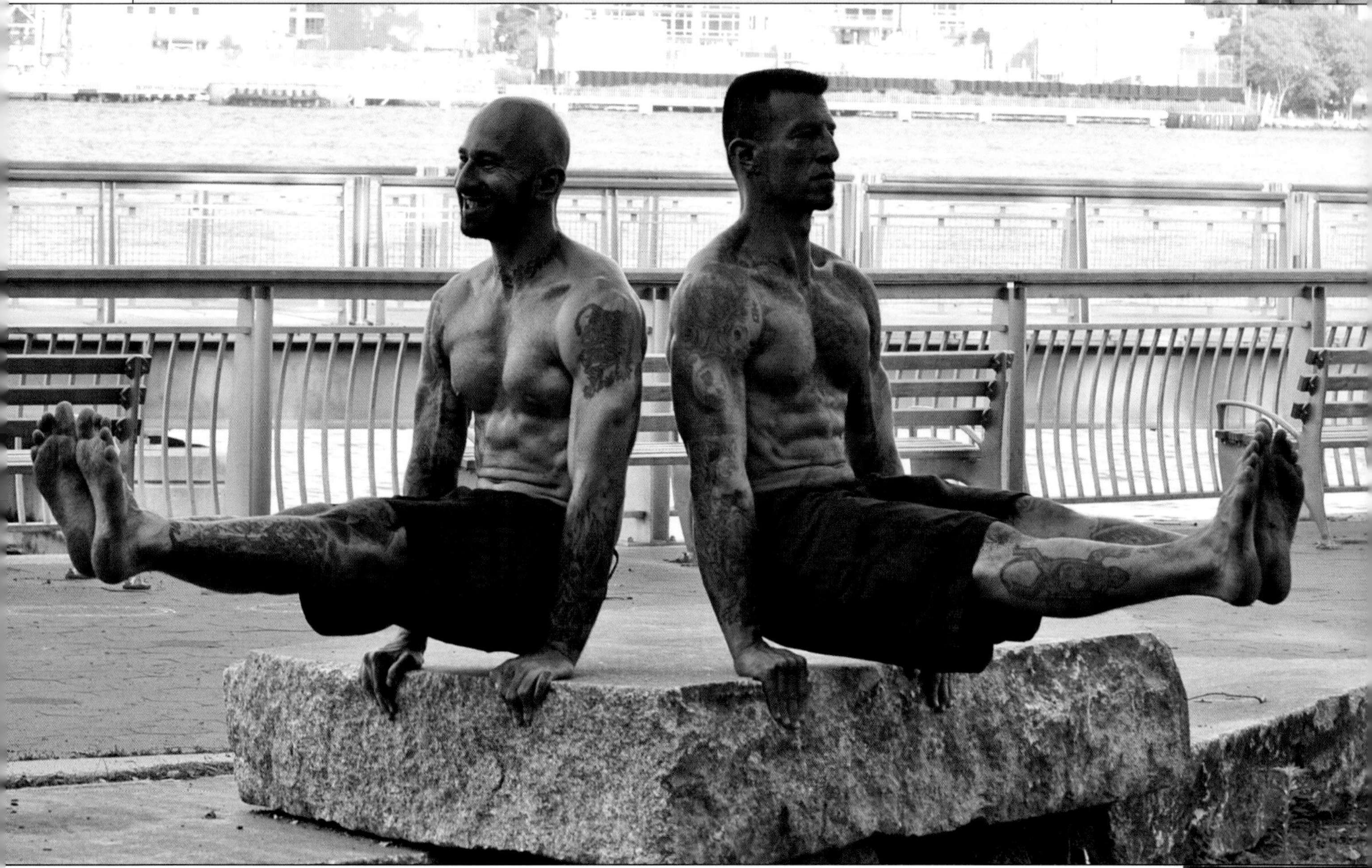

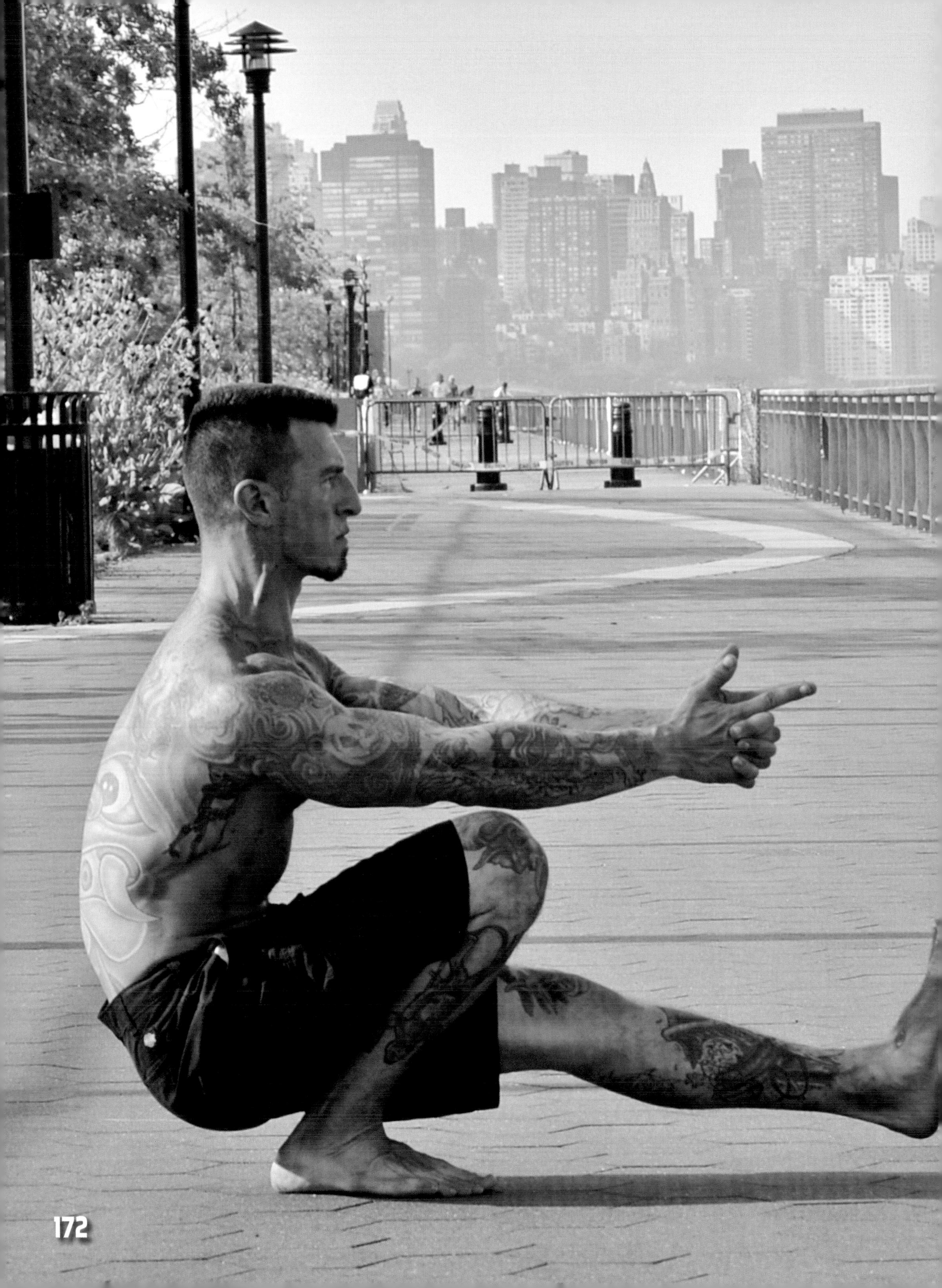

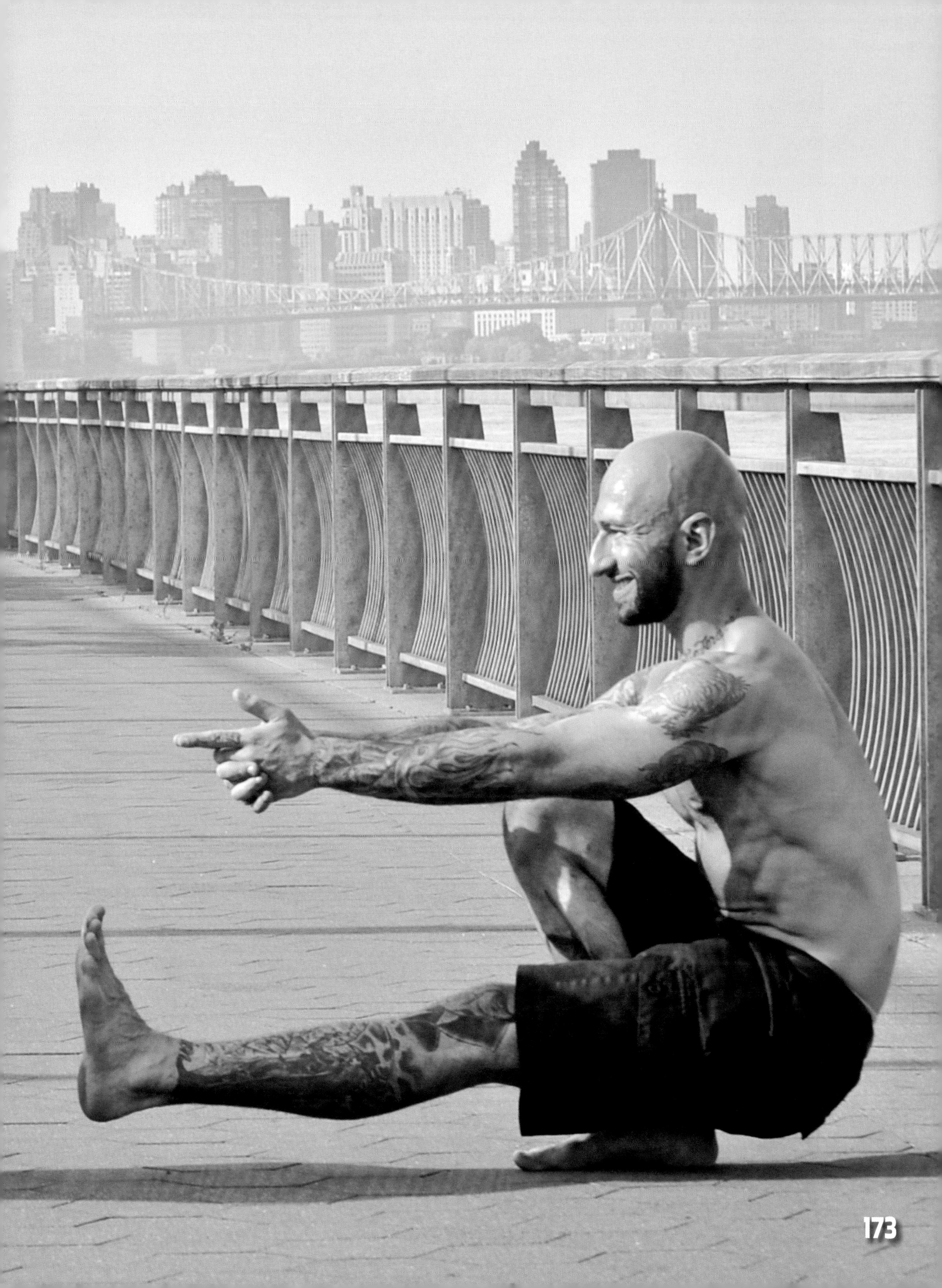

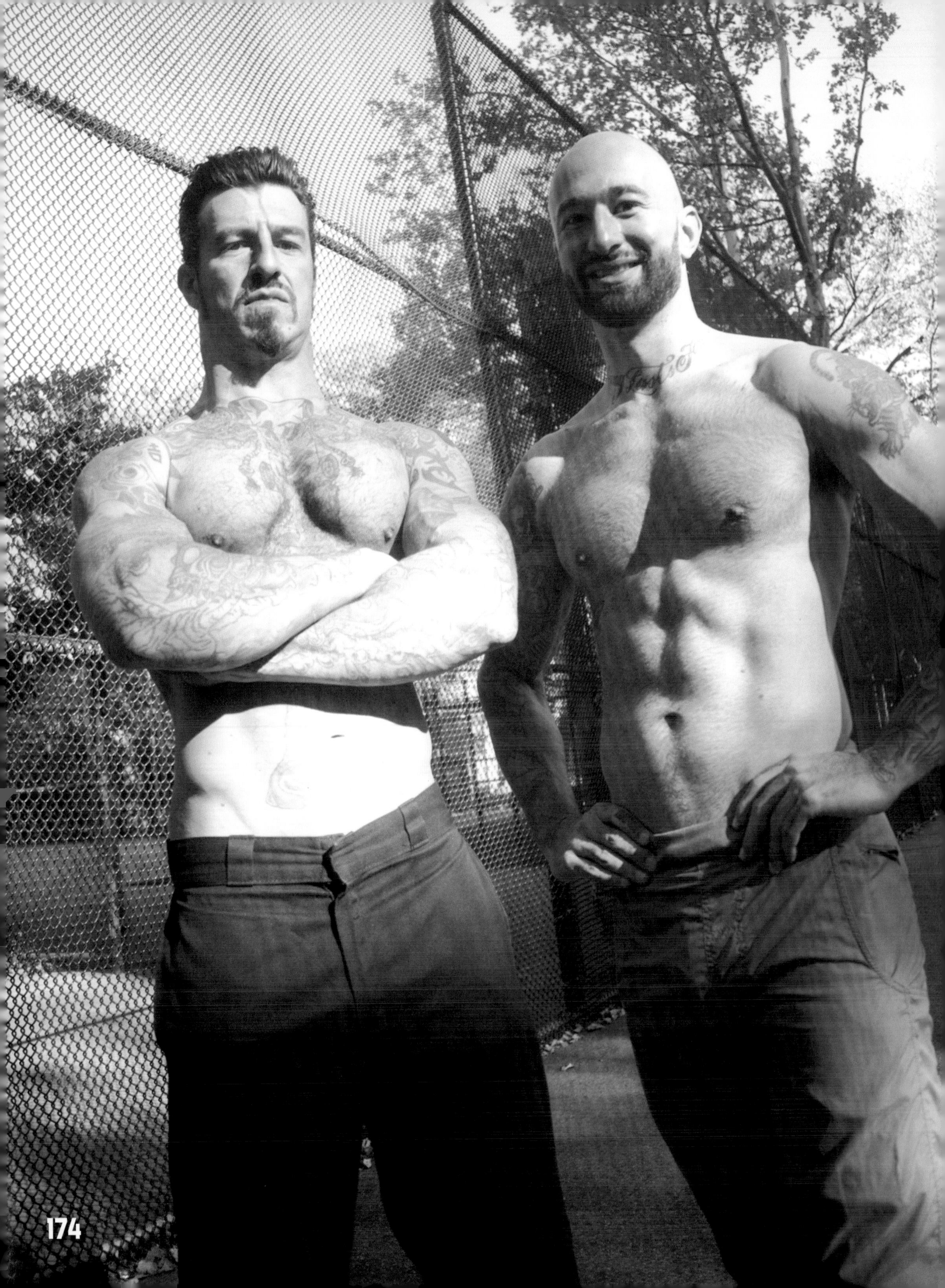

Chapter Nine:

All Together Now

Bodyweight training and strength training with weights both operate under the same principle of progressive overload. Regardless of modality, the way one grows stronger is to start with a relatively low amount of resistance and gradually add more as the body adapts to the movement.

In weight training, exercises can be learned with just an empty bar to get a feel for proper technique before progressing (adding weight). This allows the lifter to learn the form without having to overcome much resistance. Due to the nature of bodyweight training, however, learning a new exercise must be approached a bit differently. Since there is no way to do a pistol squat or one arm push-up without a significant amount of resistance, we instead must practice less challenging variations in which the body is positioned in such a way so as to create more or less favorable leverage.

Over time, progressive variations can gradually bring you closer to the full exercise. In fact, the exercises can be made harder indefinitely for as long as the body can continue to adapt. The key to pushing the limits is to realize that there are actually no limits at all!

Since you can't always add resistance to bodyweight exercises quite as gradually as sticking five more pounds on a barbell, it's okay to give yourself some leeway with form when you begin working toward new exercises that are on the fringes of your capabilities. Just don't get carried away with thinking you've mastered an exercise because you can bang out a couple sloppy reps. Once you can do a few repetitions of a new movement, focus on cleaning up your form before going for anything more difficult.

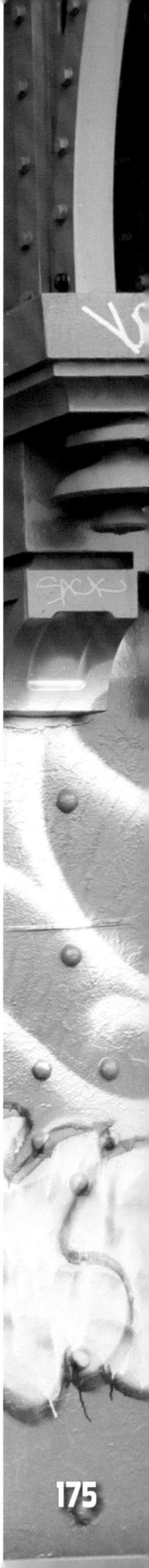

Designing Workouts

Programming is one of the most over-thought parts of working out. While I know it can be overwhelming to look through a book of exercises if you don't know where to start, it should actually be pretty simple for anyone to implement a progressive calisthenics training program. There is no magic formula that is perfect for everyone — you've got to listen to your body and be prepared to make adjustments as you go. Start exploring and see for yourself what these different exercises feel like.

If you can perform a given exercise, keep on practicing and refining it until it is no longer a challenge, then find a harder variant. If you can't perform the exercise, practice easier variations for a while to build strength, then return to the harder movement a few weeks (or months) later to assess your growth.

There are sample routines at the end of this book, but I want you to stray from them and experiment for yourself. They are only a guideline. But before all that, I need to address a few questions I expect you may be having at this point.

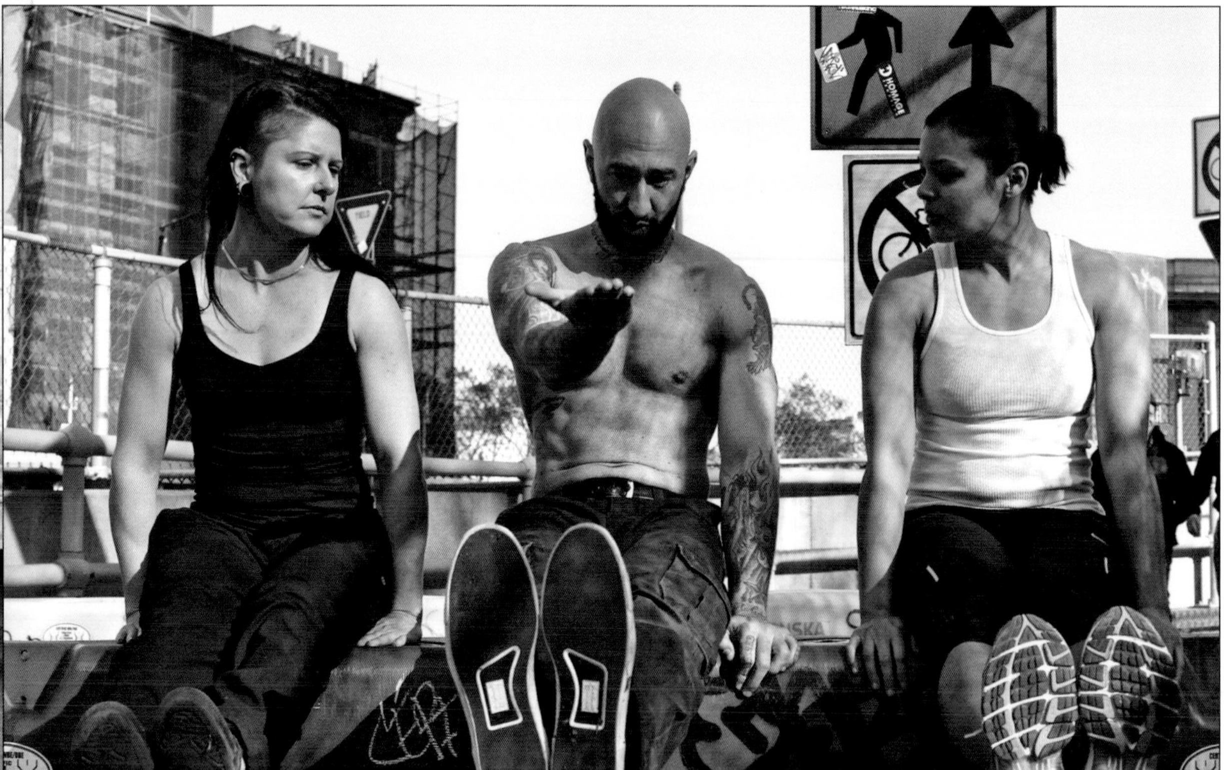

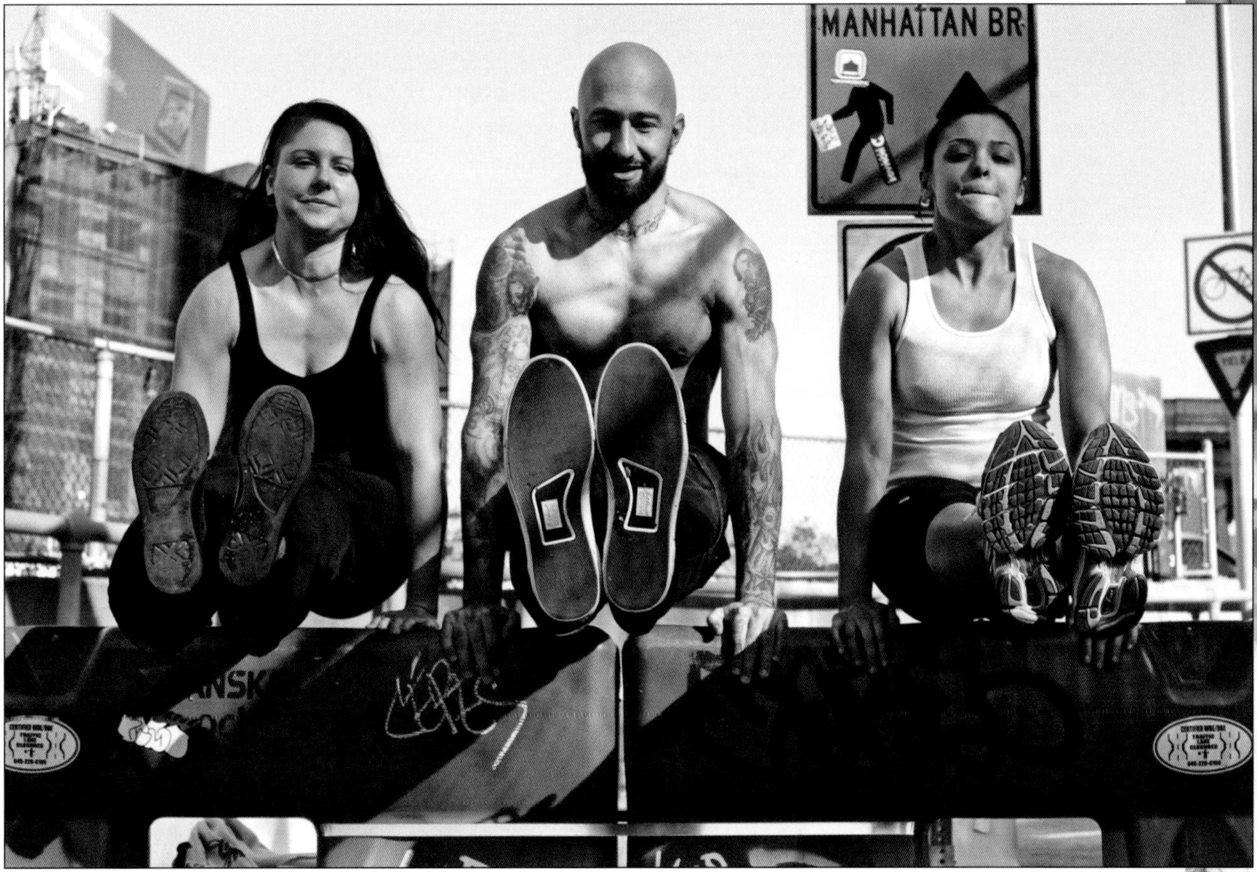

How Many Reps?

One of the most common questions I get asked it how to know when it is time to move onto a harder variation of an exercise. My answer is usually something like, "When you are ready," but most people are not satisfied with that answer. They want a rep range.

While there are general linear patterns, everyone's progress will be unique. Don't become upset if you struggle with certain exercises. We all have strengths and weaknesses and bodyweight training tends to make it pretty obvious what our shortcomings are.

As a general rule, however, the less intense an exercise is, the more reps you are going to need to be able to perform before progressing. That's why the range I'd suggest for wall push-ups is 40-50 reps before moving to knee push-ups, but the range from knee push-ups to full push-ups is 30-40. From full push-ups to close grip push-ups, the range goes down to 20-30. By the time you get to high level moves like one arm push-ups, it takes only around 5-10 reps to advance to the point where you can begin exploring plyo one-arm push-ups and eventually, the "perfect" one arm push-up (which in its idealized form is virtually unattainable).

PUSHING THE LIMITS!

Of course, each rep in a set of one arm push-ups requires a lot more strength than reps in a set of wall push-ups — so the overall output can actually be higher even though it's fewer reps. Additionally, as you build more strength you'll continue to improve on the earlier steps in the progressions. You should still use them in the same training session as a warm-up before your harder exercises, or once you have fatigued yourself practicing those more difficult moves.

Over the course of a few years, anyone can build from wall push-ups and partial squats to one arm push-ups and pistols. All that's required is patience and dedication.

Exercises	Approximate # of reps needed before moving on
Wall Push-up	40-50
Knee Push-up	30-40
Full Push-up	20-30
Close Push-up	15-20
Self Assisted One Arm Push-up	10-15
One Arm Push-up	5-10
Assisted Squats/Partial Squat	40-50
Full Squat	30-40
Close Squat	20-30
Side to Side Squat	15-20
Assisted Pistol	10-15
Pistol Squat	5-10

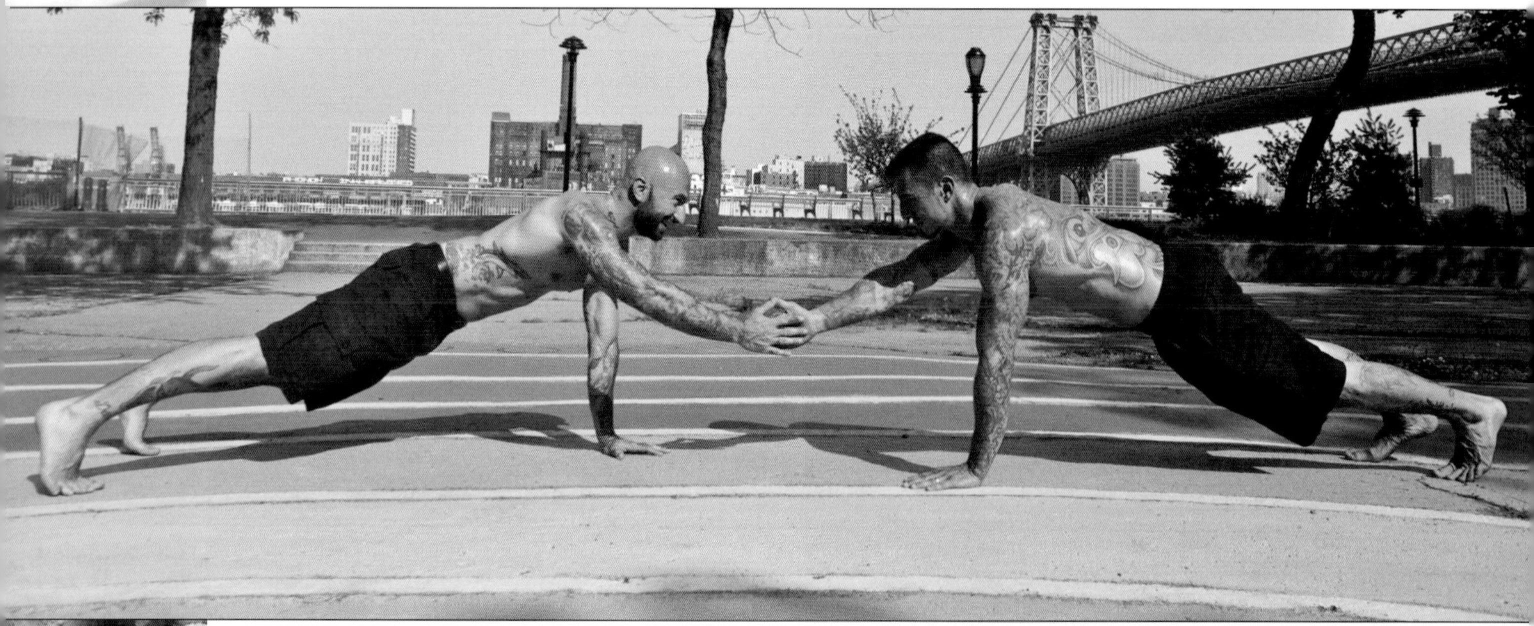

Though the sequences on the previous page are a great way to approach gradually progressing your skills, there are other steps one could take along the way, which is why I have included so many different exercises in this book. Feel free to modify the progressions using whatever variations you need to suit your needs. Strength development is not always linear and we don't all follow the same path.

How Often To Train?

This is the other big question about program design. As a general guideline, three days per week is the minimum amount of training that will allow for continuous improvement. Though age, genetics and lifestyle factors can contribute to your progress as well. Again, there is plenty of room for personal discretion here.

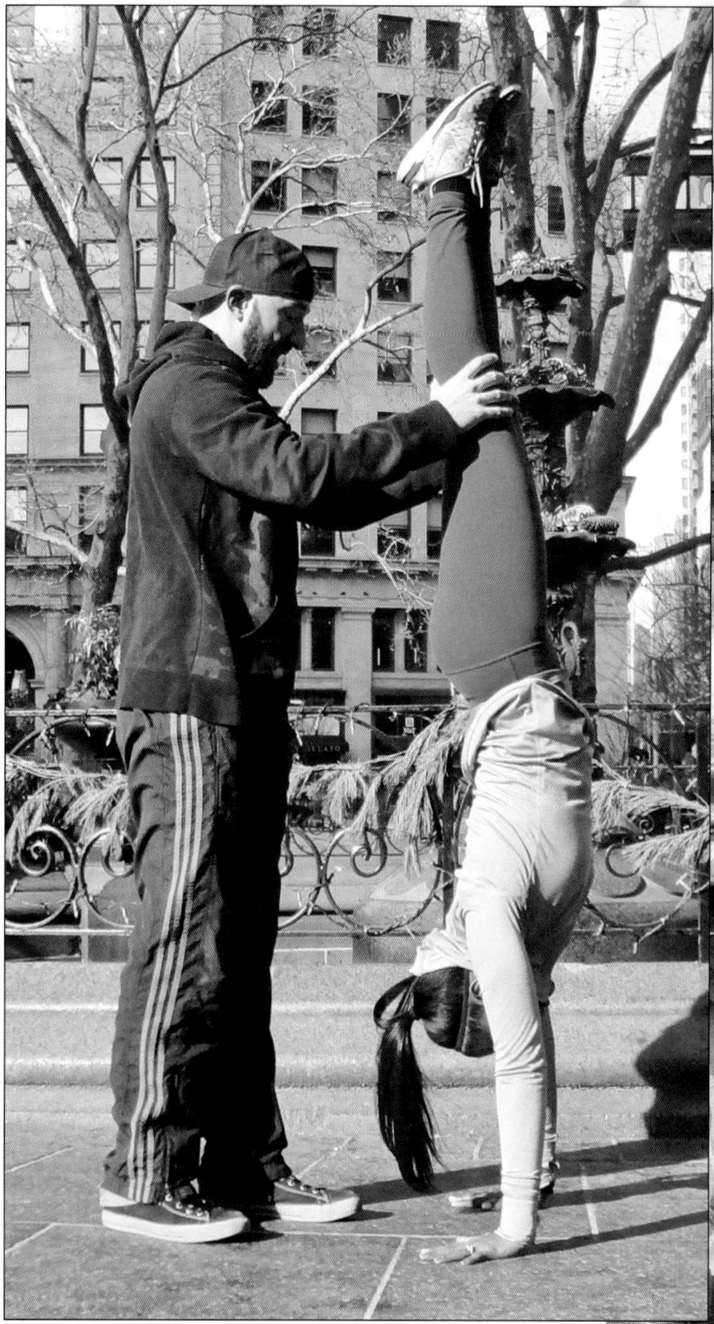

Raw beginners can train as little as once or twice per week and still make gains for the first two or three months of training, however. In fact, the difference between doing nothing and doing something is such a huge chasm, those first few workouts might leave you very sore, so it's okay to take longer rest between sessions when starting. Once you acclimate to that, you'll need to step it up to at least three days a week to experience continued growth. Of course, with improved conditioning, the body will be able to handle more work with less rest. The soreness you experience once you are in shape is rarely as severe as when you begin your training.

How To Break It Down?

Split routines are all the rage in bodybuilding, but you don't have to train different muscles on different days to get strong with your bodyweight. I recommend beginners do full body workouts every time they train, which should be three or four days a week. An every-other-day routine (or every third day in the beginning) can work really nicely as well, so it need not always be Monday, Wednesday and Friday. Don't get too hung up on the calendar.

After you've been training for a long time and can handle high amounts of volume, a split routine may be feasible. A simple two-day split consisting of alternating your upper-body and lower-body exercises works nicely, or you could try the classic three-day push, pull, legs trifecta (I like to train inversions at the end of a leg day). Some people like to train more frequently, and a three-day split allows you to spread your exercises out over the course of the week, increasing the amount of sets and reps for each movement without adding to the duration of your workouts.

Since daily strength training can be a lot for some people to handle, another option is to do strength workouts every other day with additional exercises like running, swimming or skipping rope performed on the days in between.

There are a lot of different ways to break up your training and no single method is right for everyone. In fact, the same individual may even find themselves needing to vary their approach week-to-week or month-to-month depending on how busy they may be with other aspects of their life.

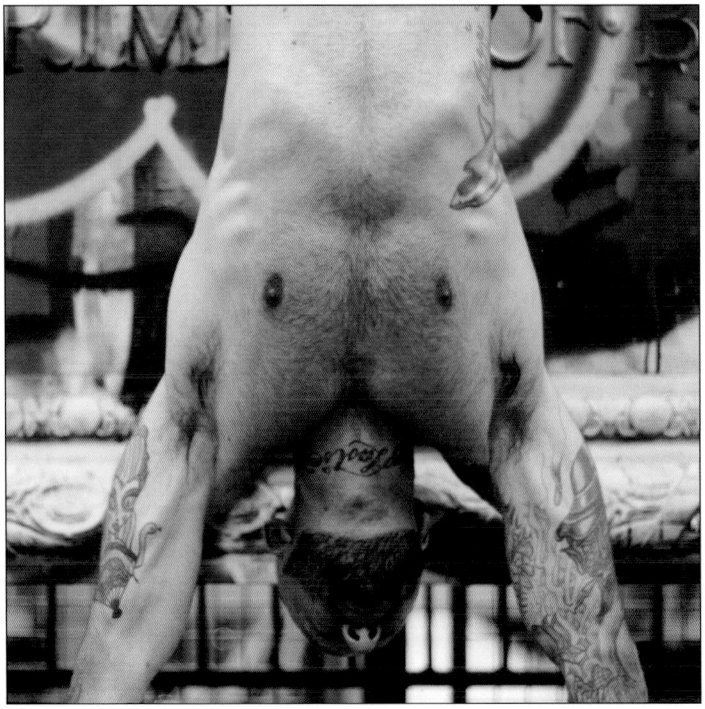

Progressive Overload And Diminishing Returns

No matter what style of training or specific program you follow, the general formula behind strength training is the same: work your muscles, give them rest and repeat.

The human body has an amazing ability to adapt to stress. Every time you work out, you are essentially injuring your muscles, then when you rest they recover and come back with a vengeance. It's a case of whatever doesn't kill 'em makes 'em stronger.

Once recovery is achieved—which could take anywhere from a day to a week depending on your level of conditioning relative to the intensity of your workout—you have a small window in which you can build on the previous session. Train again too soon and you won't be recovered enough to benefit from the next workout, wait too long and you'll have regressed back to your previous state. This is why many people fail to make progress. They simply cannot stay consistent for any significant amount of time.

On the other hand, there are people who do manage to stay consistent for years and eventually, they will also find that their progress gradually begins to slow down. It can take several years to get to this point though, and gains will still come but they will come so slowly you might not even notice if you aren't watching closely. This is simply a case of diminishing returns, a concept that applies to everything in life. Whether we're talking about working out, learning an instrument, or climbing the corporate ladder, the farther along you get on any path, the more effort it takes to keep moving forward.

When I was in school, I found the amount of work needed to simply get by and pass my classes was typically pretty low. Barring disabilities, anyone who's even remotely intelligent can get a high school diploma in America simply by showing up and applying even the slightest effort. But to get straight A's takes hours of studying and dedication.

Fitness is no different. If you're starting off in average shape, you can get in better-than-average shape in a few months by working out three times a week. (Just don't forget you have to eat less to lose weight!) However, if you've been at it a while and are already in better than average shape, it's going to take more intensity to keep progressing.

This is why we add more training days.

This is why we increase our sets and reps.

This is why we move to harder exercise variations.

This is why we keep **PUSHING THE LIMITS!**

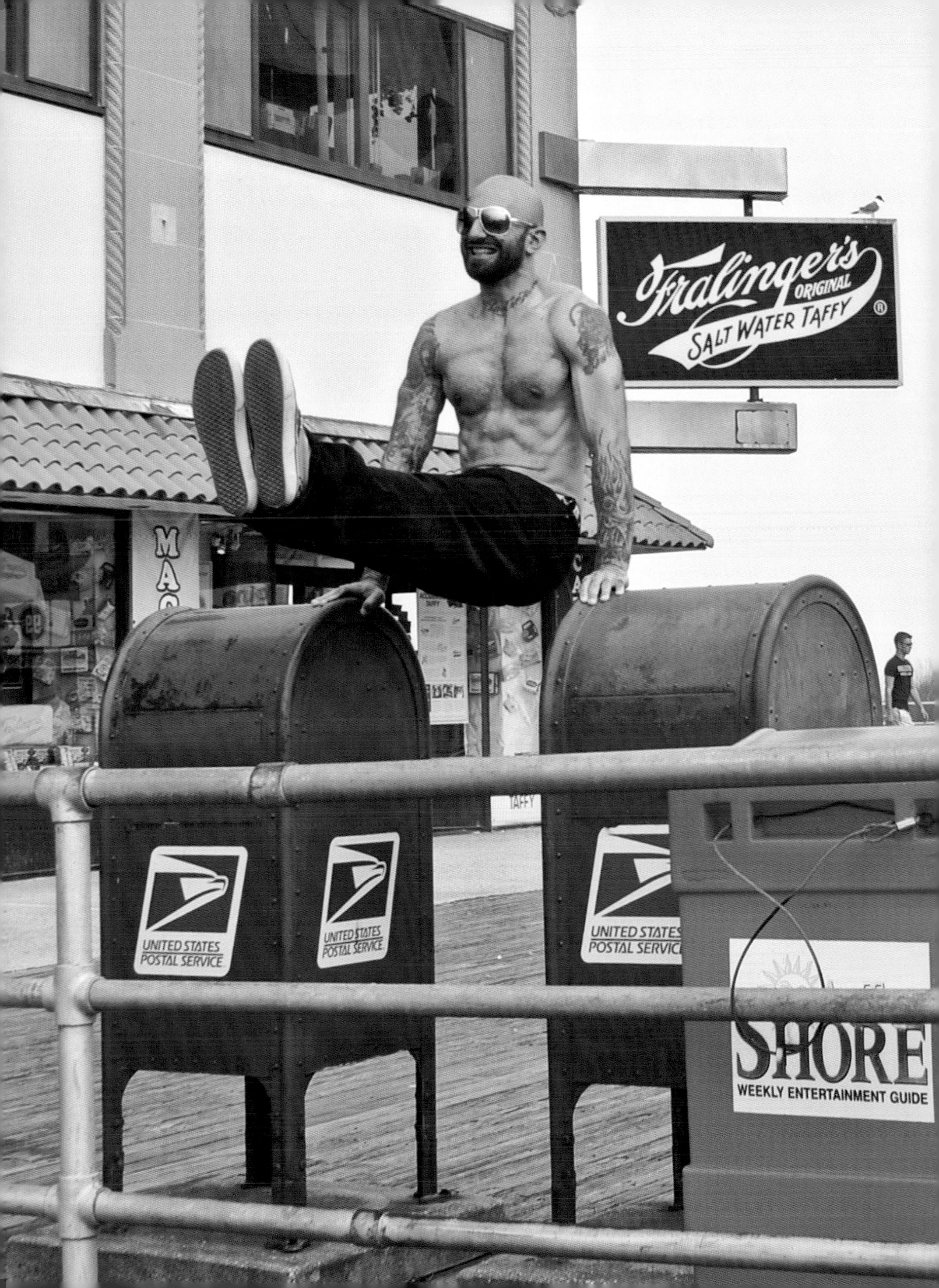
Fralinger's
ORIGINAL
SALT WATER TAFFY
UNITED STATES POSTAL SERVICE
UNITED STATES POSTAL SERVICE
UNITED STATES POSTAL SERVICE
SHORE
WEEKLY ENTERTAINMENT GUIDE

Appendix A:

Bonus Exercises

When it comes to bodyweight training, the possibilities are truly endless. With that in mind, here are some other worthwhile exercises to help supplement your training. Have fun experimenting with these bonus exercises and feel free to modify them as you see fit.

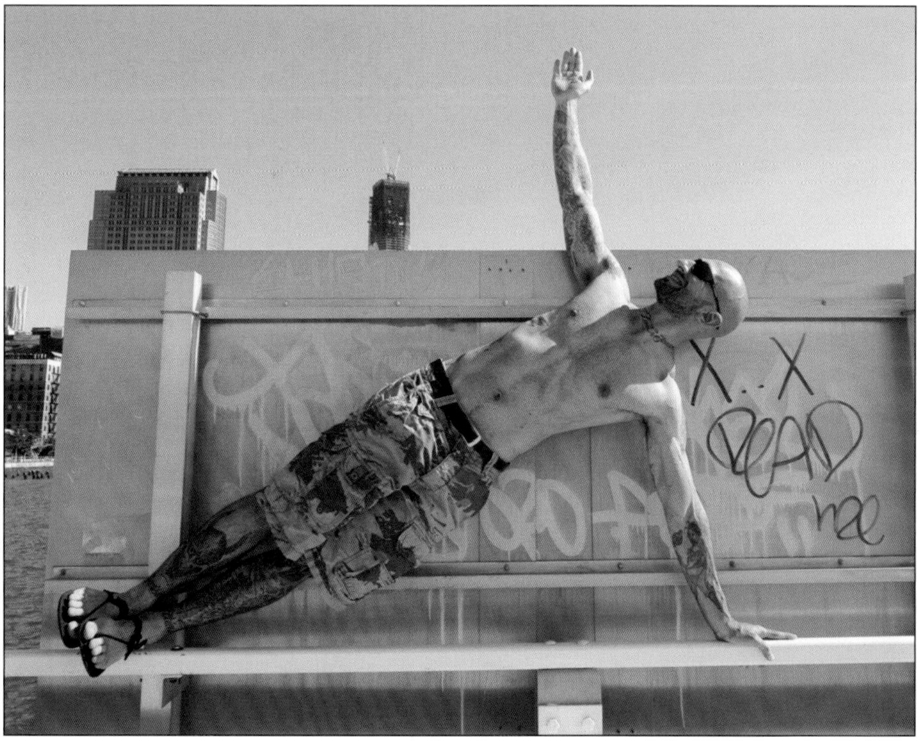

Single Leg Deadlift

Much like a pistol squat is exponentially harder than a regular two legged squat, single leg deadlifts are more challenging than you might expect. Doing a deadlift on one leg takes strength, balance and flexibility. While some may dismiss this exercise as being too easy, the one-legged bodyweight deadlift is a fantastic way to build strength and stability in your hamstrings, glutes and lower back. If done slowly and with strict attention to detail, performing a dozen or two one-legged bodyweight deadlifts can be a serious workout.

The movement of a single leg deadlift is not unlike that of a drinking bird toy. As you lean your upper body forward, reach your opposite leg out behind you. This will not only help you balance, it will also further engage your lower back as well as the leg that's in the air. It can help to touch your hand to your opposite foot at the bottom to keep from externally rotating at the hip. Watch out that you don't bend your spine on the way down, but rather take the stretch in your hamstrings.

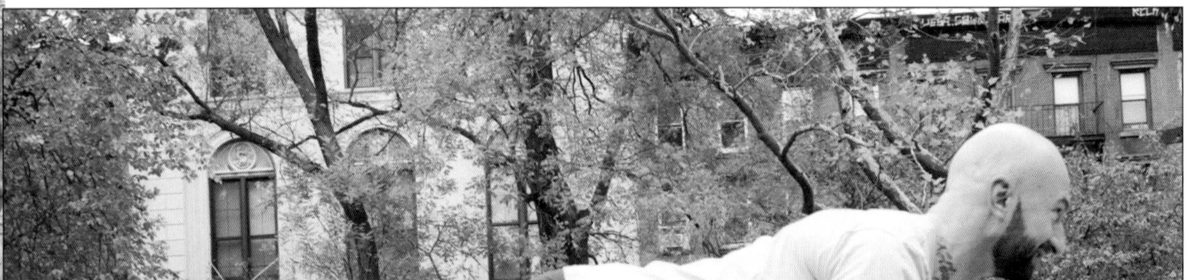

The movement of a single leg deadlift is not unlike that of a drinking bird toy. As you lean your upper body forward, reach your opposite leg out behind you.

Lying Knee Tuck

The lying knee tuck is a great beginner exercise that can serve as a gatekeeper to harder moves like the lying leg raise, L-sit and even the pistol squat.

Lie on your back with your hands by your sides and lift your feet a few inches off the ground. You may place your hands beneath your lower back for support if you need to, but do your best to minimize any arch. Think about keeping your heels relatively close to the ground as you tuck your knees all the way to your chest, allowing your lower back to come off the ground slightly at the top. Stay in control as you extend your legs back to the start position. Press your lower back down into the ground to engage your deep abdominal stabilizers.

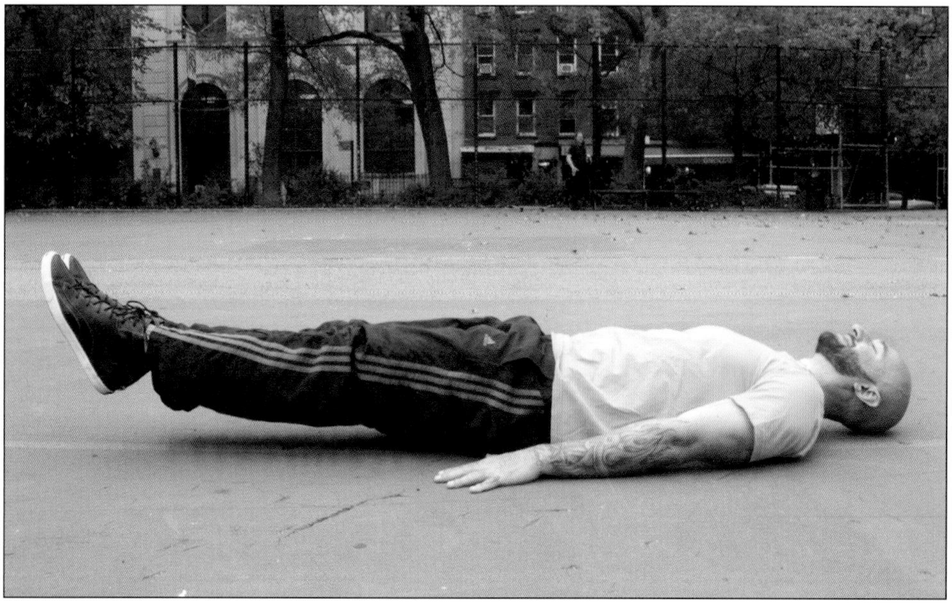

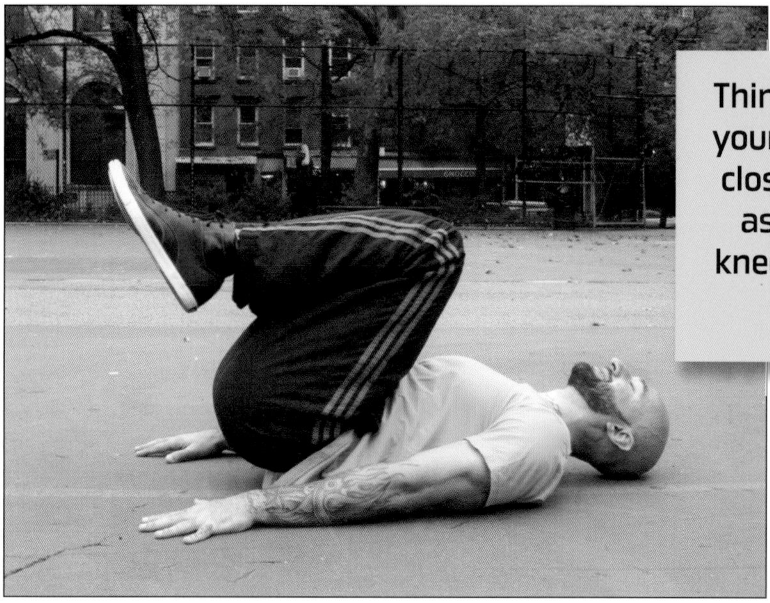

Think about keeping your heels relatively close to the ground as you tuck your knees all the way to your chest.

Lying Leg Raise

When knee tucks become easy for you, move onto lying leg raises. Start in the same position, but instead of bending your knees towards your chest, keep your legs straight and lift them up until your feet are in the air in front of your hips. Your butt might come off the floor at the top of the range of motion; this is fine. Lower back down with control and repeat. Again, try not to let your back arch at the bottom of the range of motion.

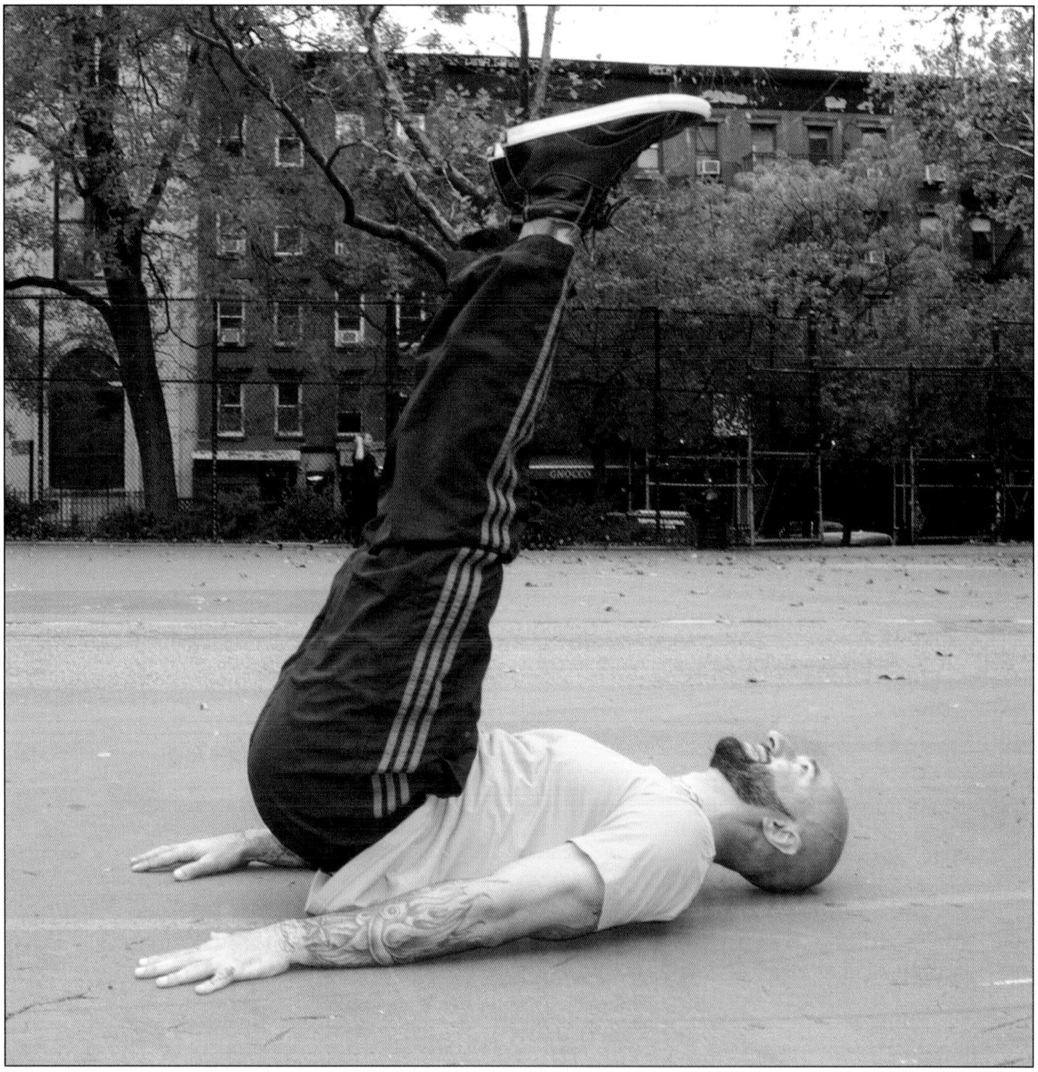

Headstand Leg Raise

Once you've gotten comfortable with both the headstand and the lying leg raise, try combining them for a new challenge. Begin in a headstand, then slowly lower your legs away from your trunk and raise them back toward the top. You'll need to lean your hips slightly in the opposite direction of your toes to keep from tipping over as you reach your legs away from your body.

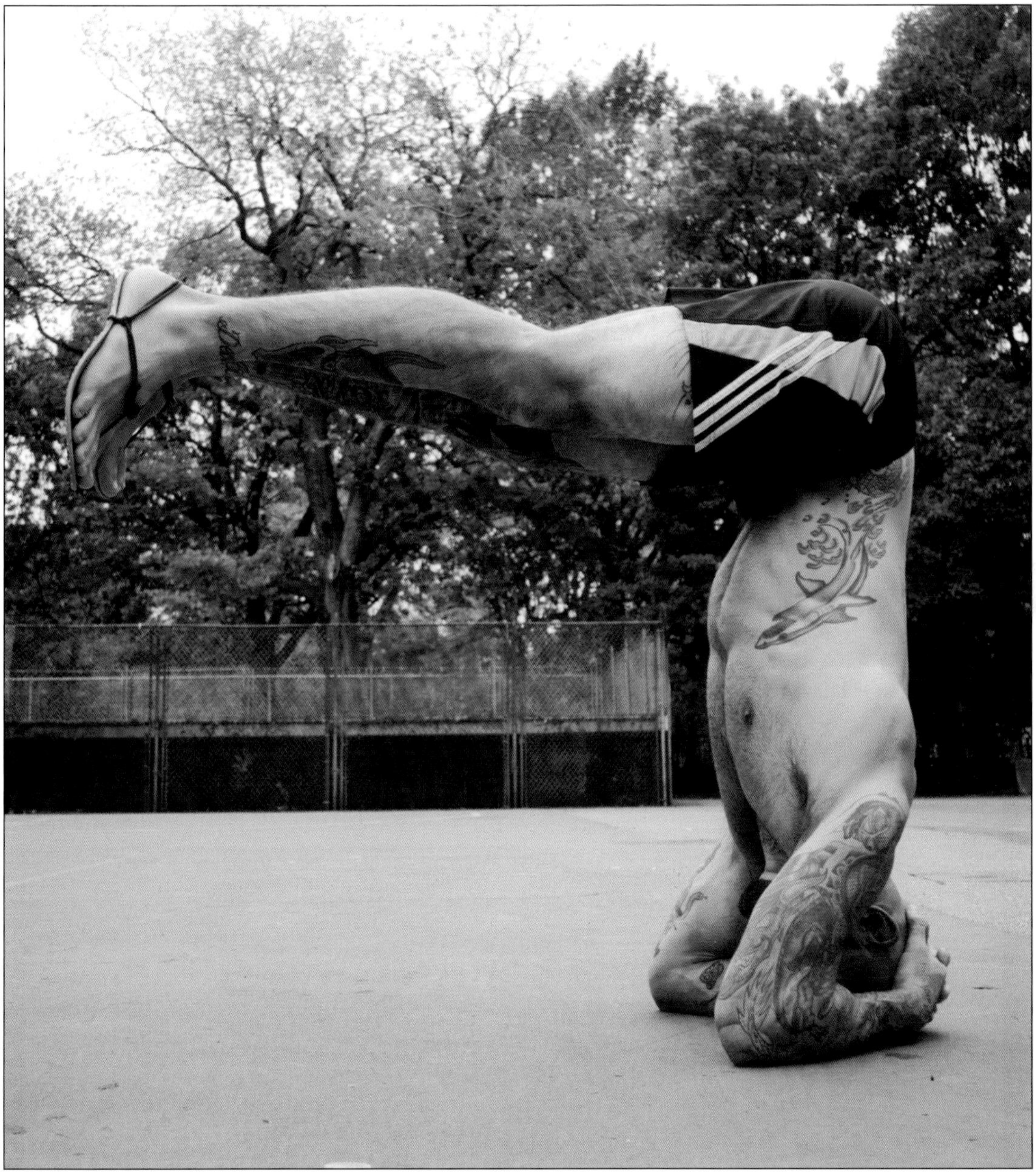

Side Plank

A familiar pose to yoga practitioners, the side plank puts more emphasis on your obliques than a standard front plank. Just like the classic version, you can perform a side plank on your palm or your elbow, and with one or two legs. As your have to support your weight on one hand, it is also more work for your shoulder and arm than a standard plank.

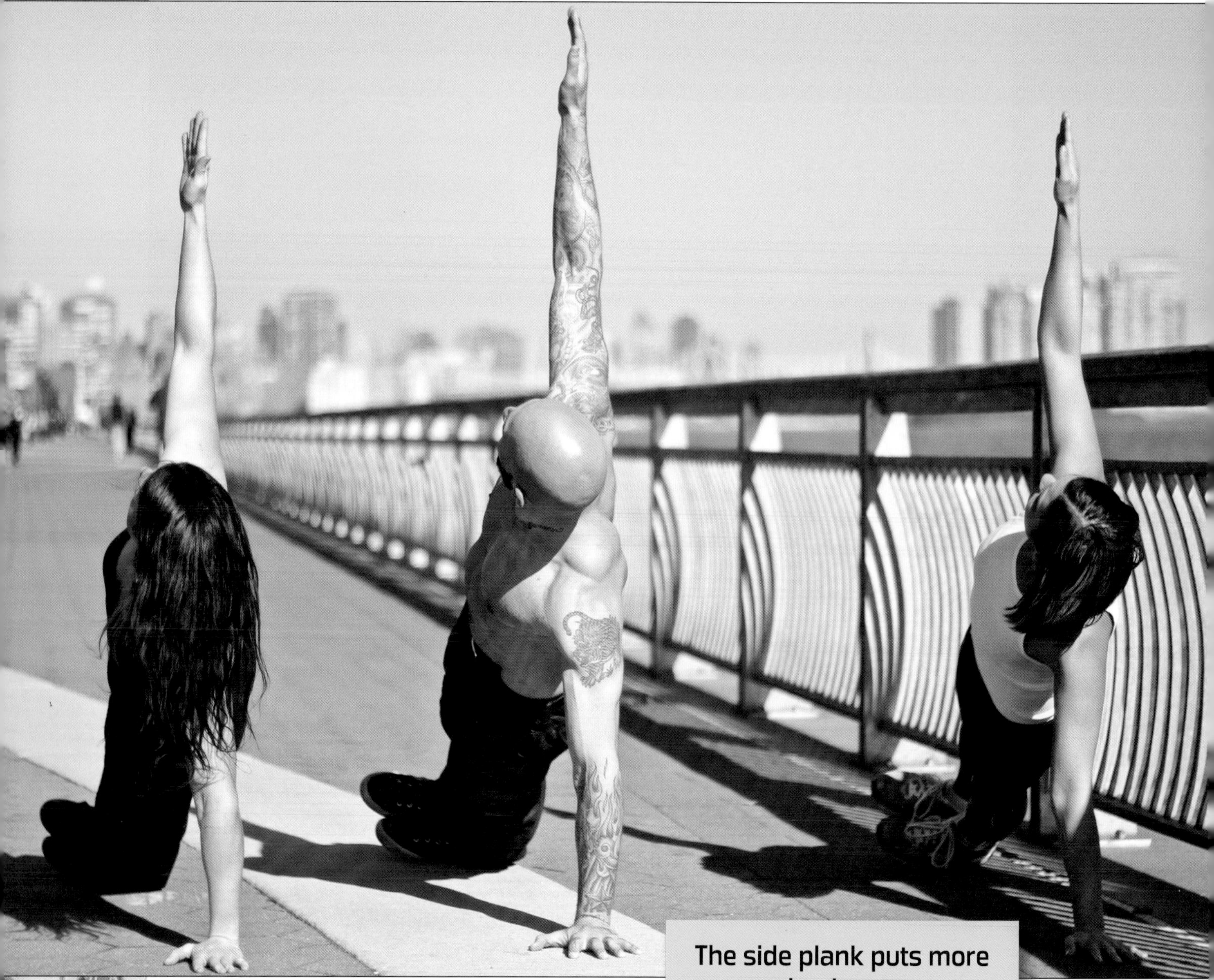

The side plank puts more emphasis on your obliques than a standard front plank.

Side Crow

Another common yoga pose, the side crow is like a frog stand except with both legs resting on one arm. Place your hands on the ground and rotate your hips a quarter turn to the side with your legs stacked on top of each other. Leverage both legs on the back of one of your triceps and slowly tip your weight off your feet. Like all isolateral moves, do your best to balance your practice by training both sides of your body evenly.

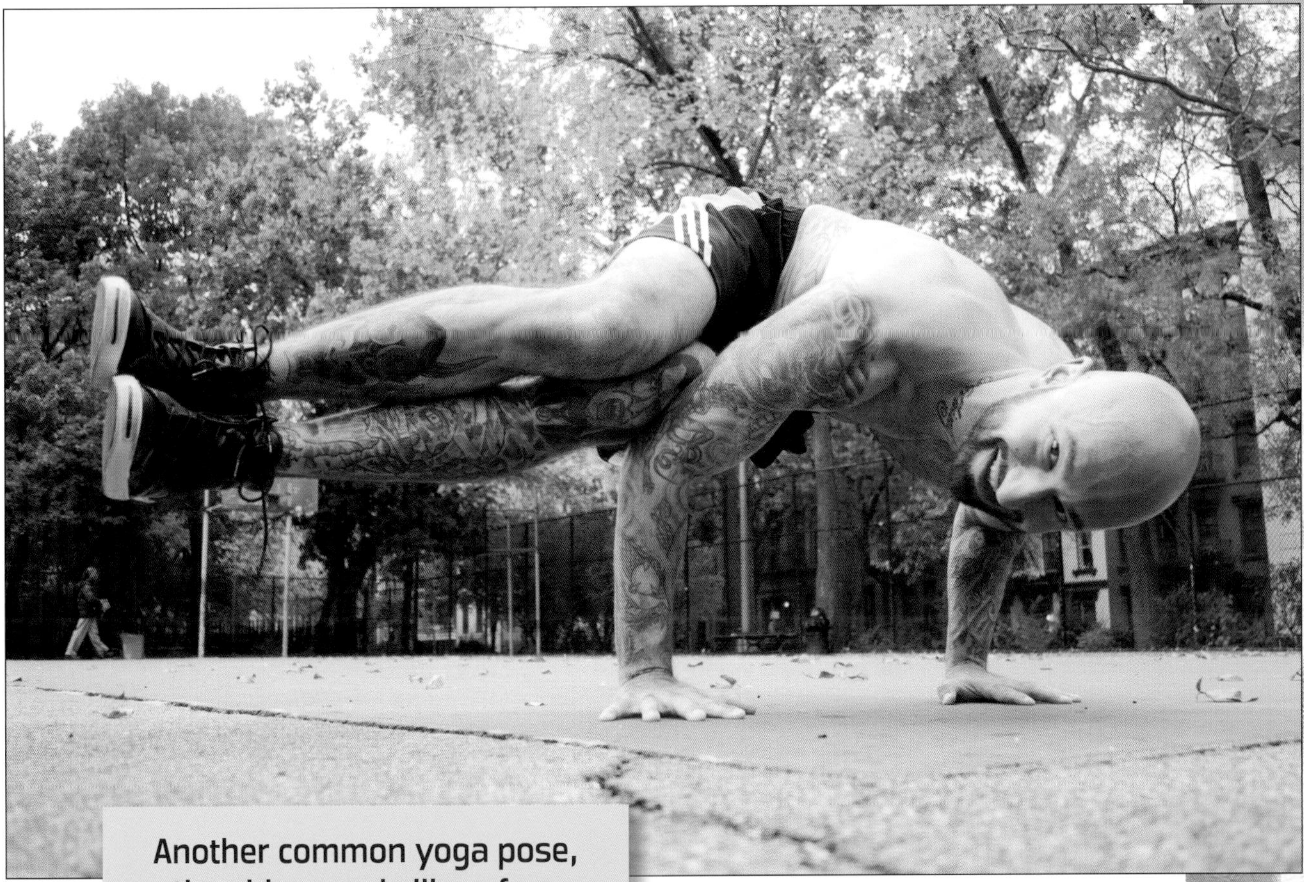

Another common yoga pose, the side crow is like a frog stand except with both legs resting on one arm.

L-Sit

In order to perform an L-sit, you'll need a strong core, strong arms and better than average flexibility in your hamstrings. The objective is to sit on the floor with your legs straight in front you like a letter "L" and lift your body off the ground onto your hands. This is one of those exercises with a very literal name.

If you can't get to this position right away, practice with your knees bent to work your way up to the full L-sit. You can gradually build towards extending your legs away from your body over time.

Keep your arms tight against your body with your elbows locked and triceps flexed. Press down with your shoulders and try to make as much space as possible between your body and the floor.

It can also be helpful to practice your L-sit between two elevated objects to allow some room to slowly work toward getting your legs parallel to the ground.

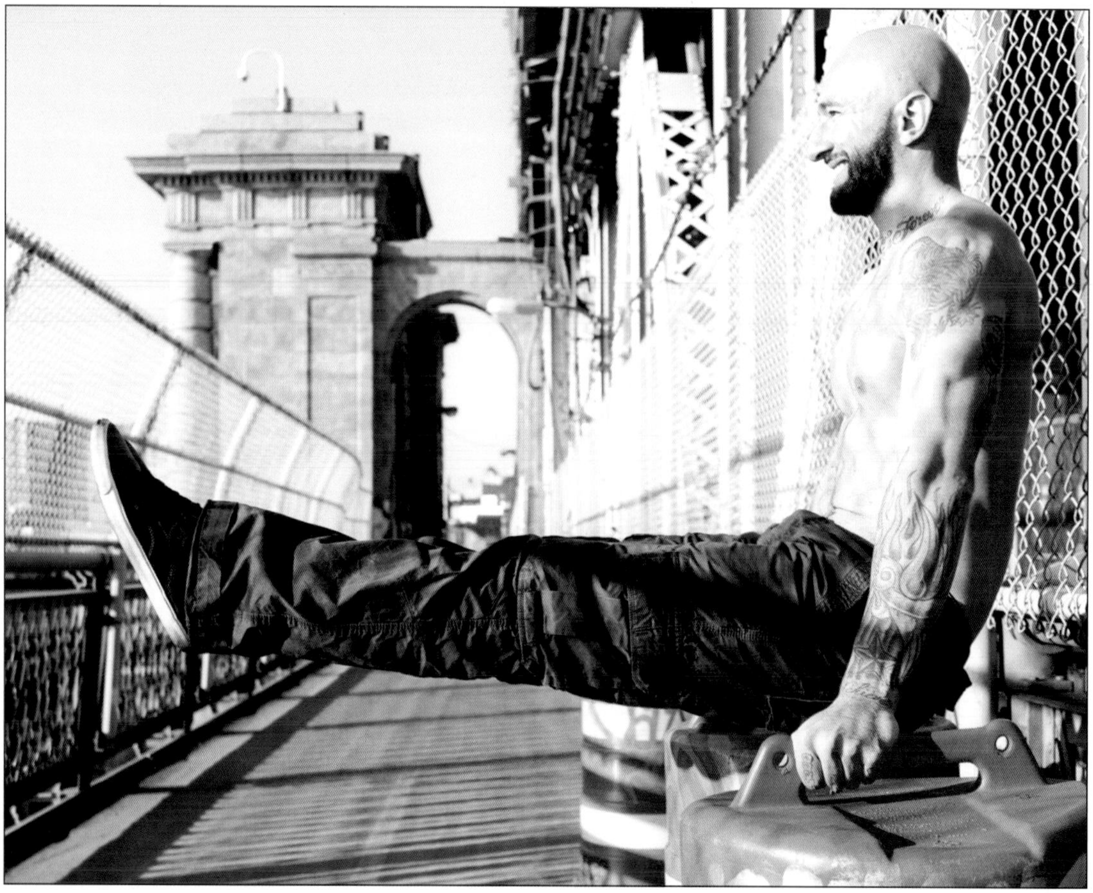

Elbow Lever

As the name implies, an elbow lever is performed by leveraging your body against one or both elbows while balancing on your hand(s) with your body stretched out and hovering over the ground. Though it looks similar to the planche, it is significantly less difficult due to the fact that your torso rests on the backs of your arms.

Make sure to keep your abs contracted and engage your lower back as you raise yourself off the floor. It is also important to pitch your upper-body forward in order to counterbalance the weight of your bottom half.

If you are struggling with the elbow lever, I recommend practicing on a bench, step or any other flat, raised object. This will allow you more room to lift your legs into position, as opposed to the limited amount of space when starting with your hands on the floor.

It may take some time to get used to the sensation of having your elbows jutting into your abdomen; beginners tend to find it especially unpleasant. With practice, however, you can eventually learn to make peace with the feeling.

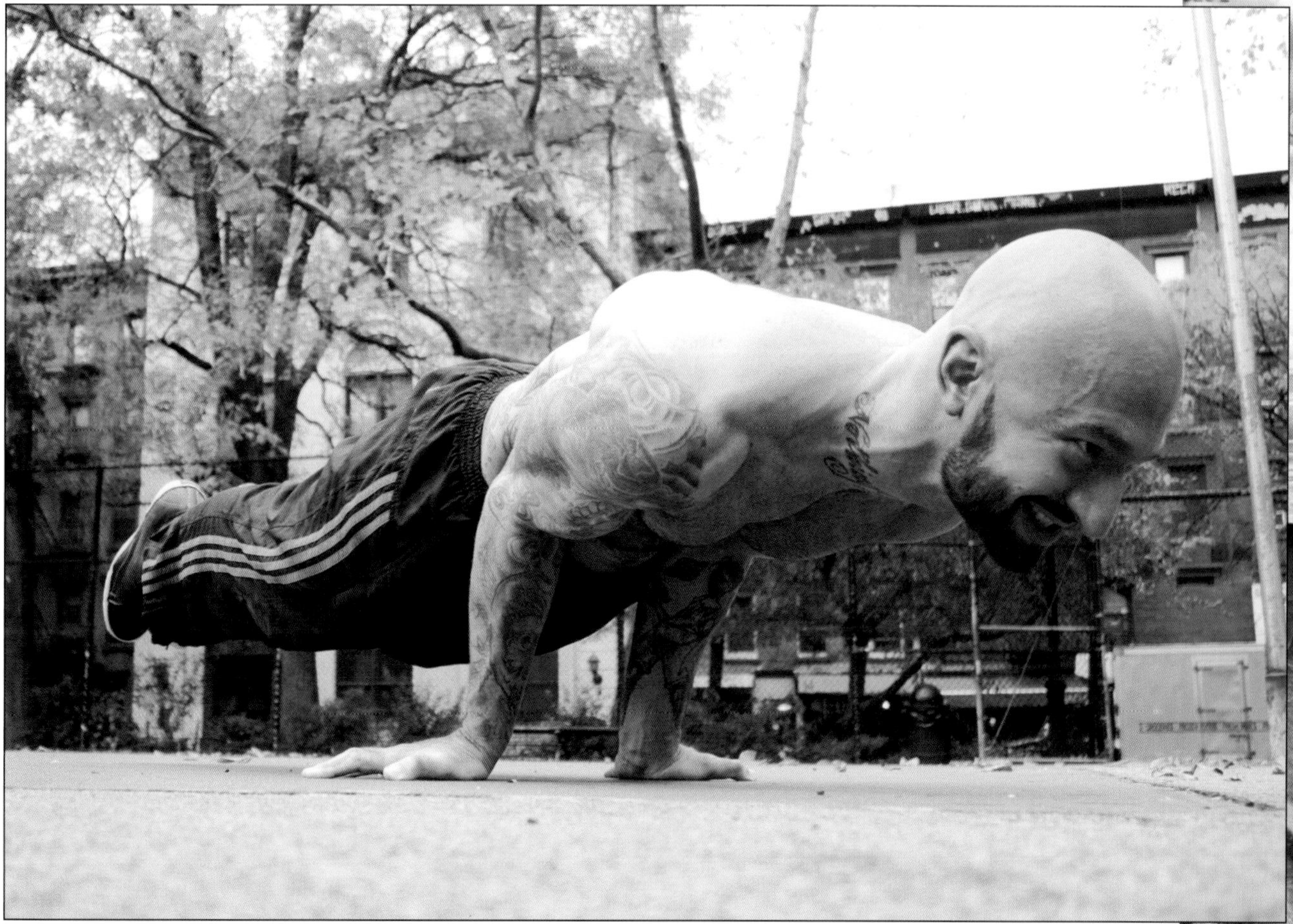

One Arm Elbow Lever

Though skilled hand-balancers have a way of making this move seem effortless, the one arm elbow lever is a very challenging feat, so be patient if you endeavor to add this one to your arsenal.

Start out by just trying to get your feet off the floor to get a feel for the balance before attempting to fully extend your body. While strength is obviously a factor in this move, the one arm elbow lever is more about balance than anything else. It may be helpful to spot yourself with your free hand in the beginning by reaching it to the side and resting one or several fingers on the ground next to you.

Holding your body in a triangular formation with your legs in a straddle can make it a bit easier to find the balance with this exercise. With practice, you'll improve to the point where you can work on bringing your body into a straight line.

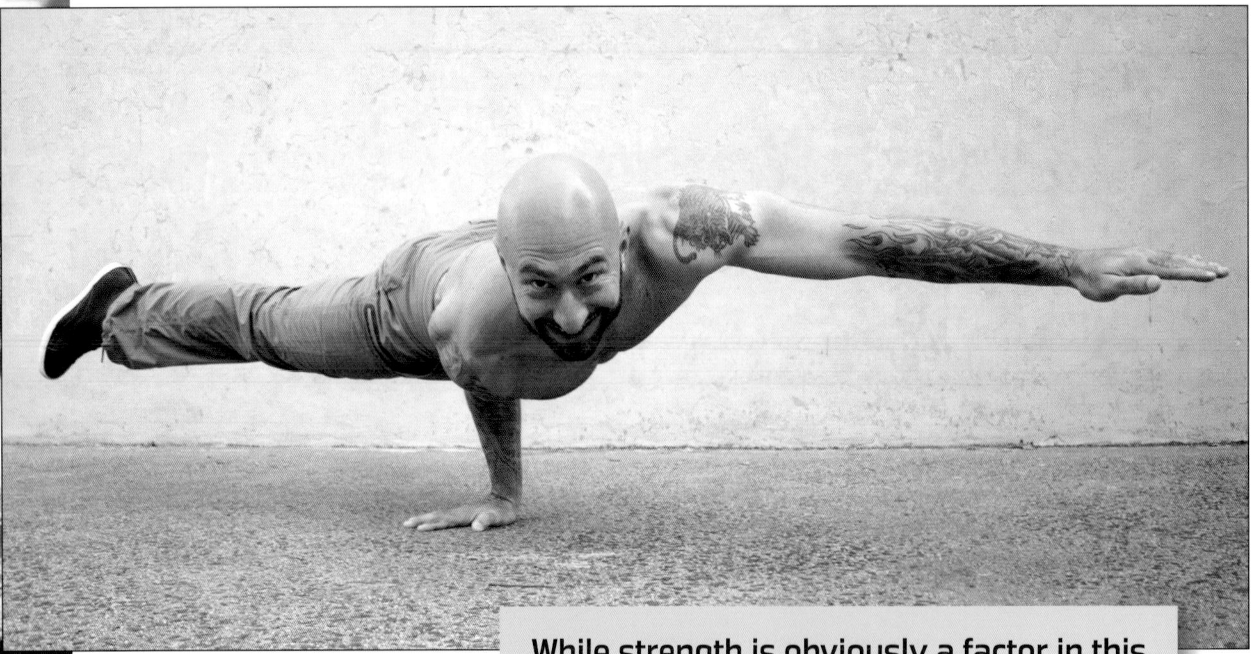

While strength is obviously a factor in this move, the one arm elbow lever is more about balance than anything else.

Tuck Planche

A less difficult variation on the gymnastics planche, the tuck planche is similar to the frog stand, except your elbows are straight and your legs are inside your arms, rather than resting on top. This subtle difference makes the exercise considerably more challenging.

Get into a deep squat and press your hands into the ground, slowly tipping your weight off of your feet while squeezing your legs up toward your chest. Allow your wrists to flex as much as possible to get your weight centered over your hands. Spread your shoulder blades apart and try to create as much space as possible between your body and the floor. This will likely be a very humbling move in the beginning. Keep at it, progressively trying to build to longer holds.

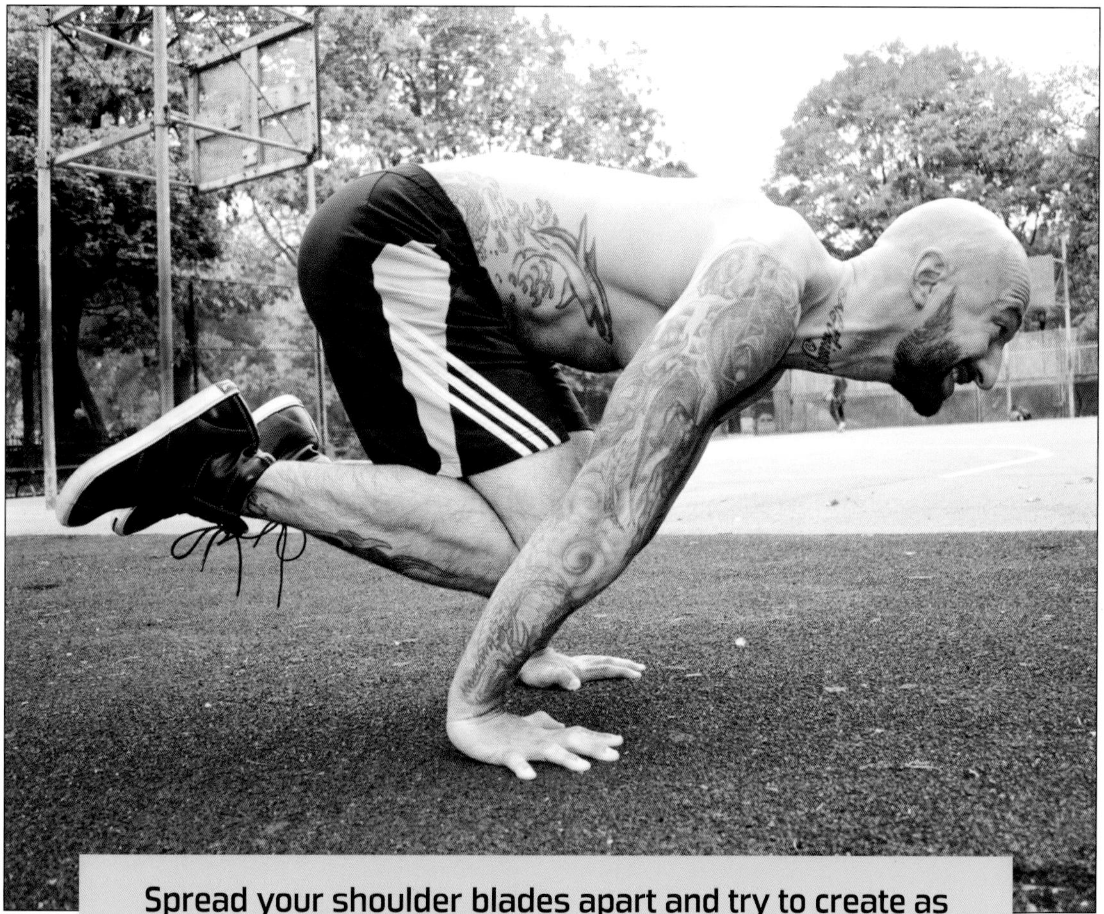

Spread your shoulder blades apart and try to create as much space as possible between your body and the floor.

Dragon Flag

A dragon flag is typically performed lying face-up on a bench or on the ground with your hands grasping a sturdy object behind you for support. From here, the objective is to lift your entire body up in a straight line, stacking it vertically over your shoulders, then slowly lower yourself back down until you're parallel to the ground and repeat. Focus on using your abs, lower back, and glutes to control the movement. Your hands are there for support, but don't pull the bench into your neck.

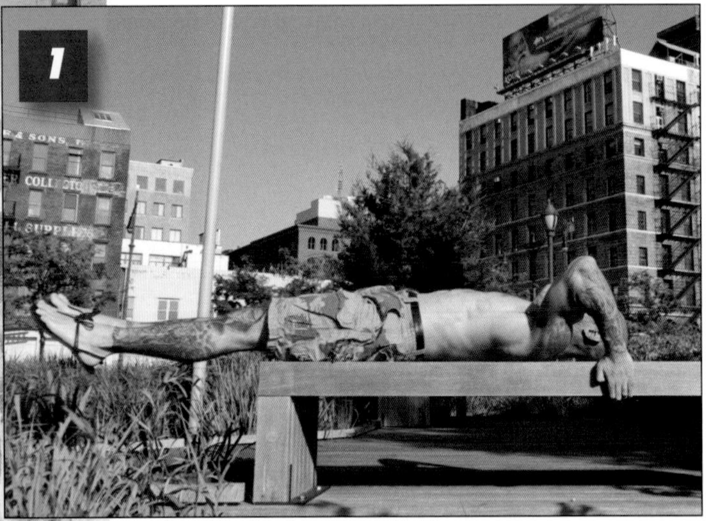

Do your best to avoid bending at the hips in order to keep your body straight from your shoulders to your toes. Your abs will have to provide extreme stabilization to do so. In fact, you'll need to engage your entire trunk musculature to maintain your form. The dragon flag emphasizes the abs, but like all the exercises in this book, it's really a full-body move.

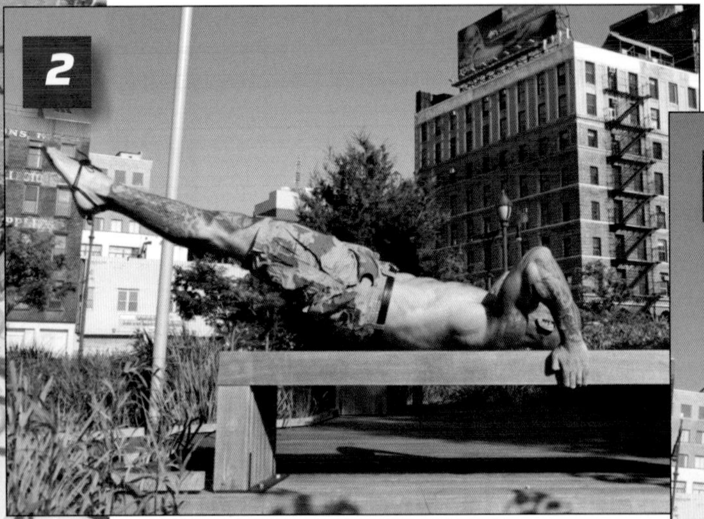

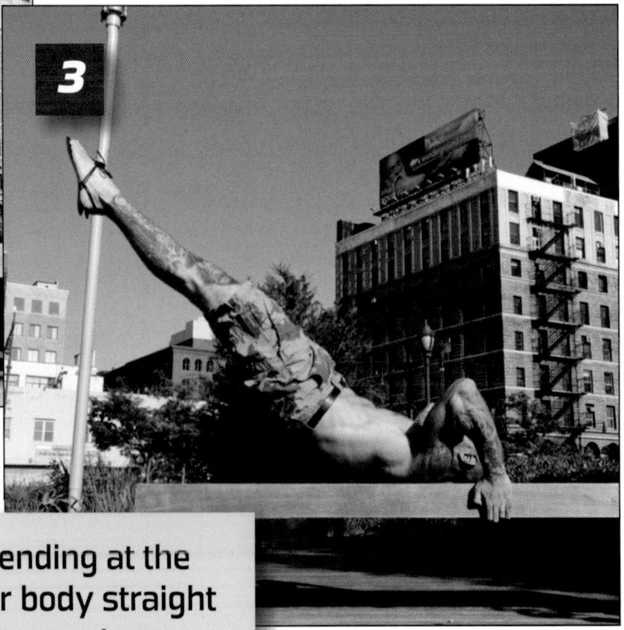

Do your best to avoid bending at the hips in order to keep your body straight from your shoulders to your toes.

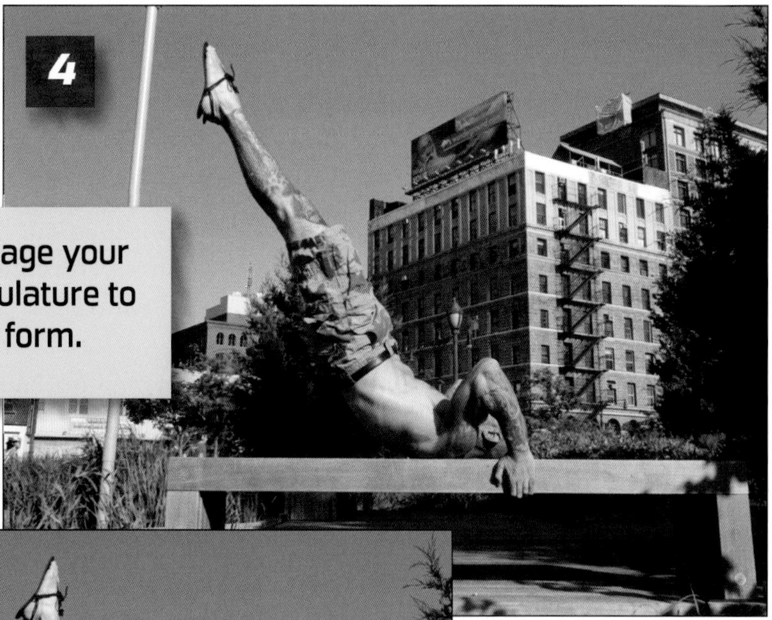

You'll need to engage your entire trunk musculature to maintain your form.

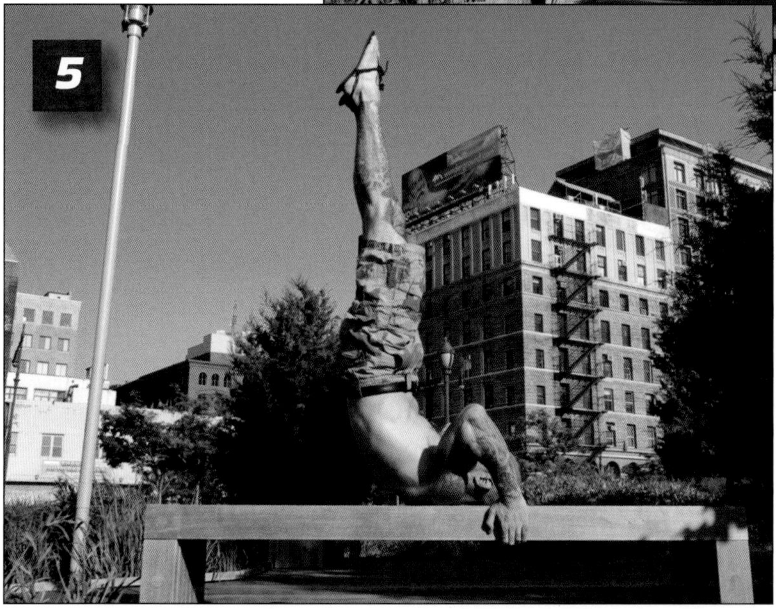

For an added challenge, you can try a dragon flag against a vertical pole.

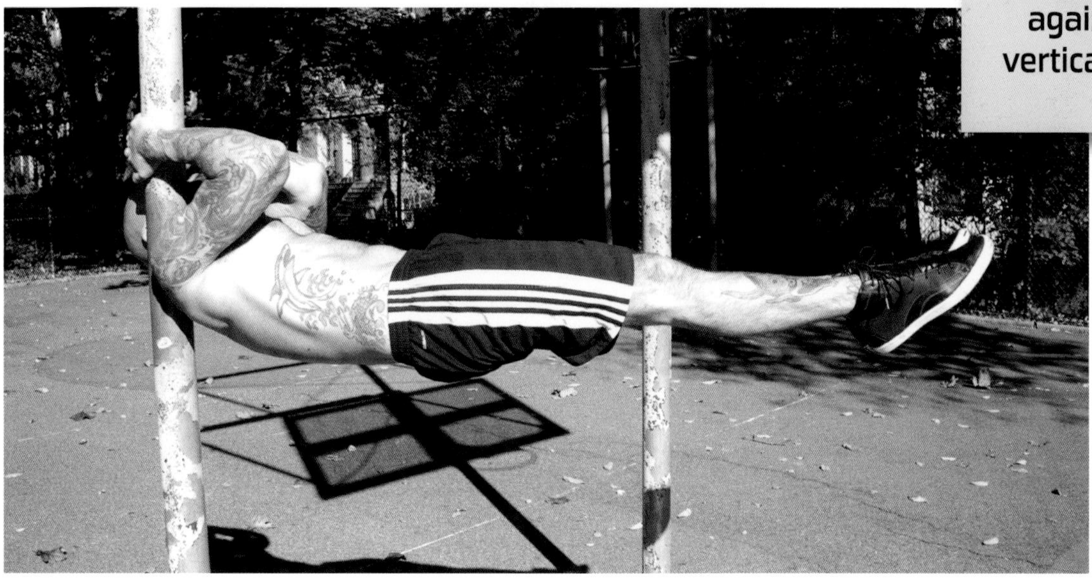

Kip-up

A bodyweight skill that involves lying on your back and explosively jumping to a standing position, the kip-up comes up in many disciplines including calisthenics, martial arts and parkour. It's a great way to work on leg power, hip drive and total body coordination. Plus if you ever fall on your butt during your training, returning to your feet via kip-up is the best way to redeem yourself.

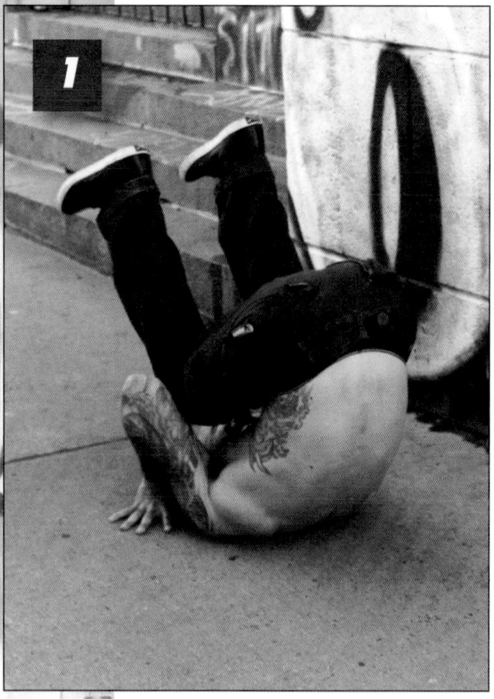

On the other hand, you'll probably look pretty dumb while trying to learn to kip-up, so if you're shy about flailing around in public, better to practice this one at home. I also recommend using a soft surface for training this exercise.

As the kip-up is a fairly advanced technique, I don't recommend working on it unless you are already fairly lean and strong (and have healthy joints). I also suggest getting comfortable with back bridges first to make sure your spine is ready.

To perform a kip-up, begin by lying on your back with your palms flat on the ground on either side of your head. From there, roll your thighs up toward your shoulders and get ready to explode from your hips.

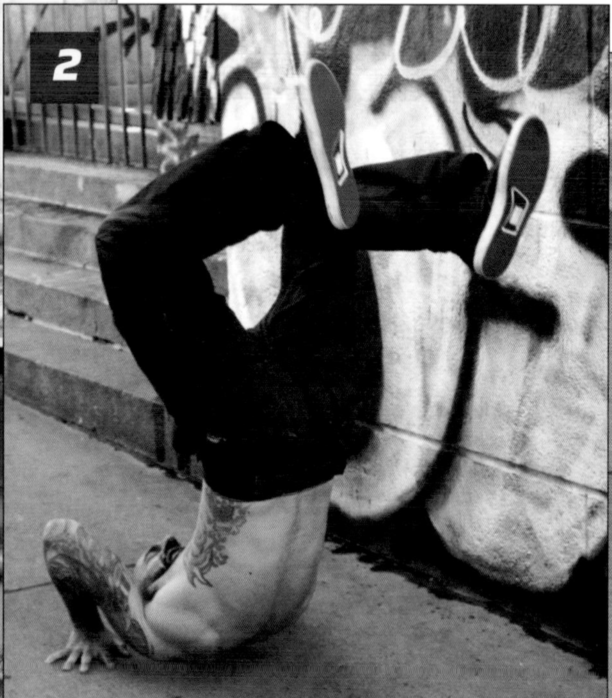

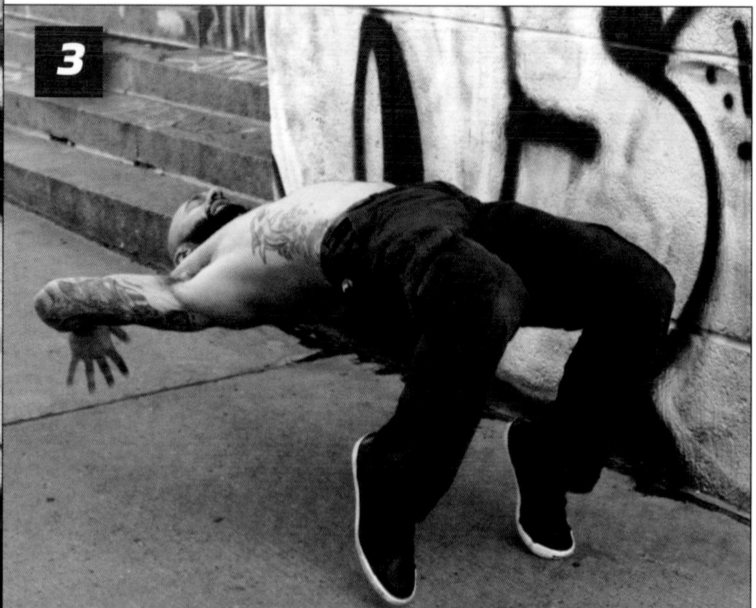

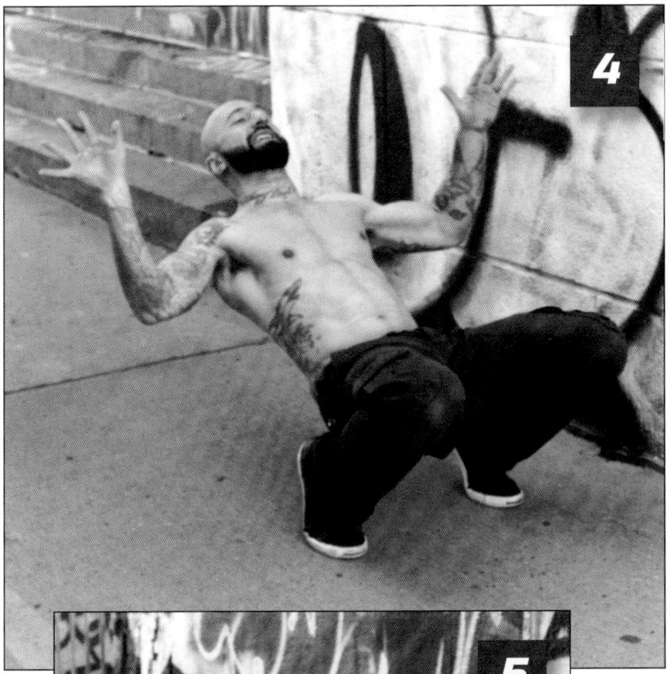

To land a successful kip-up, you'll have to kick your legs up and out as hard as you can and push off with your hands a split second later.

Think about whipping your legs around in a circle so you land toward your toes. You want to try to get your feet under your center of gravity so you don't fall backwards. Timing is crucial to landing this move and it takes a lot of trial and error. As always, be patient and keep at it. I'm still practicing toward putting more pop in my kip-up; fitness training is always a work in progress.

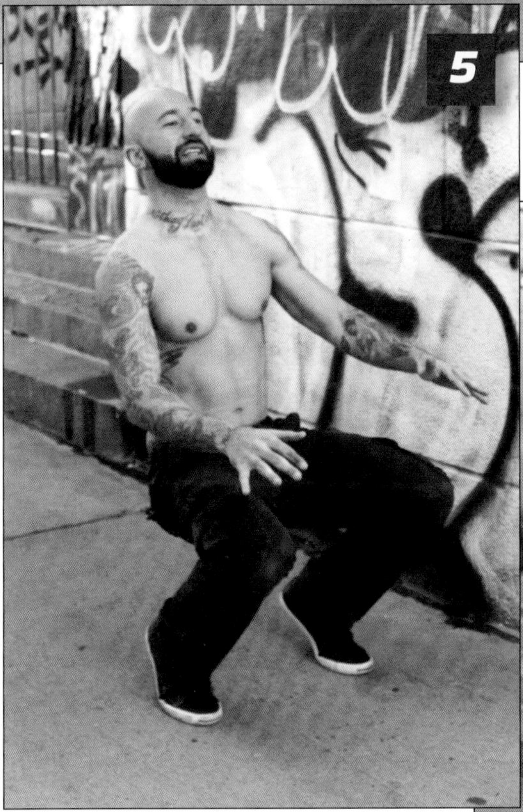

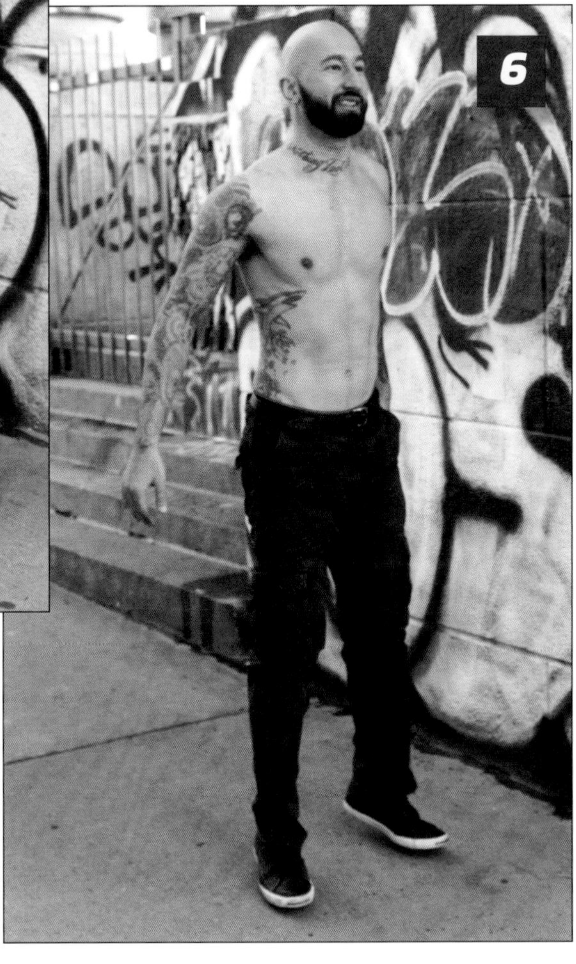

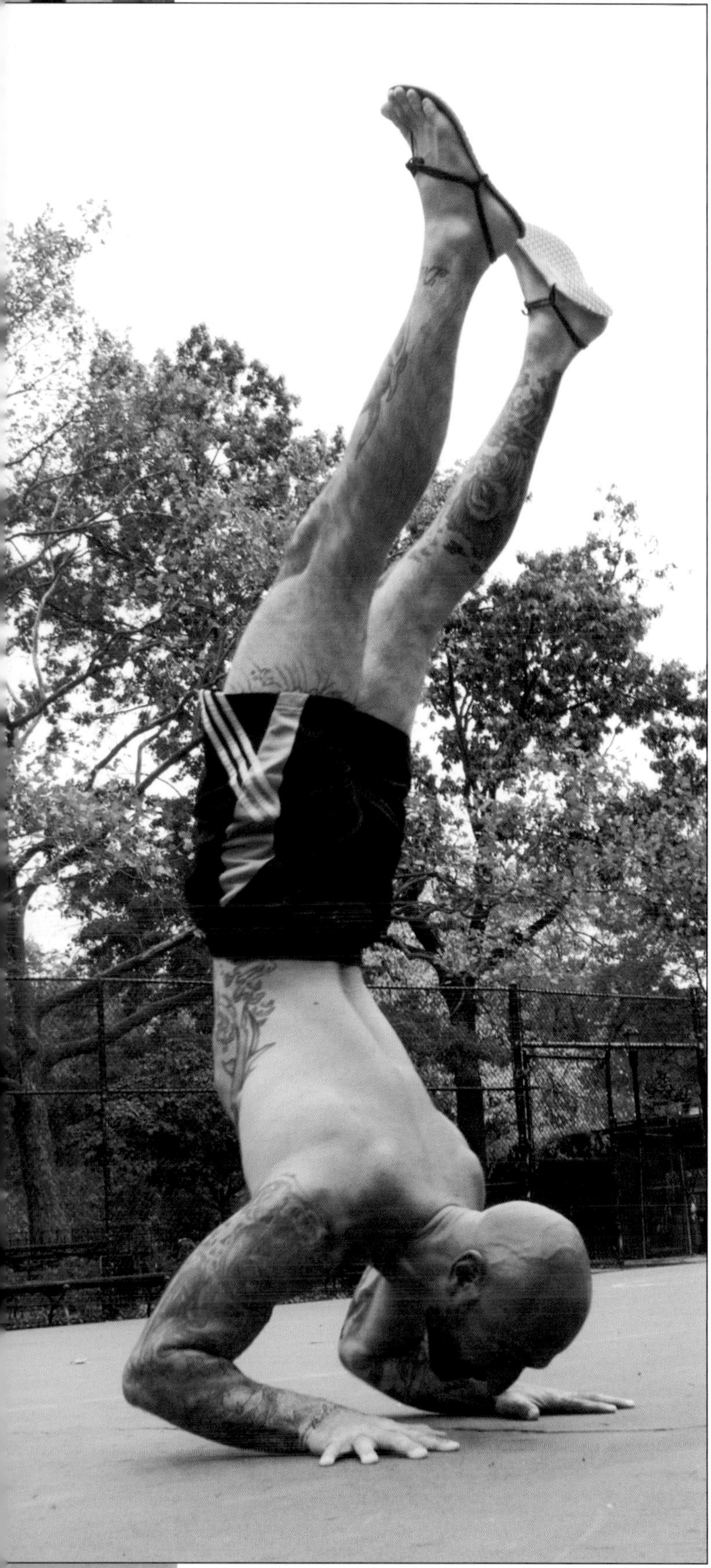

Tiger Bend

The tiger bend is the handstand push-up version of the hinge push-up, which is also sometimes called a tiger bend push-up (confusing, I know). Needless to say, this is a very advanced move. If you've gotten comfortable with normal handstand push-ups, however, you should try it on for size.

A tiger bend begins in a handstand position. From there, you slowly lower down onto your forearms, then shift your weight back to your palms and press yourself back up. Just like a standard handstand push-up, you're best off practicing against a wall for a while before you attempt to try this move freestanding.

Your bottom position should be closer to that of a scorpion pose than a straight forearm stand. If you don't allow your back to arch and your legs to dangle in front a bit, you'll continually wind up losing your balance and falling to your feet when you attempt to press yourself back to the top. You'll need to position your body a bit farther from the wall than you might think in order to allow your legs to hang forward at the bottom. Eventually you'll be ready to try a freestanding tiger bend.

As this is one of the most difficult moves in the book, expect to put in a lot of effort if you want this one in your arsenal. I recommend getting comfortable enough with the freestanding handstand push-up to do at least four or five consecutive reps before beginning to work on a freestanding tiger bend.

Pistol Press

A combination of two of my favorite exercises, this one starts off with you lowering yourself down on one leg like a pistol squat. When you get to the bottom, place the hand opposite your squatting leg on the floor and lower your face down just above your hand. Pause for a half second, press yourself back up, stand and repeat.

As the push-up portion of this exercise is slightly easier than a standard one arm push-up, it can be a useful progressive skill for someone who's close to their first one arm push-up.

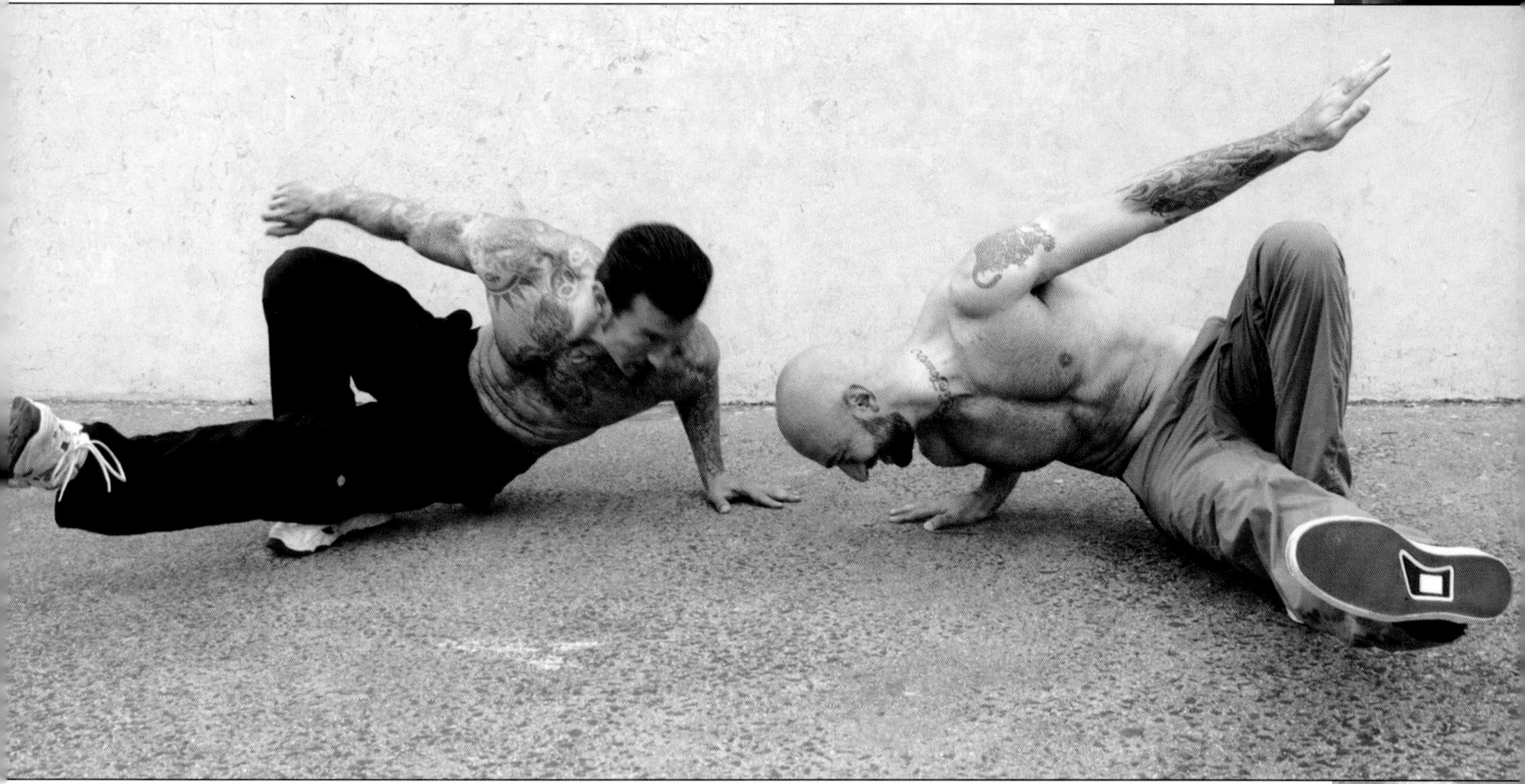

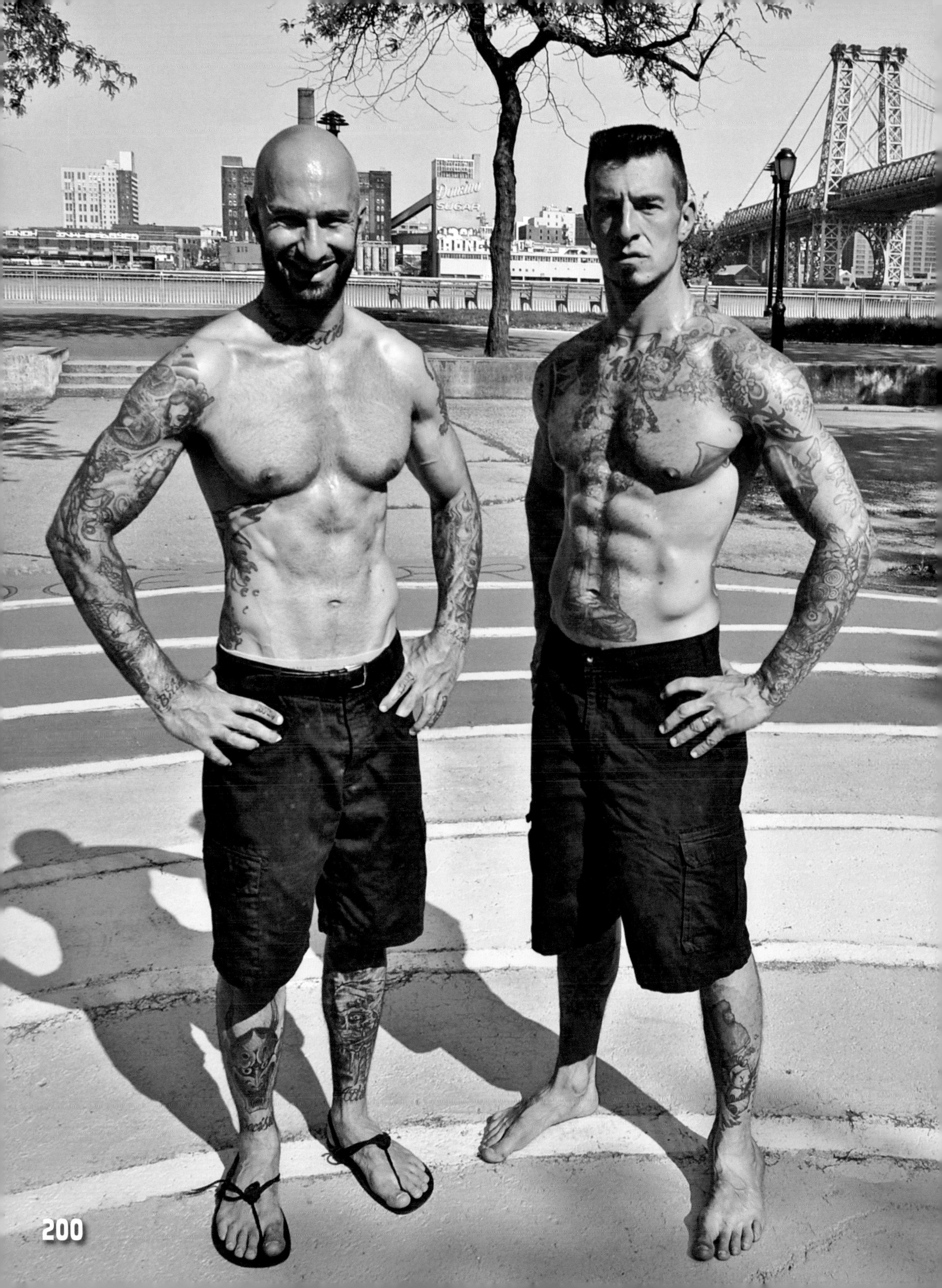
Domino
SUGAR

APPENDIX B:

Sample Routines

For all my talk about how you have to listen to your body and design your own program based on intuition, I know it's helpful to have some guidelines.

You can use the following sample routines exactly as they are, or modify them as you see fit. Just make sure you're working hard and being honest with yourself. Remember, these routines are just examples. They are not intended to be all-inclusive.

Rest as long as you need to between sets. When you can perform all exercises to completion with 30 seconds or less between sets, move on.

When you get past the first level, do one set of each of the previous levels' exercises as a warm-up.

If you cannot complete the suggested number of reps, just do as many as you can without sacrificing proper form.

Novice

Wall Push-up or Kneeling Push-up	2 sets of 30 reps
Bench Squat or Partial Squat	2 sets of 30 reps
Lying Knee Tuck	3 sets of 10 reps
Beginner Bridge	3 holds of 30 seconds
Tripod	3 holds of 30 seconds
Frog Stand	3 holds of 30 seconds

Beginner

Push-up	3 sets of 20 reps
Full Squat	3 sets of 20 reps
Split Squat or Lunge	3 sets of 10 reps (each leg)
Lying Leg Raise	3 sets of 10 reps
Straight Bridge	3 holds of 30 seconds
Headstand	3 holds of 30 seconds

Intermediate

Close Push-up	3 sets of 20 reps
Uneven Push-up	2 sets of 10 reps (each side)
Assisted Pistol	3 sets of 10 reps (each leg)
Side-to-Side Squat	3 sets of 10 reps (each leg)
Full Bridge or Neck Bridge	3 holds of 30 seconds
Elbow Lever	3 holds of 30 seconds
Handstand	3 holds of 30 seconds

Advanced

One Arm Push-up	5 sets of 5 reps (each arm)
Plyo Push-up	5 sets of 5 reps
Pistol Squat	5 sets of 5 reps (each leg)
Shrimp Squat	5 sets of 5 reps (each leg)
Headstand Leg Raise	3 sets of 10 reps
Wall Crawl	3 sets of 5 reps
One Leg Bridge	3 holds of 10 seconds (each leg)
Freestanding Handstand	3 holds of 30 seconds

Expert

One Arm Clap Push-up	3 sets of 3 reps (each side)
One Arm/One Leg Push-up	3 sets of 5 reps (each side)
One Arm/One Leg Bridge	3 holds of of 20 seconds (each side)
Pistol Squat (Hands behind back)	5 sets of 5 reps (each side)
Jumbo Shrimp	5 sets of 5 reps (each side)
Dragon Flag	5 sets of 5 reps
Tuck Planche	3 holds of 30 seconds

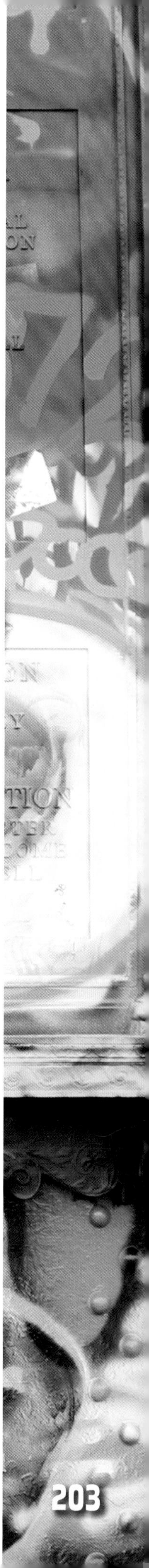

The Two Day No Equipment Split

Day 1: Squats and bridge work
Day 2: All kinds of push-ups and non-bridge inversions

One or two days of rest between each day including active recovery (swim, jog, martial arts, additional skill practice, etc.).

The Three Day No Equipment Split

Day 1: Squats
Day 2: Push-ups
Day 3: Bridges/Inversions

Use active recovery and rest days as needed.

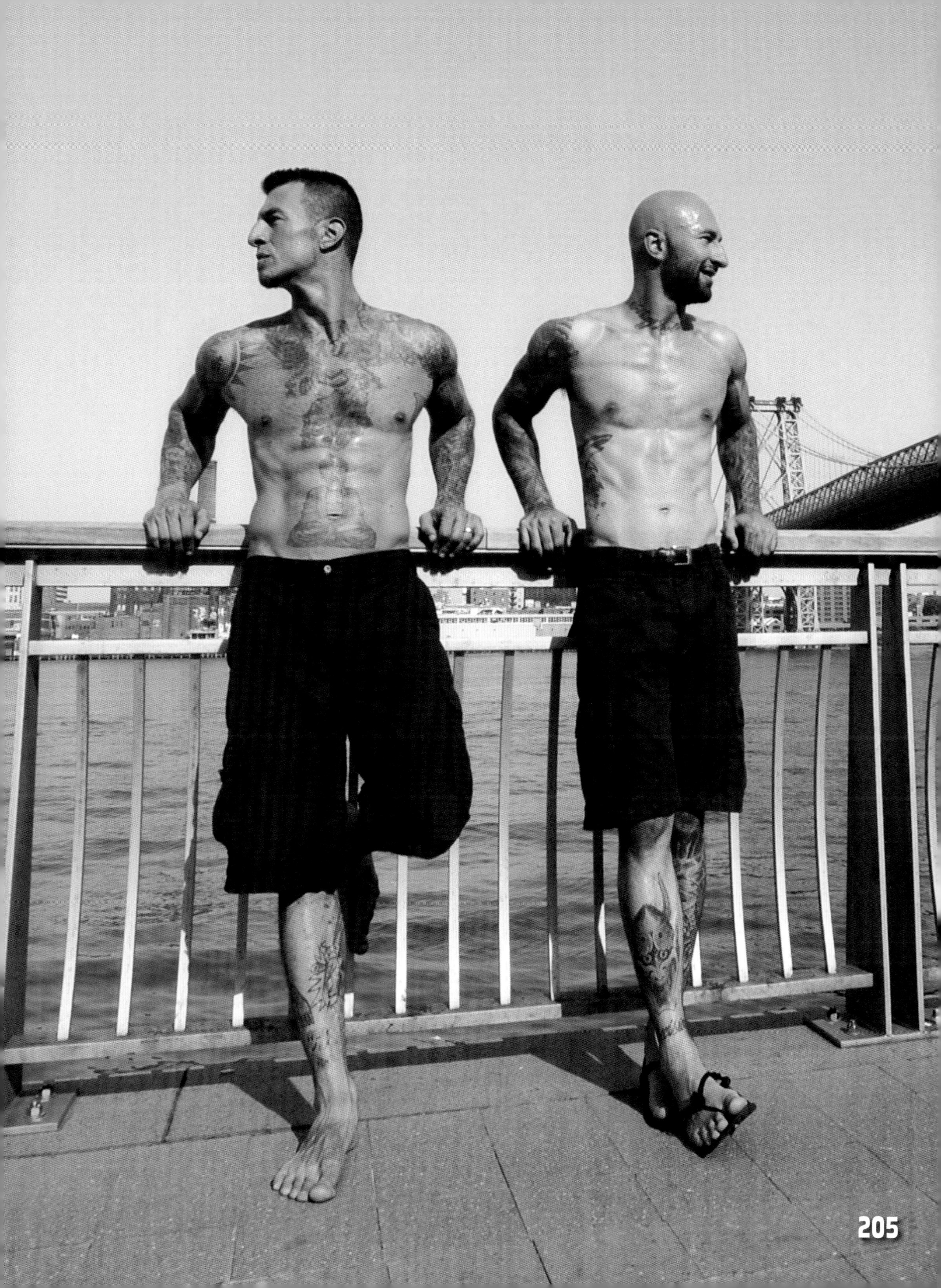

Assessing Your Strength

These assessments are based on reps performed in one continuous set. You may rest at the top position to take a breath in between reps, but the feet and/or hands may not move once the set has begun.

Men

	Push-up	Squat	One Arm Pushup	Pistol Squat
Novice	>20	>20	>1	>1
Beginner	20-39	20-50	1-3	1-3
Intermediate	40-64	51-100	4-10	4-10
Advanced	65-99	101-199	11-19	11-19
Elite	100+	200+	20+	20+

Women

	Push-up	Squat	One Arm Pushup	Pistol Squat
Novice	>1	>20	>1	>1
Beginner	1-10	20-50	>1	1-3
Intermediate	11-20	51-100	1-3	4-10
Advanced	21-30	101-199	4-9	11-19
Elite	30+	200+	10+	20+

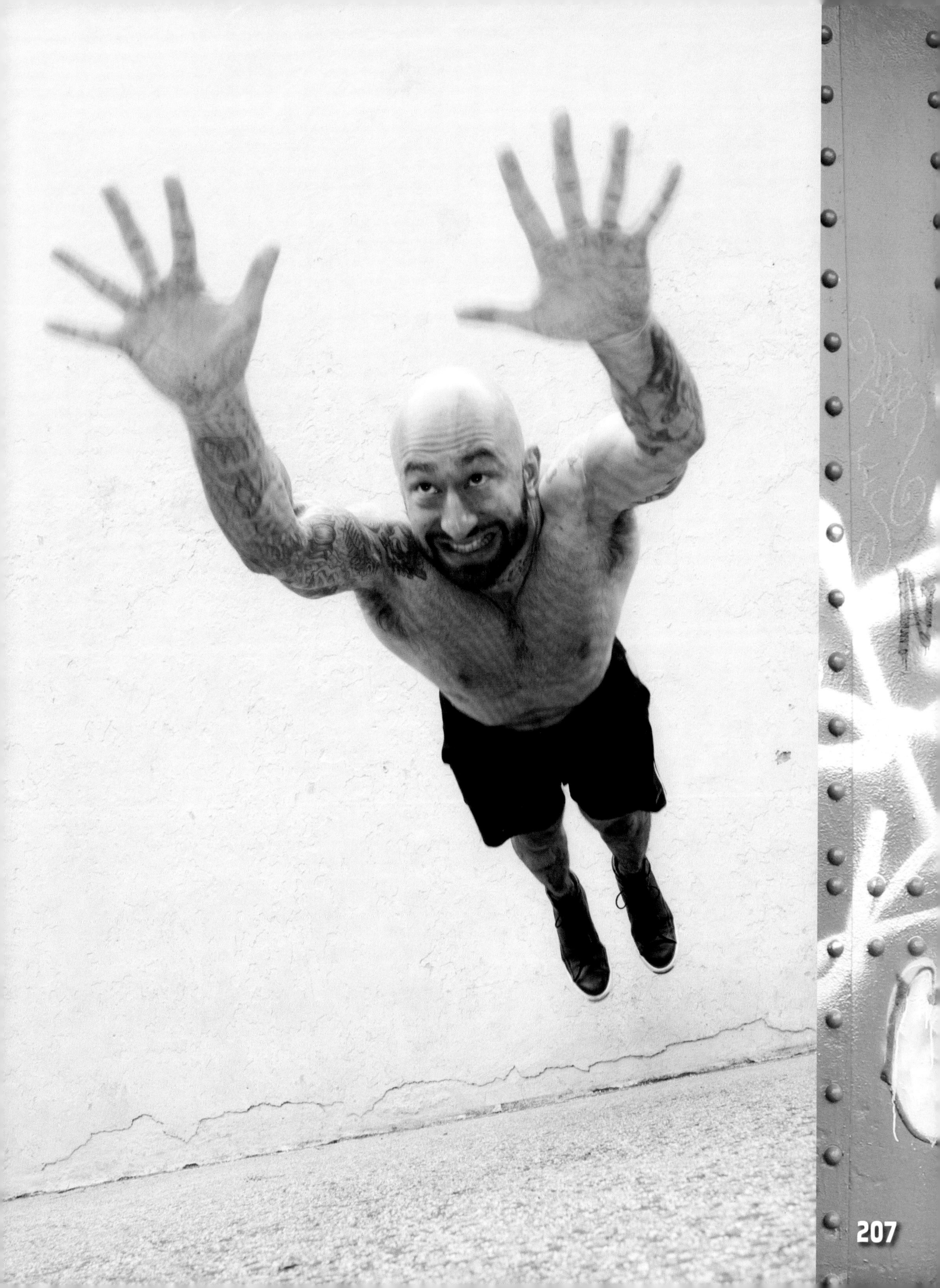

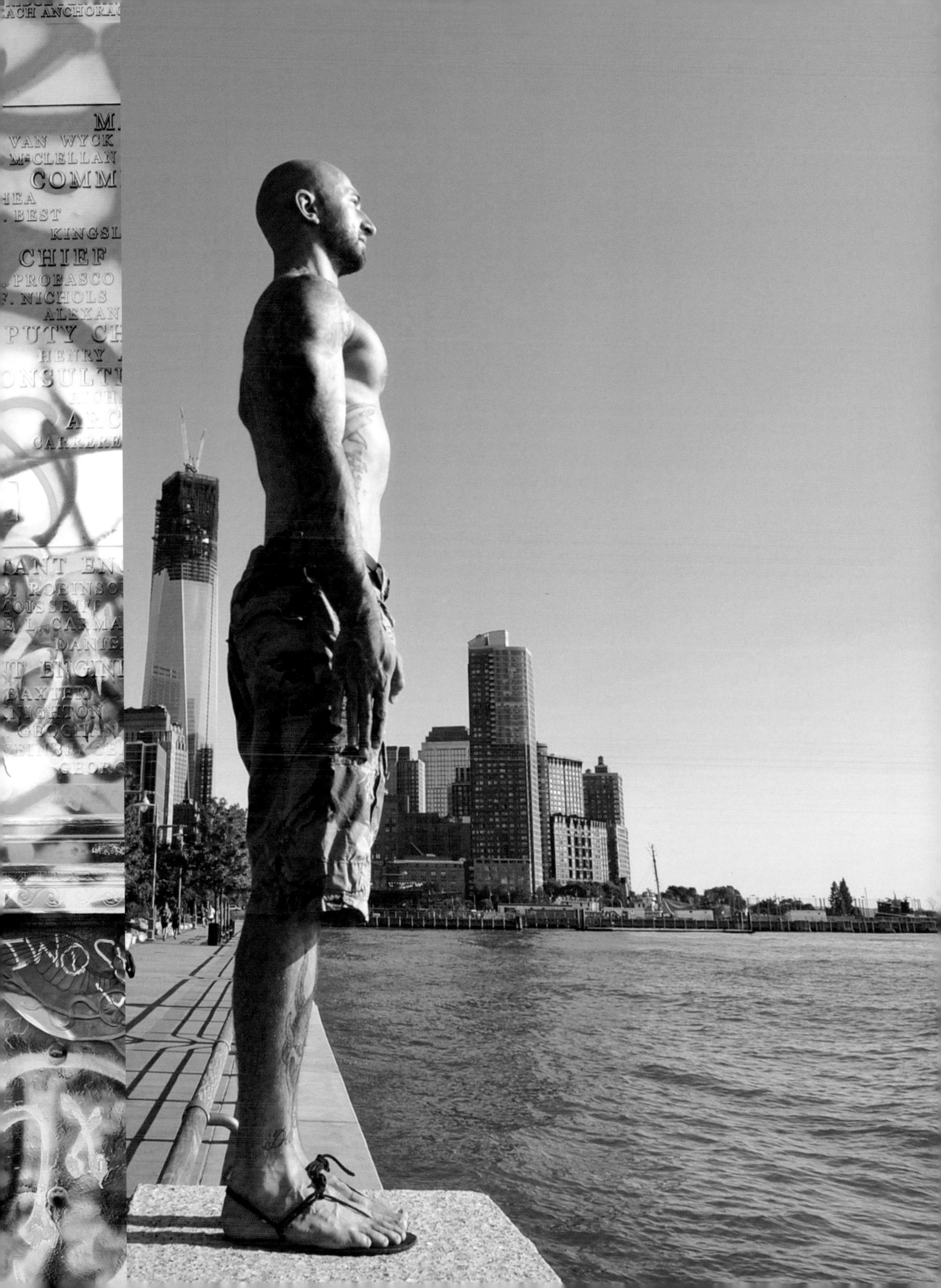
ACH ANCHORAG
M.
VAN WYCK
McCLELLAN
COMM
HEA
BEST
KINGSL
CHIEF
PROBASCO
F. NICHOLS
ALEXAN
PUTY CH
HENRY
ONSULTI
ARC
CARRÈRE
ANT EN
ROBINSO
MOISSEIFF
CARMA
DANIE
ENGINE
BAXTER
NIGHTON
GEORG

About the Author

Al Kavadlo is one of New York City's most passionate and successful personal trainers. A fixture in the ever-changing fitness scene, Al has worked with all types of clients including athletes, models and even an Olympic medalist. Al is recognized worldwide for his amazing bodyweight feats of strength and his blog (**www.AlKavadlo.com**) has become one of the most popular online resources for information about bodyweight strength training and calisthenics. Outside of fitness, Al's interests include rock music, tattoo collecting and facial hair.

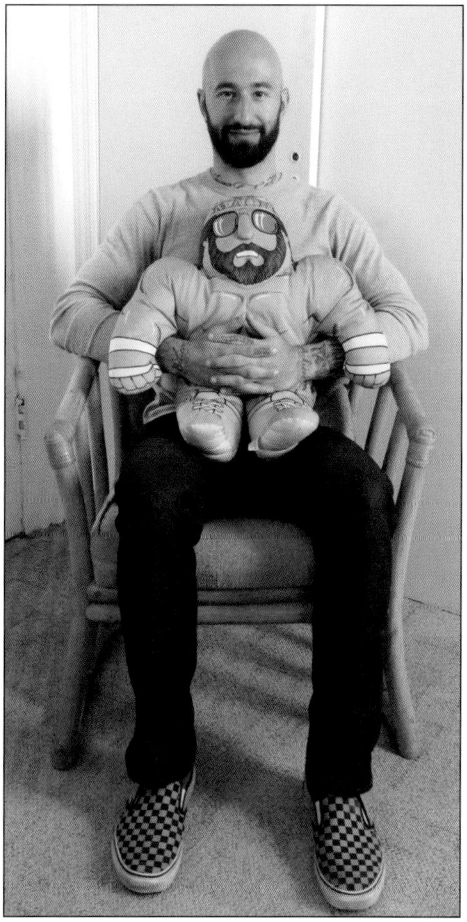

Also Available by Al Kavadlo:

Raising The Bar: The Definitive Guide to Pull-up Bar Calisthenics
(Dragon Door Publications, 2012)

We're Working Out! A Zen Approach to Everyday Fitness
(Muscle-up Publications, 2010)

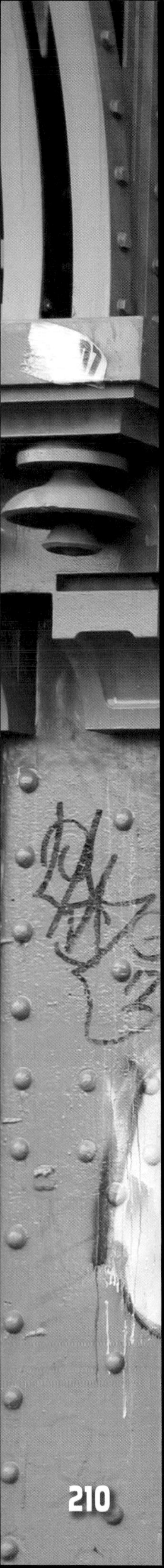

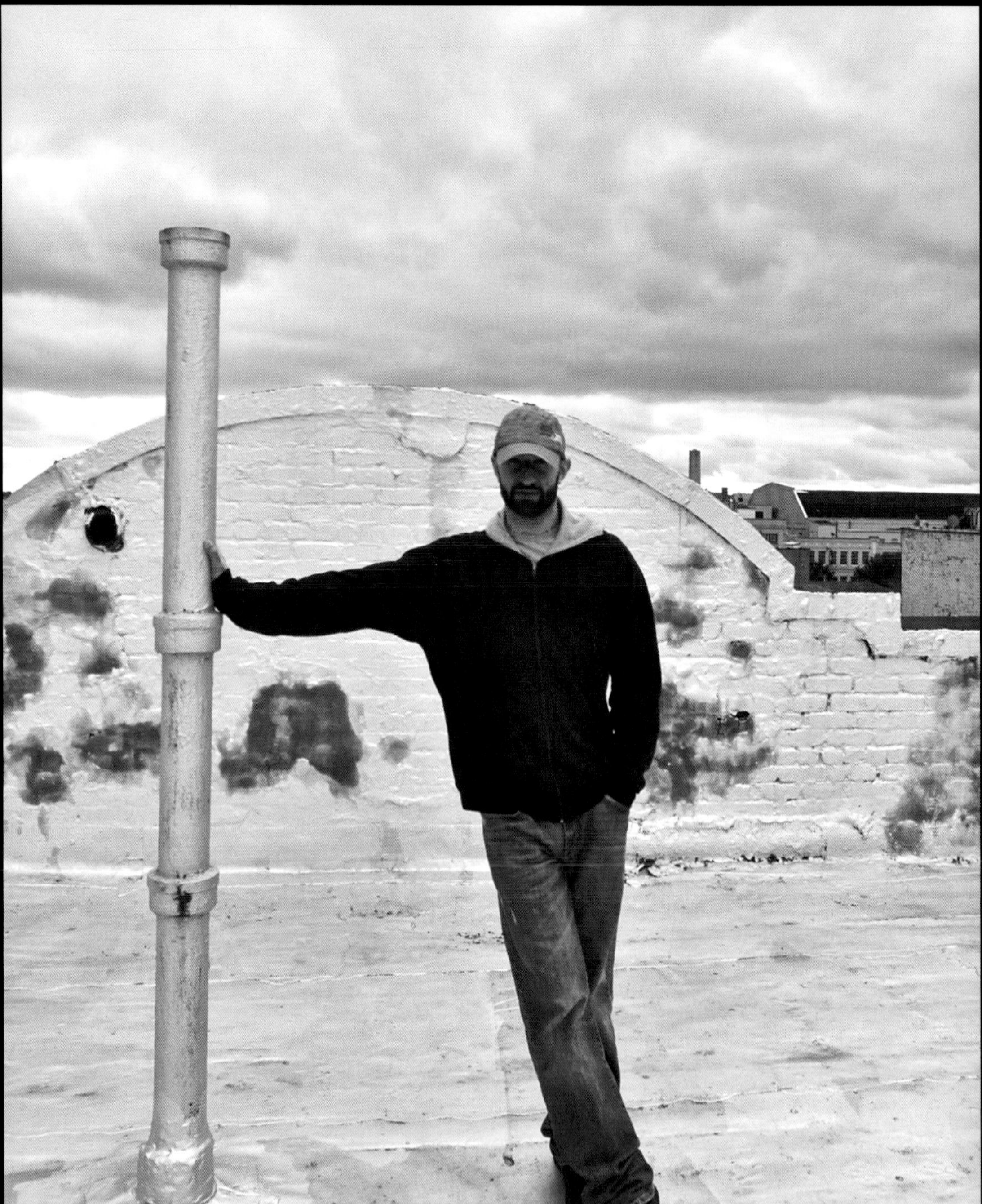

ACKNOWLEDGEMENTS

Thanks to my brother, training partner and best friend, Danny Kavadlo for all the love, support and encouragement he's given me throughout my life. This book would not have been possible without Danny's help. In addition to appearing in many of the photos, Danny took some of the photos himself, proofread my manuscript and gave me some suggestions that really improved the quality of this book. I am very lucky to have a brother like Danny.

Thanks to all the talented photographers whose photos really make this book come to life, especially Colleen Leung and Jordan Perlson, both of whom went above and beyond to capture some breathtaking images, at times putting their own safety at risk to do so. Thankfully nobody was hurt in the process.

Thanks to John Du Cane, Derek Brigham, Adrienne Harvey and the rest of the team at Dragon Door for being so great to work with and for allowing me total creative freedom (while still offering their expert feedback).

Thanks to Jason Ferruggia for writing the foreword for this book. I've been a fan of Jason's for a long time and it's an honor to have him involved.

Thanks to "Coach" Paul Wade for his unwavering support and guidance. Though we've never actually met face-to-face, Coach Wade has become one of my closest friends and confidants.

Thanks to Daniel Lucas, Keith Paine, Antonio Sini and the rest of the team at Nimble Fitness in NYC for their continued love, support and encouragement.

Last but not least, a big thank you to all the rest of my family, friends, clients, colleagues and fans who have helped foster a positive environment for me. This book would not have been possible without each and every one of you!

We're Working Out!

Al Kavadlo

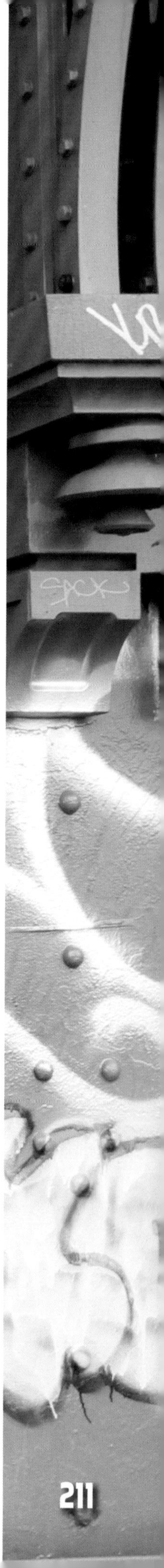

For more information on bodyweight strength training as well as free video tutorials, make sure to check out **www.AlKavadlo.com!**

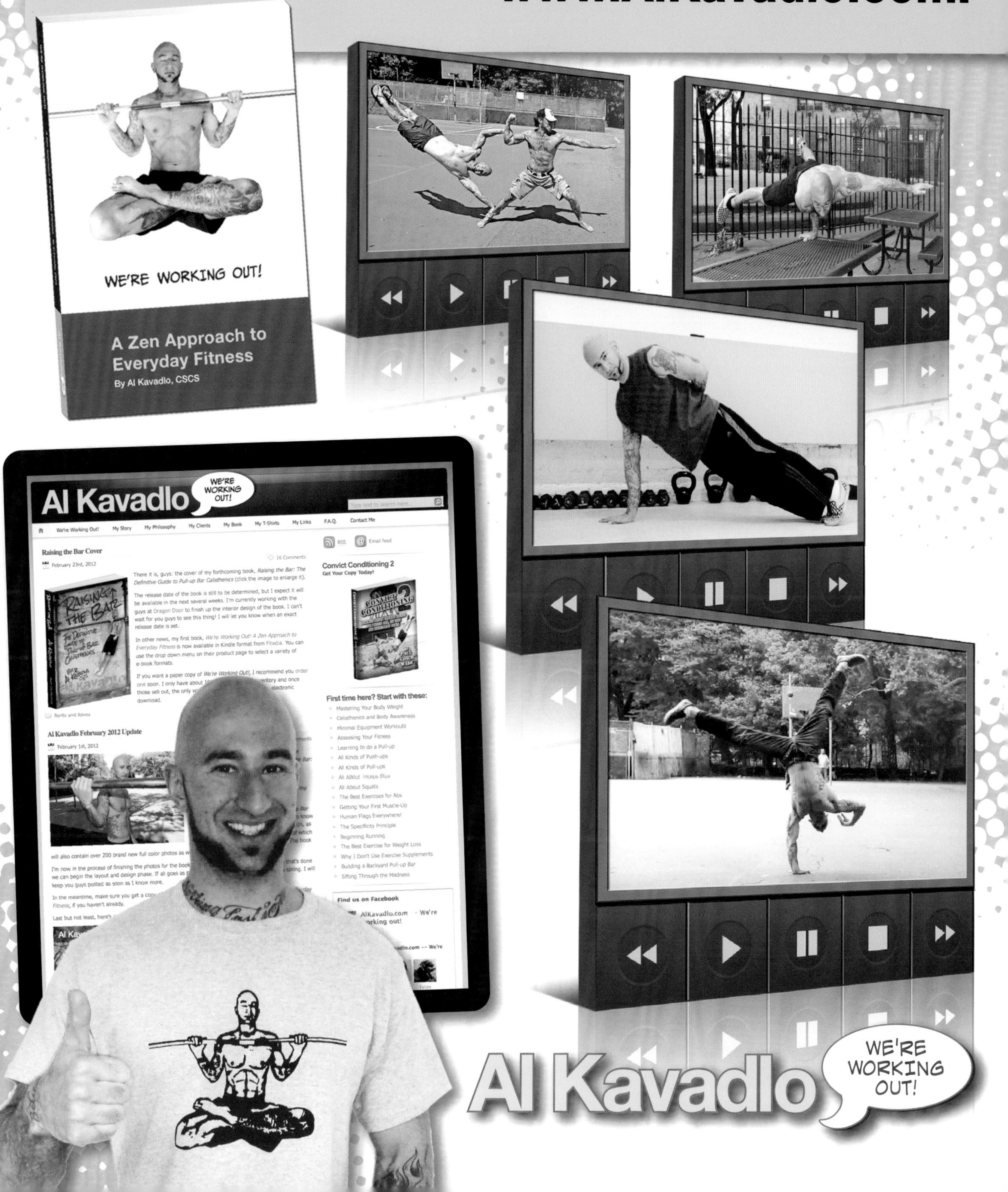

High Praise for *Raising the Bar*

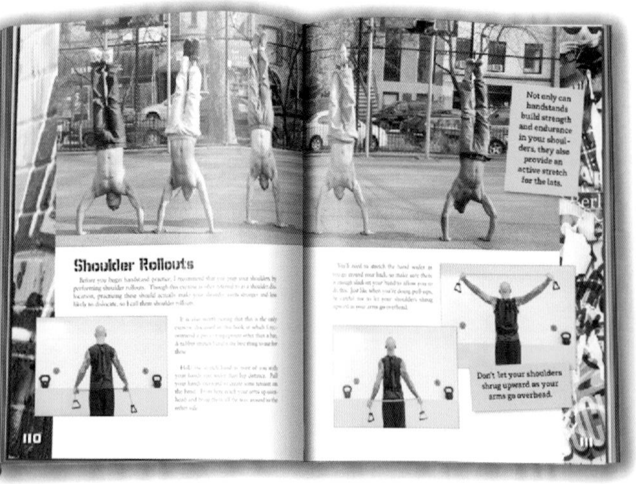

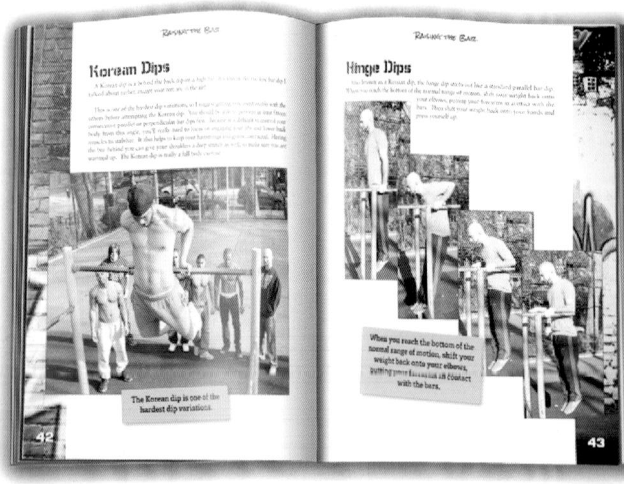

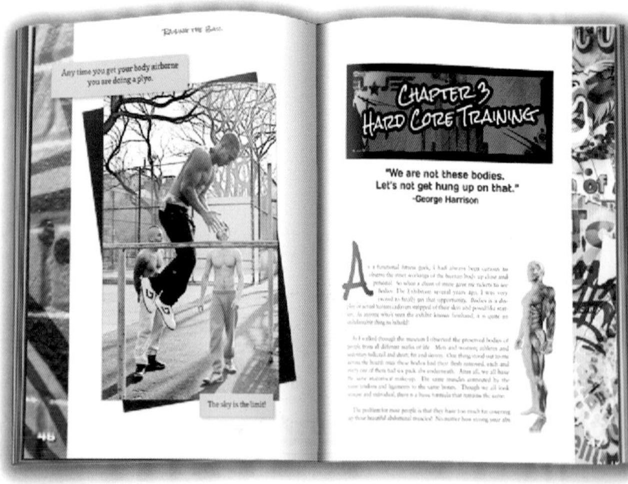

Brilliant Book—simply brilliant

"This is a fantastic book—period! Al has provided some basic cues which have made my chin ups and leg raises much easier. This is a great piece of work and EVERYONE can benefit from it—Olympic lifter, powerlifter, bodybuilder etc. You don't have to do all the moves—you can pick a couple and run with them. Al shows some great progressions and tons of different movements. I could go on and on but the best thing would be to buy the book-you wont regret it."

—Darius Rana, Sydney, Australia

Raise YOUR Bar

"Unlike much of the trash in the modern fitness industry, Al takes a structured approach to coaching and programming. *Raising The Bar* starts at a level that everyone can handle and then builds on it—it's not a random selection of exercises but a reasoned approach to improving skill in a number of key movements.

This, in my opinion, is the key to progression and Al delivers it in his own enigmatic style. And if you're in any doubt as to the effectiveness of the approach then you need to see what Al can do! You'll be blown away!"

—Matt Palfrey, Bath, UK

Best book ever written!

"As a personal trainer, I've spent years convincing my clients that they don't need any fancy, overpriced, useless junk to get a great workout. The greatness is within the simplicity. I've watched every trainer in the area mess up the concept of functional fitness with their 'ideas'. Balancing on stacks of bosu balls, using the other leg to pull on rubber bands, one arm using a shaky weight, and the other arm doing curl to presses with a half pound pink dumbbell, all while balancing a medicine ball on your nose sounds good in theory, but at the end of the day, nothing gets accomplished.

Al, just like everything else Dragon Door publishes, manages to take the simplest of tools, and make it the most important. These movements are something that everyone not only CAN do, but we are all SUPPOSED to do them. They're in our DNA. Not like all the machines and circus tricks.

Al has been a huge inspiration to me for quite sometime. This goes far beyond simple pullups and dips. This is the perfect book to go along with *The Naked Warrior, Convict Conditioning 1 & 2*, and Pavel's flexibility work. Thank you Al, for writing such an awesome book."

—Rick Chafton HKC, FMS, Crystal Lake, IL

Worth every dime

I was gun shy about spending the money. It's not the best of times. I could not afford to blow that kind of money on a stinker. Thankfully this book is anything but. I have been a life long aerial guy. I just always had this conviction that being able to push and pull my own weight around was a key survival attribute. That said, I also thought I knew it all and there was nothing left to learn about the subject. Wrong. There is, there was, and this book had it."

—Steve Shear, Lawrence, NY

A must have for any bodyweight practitioner!

"Al put together an outstanding book! It reads very easy in a way anyone could understand. He gives some awesome and doable progressions along with some of his favorite routines. If you want to become a BAR-STAR, then you need this book!"

—Tim Stovall, Evansville, IN

How basketballs, baseballs and *kissing-the-baby* all translate into greater strength gains... Page 44

How to guarantee steel rod fingers... Page 45

Do you make this stupid mistake with your push ups? This is wrong, wrong, wrong!... Page 45

How to achieve 100 consecutive one-arm pushups each side... Page 64

Going Beyond the One-Arm Pushup... Pages 68—74

Going up!— how to build elevator-cable thighs... Page 75

Where the *real* strength of an athlete lies... Page 75

Most athletic movements rely largely on this attribute... Page 76

The first thing to go as an athlete begins to age—and what you MUST protect... Page 76

THE best way to develop truly powerful, athletic legs... Page 77

The phenomenon of *Lombard's Paradox*—and it contributes to power-packed thighs... Page 78

Why bodyweight squats blow barbell squats away... Page 79

The enormous benefits of mastering the one-leg squat... Page 80

15 secrets to impeccable squatting—for greater power and strength... Pages 81—82

Transform skinny legs into pillars of power, complete with steel cord quads, rock-hard glutes and thick, shapely calves... Page 102

How to achieve one hundred perfect consecutive one-leg squats on each leg... Page 102

Going Beyond the One-Leg Squat... Pages 106—112

How to add conditioning, speed, agility and endurance to legs that are already awesome.... Page 107

How to construct a barn door back—and walk with loaded guns... Page 113

Why our culture has failed to give the pullup the respect and attention it deserves... Page 113

Benefits of the pullup—king of back exercises... Page 114

The dormant superpower for muscle growth waiting to be released if you only do this... Page 114

Why pullups are the single best exercise for building melon-sized biceps... Page 115

Why the pullup is THE safest upper back exercise... Page 115

The single most important factor to consider for your grip choice... Page 118

How to earn lats that look like wings and an upper back sprouting muscles like coiled pythons... Page 138

How to be strong enough to rip a bodybuilder's arm off in an arm wrestling match... Page 138

How to take a trip to hell—and steal a Satanic six-pack... Page 149

The 5 absolute truths that define a genuine six-pack from hell... Page 150

This is the REAL way to gain a six-pack from hell... Page 152

3 big reasons why—in prisons—leg raises have always been much more popular than sit-ups... Page 152

Why the hanging leg raise is the greatest single abdominal exercise known to man... Page 153

10 waist training secrets to help you master the hanging leg raise... Pages 154—155

How to correctly perform the greatest all-round midsection exercise in existence... Page 174

Going beyond the hanging straight leg raise... Page 178

Setting your sights on the most powerful midsection exercise possible—the V raise.... Page 178

How to develop abdominal muscles with enormous contractile power—and iron hip strength... Page 178

How to combat-proof your spine... Page 185

Why the bridge is the most important strength-building exercise in the world... Page 185

How to train your spine—as if your life depended on it... Page 185

Why you should sell your barbell set and buy a cushioned mat instead... Page 188

How to absorb punitive strikes against your spine—and bounce back smiling... Page 188

Why lower back pain is the foremost plague of athletes the world over... Page 189

Why bridging is the *ultimate* exercise for the spinal muscles... Page 189

The 4 signs of the perfect bridge... Page 191

How to master the bridge... Page 192

How to own a spine that feels like a steel whip... Page 193

How the bridging series will grant you an incredible combination of strength paired with flexibility... Page 216

Why bridging stands alone as a *total* training method that facilitates development in practically every area of fitness and health... Page 216

How to look exceptionally masculine—with broad, etched, and powerful shoulders... Page 219

Those vulnerable shoulders—why they ache and the best way to avoid or fix the pain... Page 220

How to choose authentic over *artificial* shoulder movements... Page 223

Why an understanding of *instinctive* human movement can help solve the shoulder pain problem... Page 224

Remove these two elements of pressing—and you will remove virtually all chronic shoulder problems... Page 225

The ultimate solution for safe, pain-free, powerful shoulders... Page 225

The mighty handstand pushup... Page 226

Using the handstand pushup to build *incredibly* powerful, muscularized shoulders in a short span of time... Page 225

How to strengthen the *vestibular system*—using handstand pushups... Page 225

8 secrets to help you perfect your all-important handstand pushup technique... Pages 228—229

Discover the ultimate shoulder and arm exercise... Page 248

Going beyond the one-arm handstand pushup... Page 252

The master of this old technique will have elbows strong as titanium axles... Page 255

The cast iron principles of Convict Conditioning success... Page 259

The missing "x factor" of training success... Page 259

The best ways to warm up... Page 260

How to create training momentum... Page 262

How to put strength in the bank... Page 263

This is the real way to get genuine, lasting strength and power gains... Page 265

Intensity—what it is and what it isn't... Page 265

Why "cycling" or "periodization" is unnecessary with bodyweight training... Page 266

How to make consistent progress... Page 266

---

5 powerful secrets for busting through your plateaus... Page 267

The nifty little secret of *consolidation* training... Page 268

Living by the buzzer—and the importance of regime... Page 275

5 major *Convict Conditioning* training programs... Page 276

The *New Blood* training program... Page 278

The *Good Behavior* training program... Page 279

The *Veterano* training program... Page 280

The *Solitary Confinement* training program... Page 281

The *Supermax* training program... Page 282

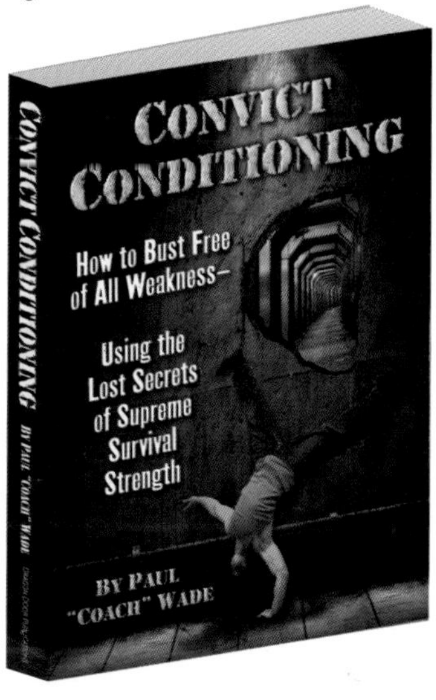

1 Beginner 2 Mid-Level 3 Advanced

Convict Conditioning

How to Bust Free of All Weakness—Using the Lost Secrets of Supreme Survival Strength

By Paul "Coach" Wade

#B41 $39.95

Paperback 8.5 x 11 320 pages

191 photos, charts and illustrations

www.dragondoor.com

1-800-899-5111

Dragon Door

Order *Convict Conditioning* online:

www.dragondoor.com/B41

Dragon Door Customer Acclaim for Paul Wade's *Convict Conditioning*

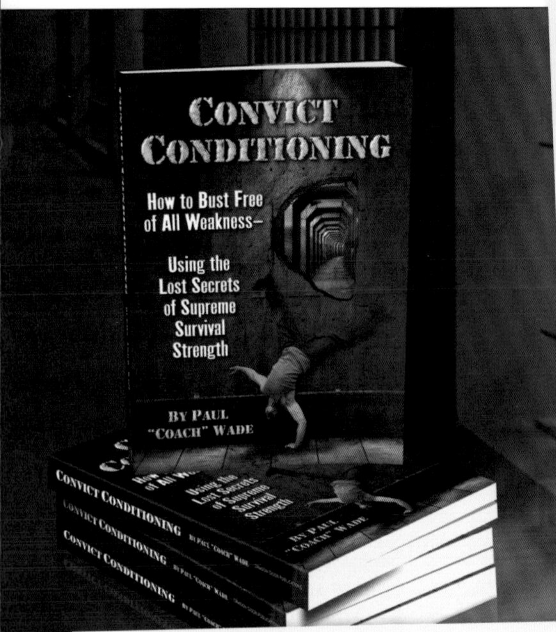

A Strength Training Guide That Will Never Be Duplicated!

"I knew within the first chapter of reading this book that I was in for something special and unique. The last time I felt this same feeling was when reading ***Power to the People!*** To me this is the Body Weight equivalent to Pavel's masterpiece.

Books like this can never be duplicated. Paul Wade went through a unique set of circumstances of doing time in prison with an 'old time' master of calisthenics. Paul took these lessons from this 70 year old strong man and mastered them over a period of 20 years while 'doing time'. He then taught these methods to countless prisoners and honed his teaching to perfection.

I believe that extreme circumstances like this are what it takes to create a true masterpiece. I know that 'masterpiece' is a strong word, but this is as close as it gets. No other body weight book I have read (and I have a huge fitness library)...comes close to this as far as gaining incredible strength from body weight exercise.

Just like Power to the People, I am sure I will read this over and over again...mastering the principles that Paul Wade took 20 years to master.

Outstanding Book!"***—Rusty Moore - Fitness Black Book*** *- Seattle, WA*

Brutal Elegance.

"I have been training and reading about training since I first joined the US Navy in the 1960s. I thought I'd seen everything the fitness world had to offer. Sometimes twice. But I was wrong. This book is utterly iconoclastic.

The author breaks down all conceivable body weight exercises into six basic movements, each designed to stimulate different vectors of the muscular system. These six are then elegantly and very intelligently broken into ten progressive techniques. You master one technique, and move on to the next.

The simplicity of this method belies a very powerful and complex training paradigm, reduced into an abstraction that obviously took many years of sweat and toil to develop.

Trust me. Nobody else worked this out. This approach is completely unique and fresh.

I have read virtually every calisthenics book printed in America over the last 40 years, and instruction like this can't be found anywhere, in any one of them. ***Convict Conditioning*** is head and shoulders above them all. In years to come, trainers and coaches will all be talking about 'progressions' and 'progressive calisthenics' and claim they've been doing it all along. But the truth is that Dragon Door bought it to you first. As with kettlebells, they were the trail blazers.

Who should purchase this volume? Everyone who craves fitness and strength should. Even if you don't plan to follow the routines, the book will make you think about your physical prowess, and will give even world class experts food for thought. At the very least if you find yourself on vacation or away on business without your barbells, this book will turn your hotel into a fully equipped gym.

I'd advise any athlete to obtain this work as soon as possible."***—Bill Oliver*** *- Albany, NY, United States*

A must for all martial artists

"As a dedicated martial artist for more than seven years, this book is exactly what I've been looking for.

For a while now I have trained with machines at my local gym to improve my muscle strength and power and get to the next level in my training. I always felt that the modern health club, technology based exercise jarred with my martial art though, which only required body movement.

Finally this book has come along. At last I can combine perfect body movement for martial skill with perfect body exercise for ultimate strength.

All fighting arts are based on body movement. This book is a complete textbook on how to max out your musclepower using only body movement, as different from dumbbells, machines or gadgets. For this reason it belongs on the bookshelf of every serious martial artist, male and female, young and old."***—Gino Cartier*** *- Washington DC*

I've packed all of my other training books away!

"I read CC in one go. I couldn't put it down. I have purchased a lot of bodyweight training books in the past, and have always been pretty disappointed. They all seem to just have pictures of different exercises, and no plan whatsoever on how to implement them and progress with them. But not with this one. The information in this book is AWESOME! I like to have a clear, logical plan of progression to follow, and that is what this book gives. I have put all of my other training books away. CC is the only system I am going to follow. This is now my favorite training book ever!"***—Lyndan*** *- Australia*

More Dragon Door Customer Acclaim for *Convict Conditioning*

Fascinating Reading and Real Strength

"Coach Wade's system is a real eye opener if you've been a lifetime iron junkie. Wanna find out how really strong (or weak) you are? Get this book and begin working through the 10 levels of the 6 power exercises. I was pleasantly surprised by my ability on a few of the exercises...but some are downright humbling. If I were on a desert island with only one book on strength and conditioning this would be it. (Could I staple Pavel's "Naked Warrior" to the back and count them as one???!) Thanks Dragon Door for this innovative new author."—***Jon Schultheis***, *RKC (2005) - Keansburg, NJ*

A lifetime of lifting...and continued learning.

"I have been working out diligently since 1988 and played sports in high school and college before that. My stint the Army saw me doing calisthenics, running, conditioning courses, forced marches, etc. There are many levels of strength and fitness. I have been as big as 240 in my powerlifting/strongman days and as low as 185-190 while in the Army. I think I have tried everything under the sun: the high intensity of Arthur Jones and Dr. Ken, the Super Slow of El Darden, and the brutality of Dinosaur Training Brooks Kubic made famous.

This is one of the BEST books I've ever read on real strength training which also covers other just as important aspects of health; like staying injury free, feeling healthy and becoming flexible. It's an excellent book. He tells you the why and the how with his progressive plan. This book is a GOLD MINE and worth 100 times what I paid for it!"
—***Horst*** *- Woburn, MA*

Single best strength training book ever!

"I just turned 50 this year and I have tried a little bit of everything over the years: martial arts, swimming, soccer, cycling, free weights, weight machines, even yoga and Pilates. I started using ***Convict Conditioning*** right after it came out. I started from the beginning, like Coach Wade says, doing mostly step one or two for five out of the six exercises. I work out 3 to 5 times a week, usually for 30 to 45 minutes.

Long story short, my weight went up 14 pounds (I was not trying to gain weight) but my body fat percentage dropped two percent. That translates into approximately 19 pounds of lean muscle gained in two months! I've never gotten this kind of results with anything else I've ever done. Now I have pretty much stopped lifting weights for strength training. Instead, I lift once a week as a test to see how much stronger I'm getting without weight training. There are a lot of great strength training books in the world (most of them published by Dragon Door), but if I had to choose just one, this is the single best strength training book ever. BUY THIS BOOK. FOLLOW THE PLAN. GET AS STRONG AS YOU WANT. "—***Wayne*** *- Decatur, GA*

This book sets the standard, ladies and gentlemen

"It's difficult to describe just how much this book means to me. I've been training hard since I was in the RAF nearly ten years ago, and to say this book is a breakthrough is an understatement. How often do you really read something so new, so fresh? This book contains a complete new system of calisthenics drawn from American prison training methods. When I say 'system' I mean it. It's complete (rank beginner to expert), it's comprehensive (all the exercises and photos are here), it's graded (progressions from exercise to exercise are smooth and pre-determined) and it's totally original. Whether you love or hate the author, you have to listen to him. And you will learn something. This book just makes SENSE. In twenty years people will still be buying it."—Andy McMann - Ponty, Wales, GB

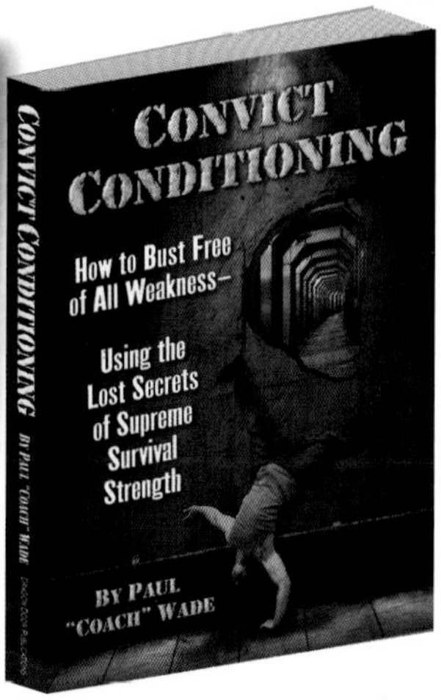

Convict Conditioning
How to Bust Free of All Weakness—Using the Lost Secrets of Supreme Survival Strength
By Paul "Coach" Wade
#B41 $39.95
Paperback 8.5 x 11 320 pages
191 photos, charts and illustrations

1 Beginner 2 Mid-Level 3 Advanced

Best bodyweight training book so far!

"I'm a martial artist and I've been training for years with a combination of weights and bodyweight training and had good results from both (but had the usual injuries from weight training). I prefer the bodyweight stuff though as it trains me to use my whole body as a unit, much more than weights do, and I notice the difference on the mat and in the ring. Since reading this book I have given the weights a break and focused purely on the bodyweight exercise progressions as described by 'Coach' Wade and my strength had increased more than ever before. So far I've built up to 12 strict one-leg squats each leg and 5 uneven pull ups each arm.

I've never achieved this kind of strength before - and this stuff builds solid muscle mass as well. It's very intense training. I am so confident in and happy with the results I'm getting that I've decided to train for a fitness/bodybuilding comp just using his techniques, no weights, just to show for real what kind of a physique these exercises can build. In sum, I cannot recommend 'Coach' Wade's book highly enough - it is by far the best of its kind ever!"—***Mark Robinson*** *- Australia, currently living in South Korea*

The Experts Give High Praise to *Convict Conditioning 2*

"Coach Paul Wade has outdone himself. His first book *Convict Conditioning* is to my mind THE BEST book ever written on bodyweight conditioning. Hands down. Now, with the sequel *Convict Conditioning 2*, Coach Wade takes us even deeper into the subtle nuances of training with the ultimate resistance tool: our bodies.

In plain English, but with an amazing understanding of anatomy, physiology, kinesiology and, go figure, psychology, Coach Wade explains very simply how to work the smaller but just as important areas of the body such as the hands and forearms, neck and calves and obliques in serious functional ways.

His minimalist approach to exercise belies the complexity of his system and the deep insight into exactly how the body works and the best way to get from A to Z in the shortest time possible.

I got the best advice on how to strengthen the hard-to-reach extensors of the hand right away from this exercise Master I have ever seen. It's so simple but so completely functional I can't believe no one else has thought of it yet. Just glad he figured it out for me.

Paul teaches us how to strengthen our bodies with the simplest of movements while at the same time balancing our structures in the same way: simple exercises that work the whole body.

And just as simply as he did with his first book. His novel approach to stretching and mobility training is brilliant and fresh as well as his take on recovery and healing from injury. Sprinkled throughout the entire book are too-many-to-count insights and advice from a man who has come to his knowledge the hard way and knows exactly of what he speaks.

This book is, as was his first, an amazing journey into the history of physical culture disguised as a book on calisthenics. But the thing that Coach Wade does better than any before him is his unbelievable progressions on EVERY EXERCISE and stretch! He breaks things down and tells us EXACTLY how to proceed to get to whatever level of strength and development we want. AND gives us the exact metrics we need to know when to go to the next level.

Adding in completely practical and immediately useful insights into nutrition and the mindset necessary to deal not only with training but with life, makes this book a classic that will stand the test of time.

Bravo Coach Wade, Bravo." **—Mark Reifkind, Master RKC,** author of ***Mastering the HardStyle Kettlebell Swing***

"I've been lifting weights for over 50 years and have trained in the martial arts since 1965. I've read voraciously on both subjects, and written dozens of magazine articles and many books on the subjects. This book and Wade's first, *Convict Conditioning*, are by far the most commonsense, information-packed, and result producing I've read. These books will truly change your life.

Paul Wade is a new and powerful voice in the strength and fitness arena, one that is commonsense, inspiring, and in your face. His approach to maximizing your body's potential is not the same old hackneyed material you find in every book and magazine piece that pictures steroid-bloated models screaming as they curl weights. Wade's stuff has been proven effective by hard men who don't tolerate fluff. It will work for you, too—guaranteed.

As an ex-cop, I've gone mano-y-mano with ex-cons that had clearly trained as Paul Wade suggests in his two *Convict Conditioning* books. While these guys didn't look like steroid-fueled bodybuilders (actually, there were a couple who did), all were incredibly lean, hard and powerful. Wade blows many commonly held beliefs about conditioning, strengthening, and eating out of the water and replaces them with result-producing information that won't cost you a dime." **—Loren W. Christensen,** author of ***Fighting the Pain Resistant Attacker,*** and many other titles

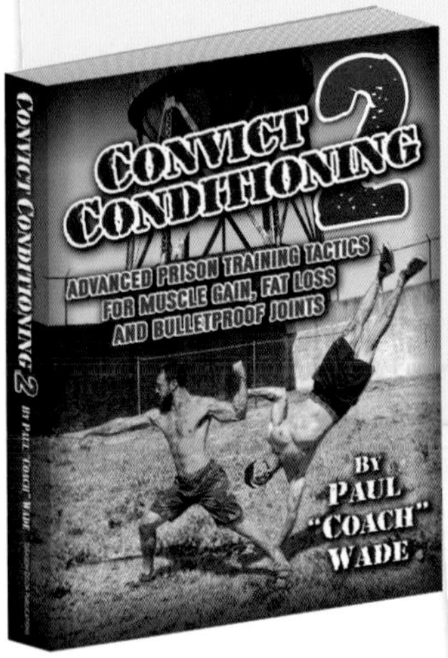

Convict Conditioning 2

Advanced Prison Training Tactics for Muscle Gain, Fat Loss and Bulletproof Joints

By Paul "Coach" Wade

#B59 $39.95

Paperback 8.5 x 11 354 pages
261 photos, charts and illustrations

2 Mid-Level
3 Advanced

"The overriding principle of *Convict Conditioning 2* is 'little equipment-big rewards'. For the athlete in the throwing and fighting arts, the section on Lateral Chain Training, Capturing the Flag, is a unique and perhaps singular approach to training the obliques and the whole family of side muscles. This section stood out to me as ground breaking and well worth the time and energy by anyone to review and attempt to complete. Literally, this is a new approach to lateral chain training that is well beyond sidebends and suitcase deadlifts.

The author's review of passive stretching reflects the experience of many of us in the field. But, his solution might be the reason I am going to recommend this work for everyone: The Trifecta. This section covers what the author calls The Functional Triad and gives a series of simple progressions to three holds that promise to oil your joints. It's yoga for the strength athlete and supports the material one would find, for example, in Pavel's *Loaded Stretching*.

I didn't expect to like this book, but I come away from it practically insisting that everyone read it. It is a strongman book mixed with yoga mixed with street smarts. I wanted to hate it, but I love it." **—Dan John,** author of *Don't Let Go* and co-author of *Easy Strength*

"*Convict Conditioning* is one of the most influential books I ever got my hands on. *Convict Conditioning 2* took my training and outlook on the power of bodyweight training to the 10th degree—from strengthening the smallest muscles in a maximal manner, all the way to using bodyweight training as a means of healing injuries that pile up from over 22 years of aggressive lifting.

I've used both *Convict Conditioning* and *Convict Conditioning 2* on myself and with my athletes. Without either of these books I can easily say that these boys would not be the BEASTS they are today. Without a doubt *Convict Conditioning 2* will blow you away and inspire and educate you to take bodyweight training to a whole NEW level." **—Zach Even-Esh,** Underground Strength Coach

www.dragondoor.com
1·800·899·5111

Dragon Door

Order *Convict Conditioning 2* online:
www.dragondoor.com/B59

—Table of Contents—

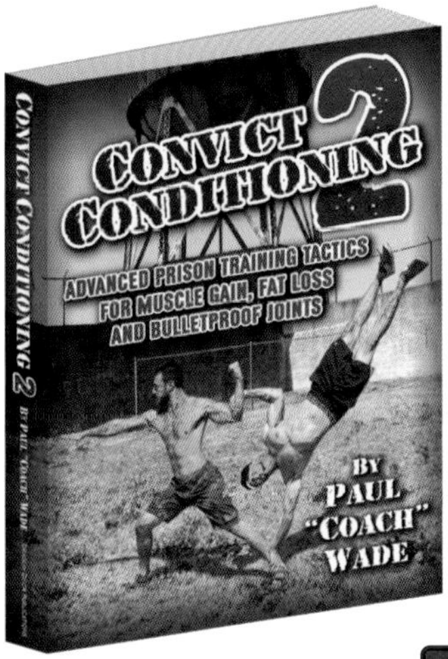

Convict Conditioning 2

Advanced Prison Training Tactics for Muscle Gain, Fat Loss and Bulletproof Joints

By Paul "Coach" Wade

#B59 $39.95

Paperback 8.5 x 11 354 pages
261 photos, charts and illustrations

2 Mid-Level
3 Advanced

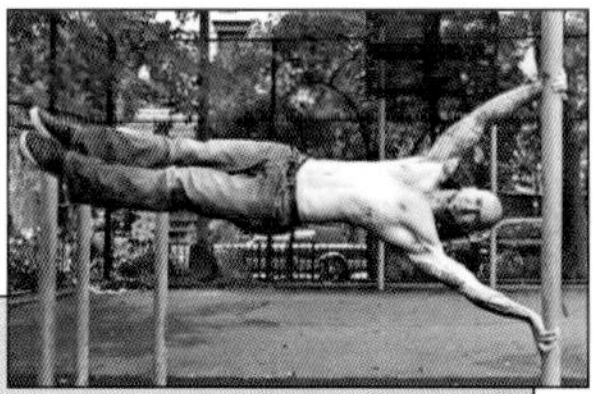

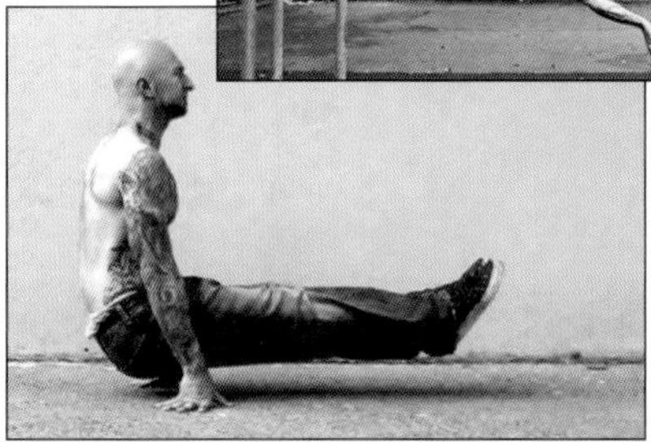

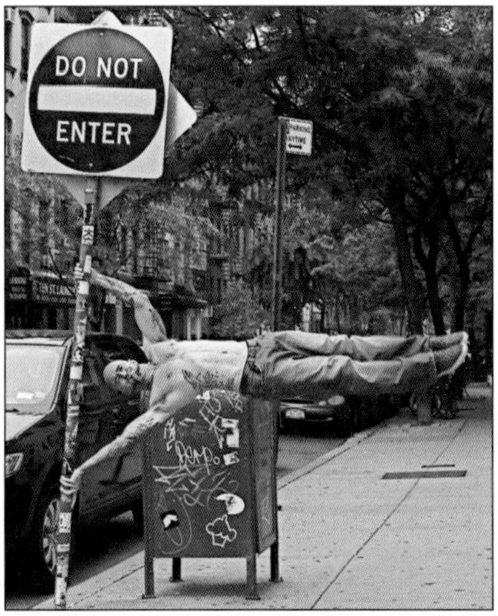

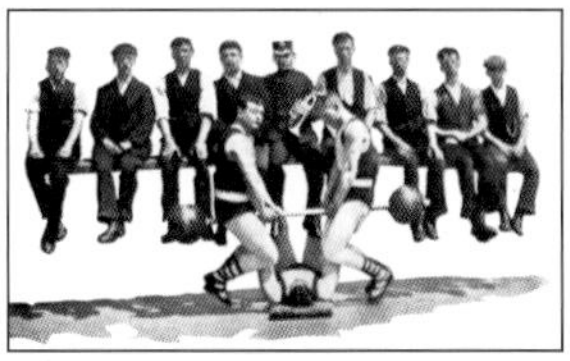

GET DYNAMIC, CHISELLED, POWER-JACK LEGS AND DEVELOP EXPLOSIVE LOWER-BODY STRENGTH—WITH PAUL "COACH" WADE'S ULTIMATE BODYWEIGHT SQUAT COURSE

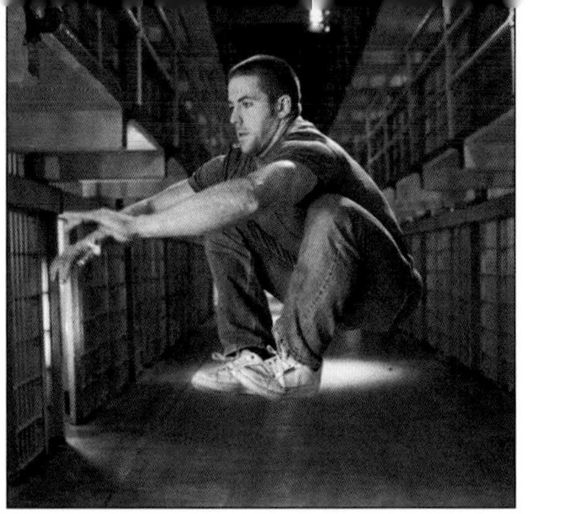

Paul Wade's *Convict Conditioning Ultimate Bodyweight Squat Course* explodes out of the cellblock to teach you in absolute detail how to progress from the ease of a simple shoulderstand squat—to the stunning "1-in-10,000" achievement of the prison-style one-leg squat. Ten progressive steps guide you to bodyweight squat mastery. Do it—and become a Bodyweight Squat Immortal.

This home-study course in ultimate survival strength comes replete with bonus material not available in **Paul Wade's** original *Convict Conditioning* book—and numerous key training tips that refine and expand on the original program.

A heavily and gorgeously-illustrated 80-plus-page manual gives you the entire film script to study at your leisure, with brilliant, precise photographs to remind you of the essential movements you absorbed in the DVD itself.

Paul Wade adds a bonus **Ten Commandments for Perfect Bodyweight Squats**—which is worth the price of admission alone. And there's the additional bonus of **5 major Variant drills** to add explosivity, fun and super-strength to your core practice.

Whatever you are looking for from your bodyweight squats—be it supreme functional strength, monstrous muscle growth or explosive leg power—it's yours for the progressive taking with *Convict Conditioning, Volume 2: The Ultimate Bodyweight Squat Course.*

WHY EVERY SELF-RESPECTING MAN WILL BE RELIGIOUS ABOUT HIS SQUATS...

Leg training is vital for every athlete. A well-trained, muscular upper body teetering around on skinny stick legs is a joke. Don't be that joke! The mighty squat is the answer to your prayers. Here's why:

- Squats train virtually every muscle in the lower body, from quads and glutes to hips, lower back and even hamstrings.
- Squat deep—as we'll teach you—and you will seriously increase your flexibility and ankle strength.
- All functional power is transmitted through the legs, so without strong, powerful legs you are *nothing*—that goes for running, jumping and combat sports as much as it does for lifting heavy stuff.

ARE YOU FAILING TO BUILD MONSTROUS LEGS FROM SQUATS—BECAUSE OF THESE MISTAKES?

Most trainees learn how to squat on two legs, and then make the exercise harder by slapping a barbell across their back. In prison, this way of adding strength wasn't always available, so cell trainees developed ways of progressing using only bodyweight versus gravity. The best way to do this is to learn how to squat all the way down to the ground and back up on just one leg.

Not everybody who explores prison training will have the dedication and drive to achieve strength feats like the one-arm pullup, but the legs are much stronger than the arms. If you put in the time and work hard, the one-leg squat will be within the reach of almost every athlete who pays their dues.

But the one-leg squat still requires very powerful muscles and tendons, so you don't want to jump into one-leg squatting right away. You need to build the joint strength and muscle to safely attempt this great exercise. Discover how to do that safely, using ten steps, ten progressively harder squat exercises.

IN THE STRENGTH GAME, FOOLS RUSH IN WHERE ANGELS FEAR TO TREAD

The wise old Chinese man shouted to his rickshaw driver: "Slow down, young man, I'm in a hurry!" If ever a warning needed to be shouted to our nation of compulsive strength-addicts, this would be it. You see them everywhere: the halt, the lame, the jacked-up, the torn, the pain-ridden—the former glory-seekers who have been reduced to sad husks of their former selves by rushing helter-skelter into heavy lifting without having first built a firm foundation.

Paul Wade reveals the ten key points of perfect squat form. The aspects of proper form apply to all your squats, and they'll not only unlock the muscle and power-building potential of each rep you do, but they'll also keep you as safe as you can be.

Bodyweight training is all about improving strength and health, not building up a list of injuries or aches and pains. They are so fundamental, we call them the Ten Commandments of good squat form.

Obey the Ten Commandments, follow the brilliantly laid out progressions religiously and you simply CANNOT fail to get stronger and stronger and stronger and stronger and stronger—surely, safely and for as long as you live...

COMPLEX MADE SIMPLE

Having read both *Convict Conditioning* and *Convict Conditioning 2*, the complementary DVD series is an excellent translation of the big six movement progressions into a simple to follow DVD. The demonstration of movement progression through the 10 levels is well described and easy to follow.
As a Physical Therapist it is a very useful way to teach safe progressions to patients/clients and other professionals. I have already used Volume I (the push up progression) to teach high school strength coaches how to safely progress athletes with pressing activity and look forward to using volume 2 with these same coaches. I think anyone who studies movement realizes very few athletes can properly squat with two legs, let alone one.

You will not find an easier way to teach the squat. Well done again Paul. Look forward to the rest of the series."
—Andrew Marchesi PT/MPT, FAFS, Scottsdale, AZ

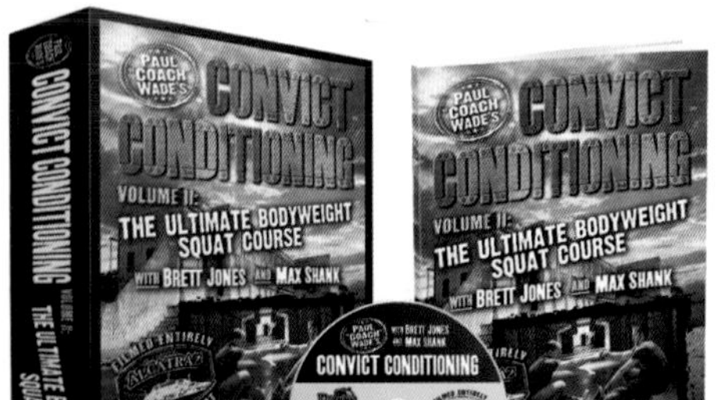

1 Beginner
2 Mid-Level
3 Advanced

Convict Conditioning
Volume 2: The Ultimate Bodyweight Squat Course
By Paul "Coach" Wade featuring Brett Jones and Max Shank
#DV084 $69.95
DVD 56 minutes with full color Companion Manual, 88 pages

NAVY SEAL ON THE ROAD

"My whole team uses it. We can work out effectively anywhere and I mean anywhere!"
—Tyler Archer, Navy

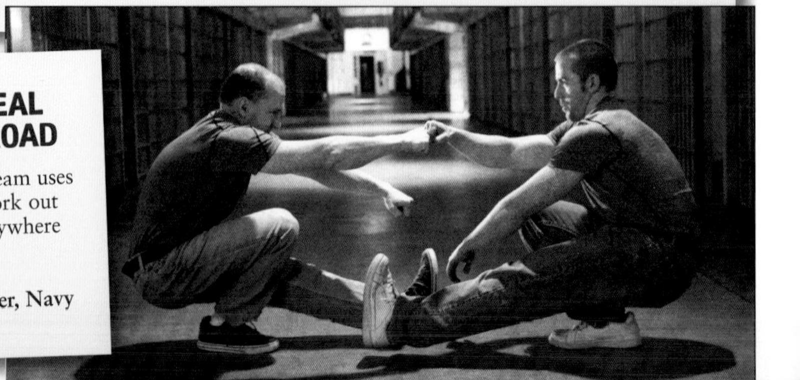

www.dragondoor.com
1-800-899-5111

Dragon Door

Order *CC Ultimate Squat* online:
www.dragondoor.com/DV084

Demonic Abs Are a Man's Best Friend—Discover How to Seize a Six-Pack from Hell and OWN the World... Leg Raises

Paul Wade's *Convict Conditioning 3, Leg Raises: Six Pack from Hell* teaches you in absolute detail how to progress from the ease of a simple Knee Tuck—to the magnificent, "1-in-1,000" achievement of the Hanging Straight Leg Raise. Ten progressive steps guide you to inevitable mastery of this ultimate abs exercise. Do it, seize the knowledge—but beware—the Gods will be jealous!

This home-study course in ultimate survival strength comes replete with bonus material not available in **Paul Wade's** original *Convict Conditioning* book—and numerous key training tips that refine and expand on the original program.

Prowl through the heavily and gorgeously-illustrated 80-plus-page manual and devour the entire film script at your animal leisure. Digest the brilliant, precise photographs and reinforce the raw benefits you absorbed from the DVD.

Paul Wade adds a bonus **Ten Commandments for Perfect Bodyweight Squats**—which is worth the price of admission alone. And there's the additional bonus of **4 major Variant drills** to add explosivity, fun and super-strength to your core practice.

Whatever you are looking for when murdering your abs—be it a fist-breaking, rock-like shield of impenetrable muscle, an uglier-is-more-beautiful set of rippling abdominal ridges, or a monstrous injection of lifting power—it's yours for the progressive taking with *Convict Conditioning, Volume 3, Leg Raises: Six Pack from Hell*

Prison-Style Midsection Training—for an All Show AND All Go Physique

When convicts train their waists, they want real, noticeable results—and by "results" we don't mean that they want cute, tight little defined abs. We mean that they want thick, strong, muscular midsections. They want *functionally* powerful abs and hips they can use for heavy lifting, kicking, and brawling. They want guts so strong from their training that it actually hurts an attacker to punch them in the belly. Prison abs aren't about all show, no go—a prison-built physique has to be all show and all go. Those guys don't just want six-packs—they want six-packs from Hell.

And, for the first time, we're going to show you how these guys get what they want. We're not going to be using sissy machines or easy isolation exercises—we're going straight for the old school secret weapon for gut training; progressive leg raises.

If you want a six-pack from Hell, the first thing you need to do is focus your efforts. If a weightlifter wanted a very thick, powerful chest in a hurry, he wouldn't spread his efforts out over a dozen exercises and perform them gently all day long. No—he'd pick just one exercise, probably the bench press, and just focus on getting stronger and stronger on that lift until he was monstrously strong. When he reached this level, and his pecs were thick slabs of meat, only then would he maybe begin sculpting them with minor exercises and higher reps.

It's no different if you want a mind-blowing midsection. Just pick one exercise that hits all the muscles in the midsection—the hip flexors, the abs, the intercostals, the obliques—then blast it.

And the one exercise we're going to discover is the best midsection exercise known to man, and the most popular amongst soldiers, warriors, martial artists and prison athletes since men started working out—the leg raise.

You'll discover ten different leg raise movements, each one a little harder than the last. You'll learn how to get the most out of each of these techniques, each of these ten steps, before moving up to the next step. By the time you get through all ten steps and you're working with the final Master Step of the leg raise series, you'll have a solid, athletic, stomach made of steel, as well as powerful hips and a ribcage armored with dense muscle. You'll have abs that would've made Bruce Lee take notice!

The Ten Commandments You Must Obey to Earn a Real Monster of an Athletic Core

Paul Wade gives you ten key points, the "Ten Commandments" of leg raises, that will take your prison-style core training from just "okay" to absolutely phenomenal. We want the results to be so effective that they'll literally shock you. This kind of accelerated progress can be achieved, but if you want to achieve it you better listen carefully to these ten key pointers you'll discover with the DVD.

Bodyweight mastery is a lot like high-level martial arts. It's more about *principles* than individual techniques. Really study and absorb these principles, and you'll be on your way to a six-pack from Hell in no time.

The hanging straight leg raise, performed strictly and for reps, is the Gold Standard of abdominal strength techniques. Once you're at the level where you can throw out sets of twenty to thirty rock solid reps of this exercise, your abs will be thick and strong, but more importantly, they'll be functional—not just a pretty six-pack, but a real monster of an athletic core, which is capable of developing high levels of force.

Hanging will work your serratus and intercostals, making these muscles stand out like fingers, and your obliques and flank muscles will be tight and strong from holding your hips in place. Your lumbar spine will achieve a gymnastic level of flexibility, like fluid steel, and your chances of back pain will be greatly reduced.

The bottom line: If you want to be stronger and more athletic than the next guy, you need the edge that straight leg raises can give you.

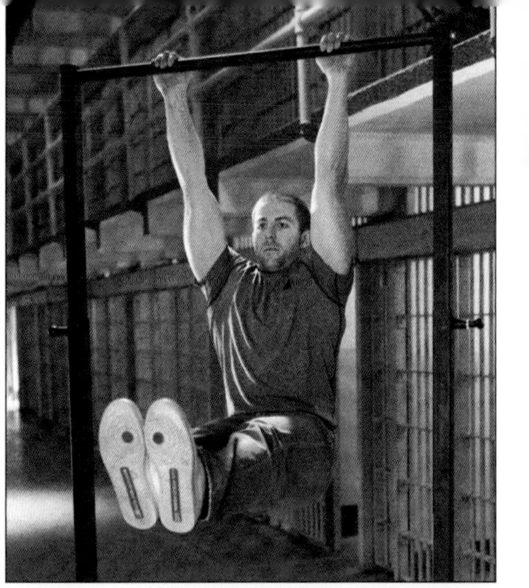

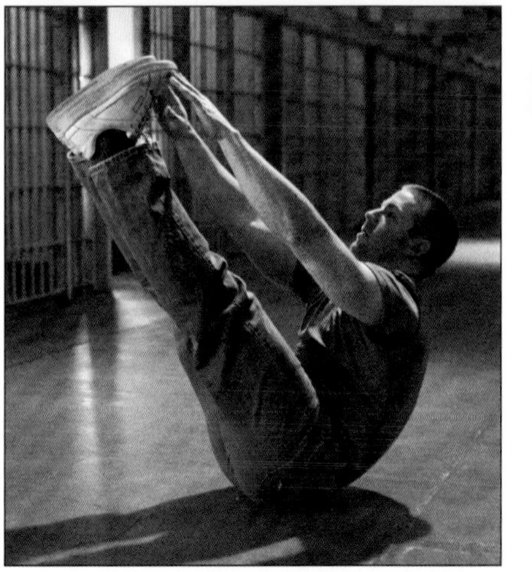

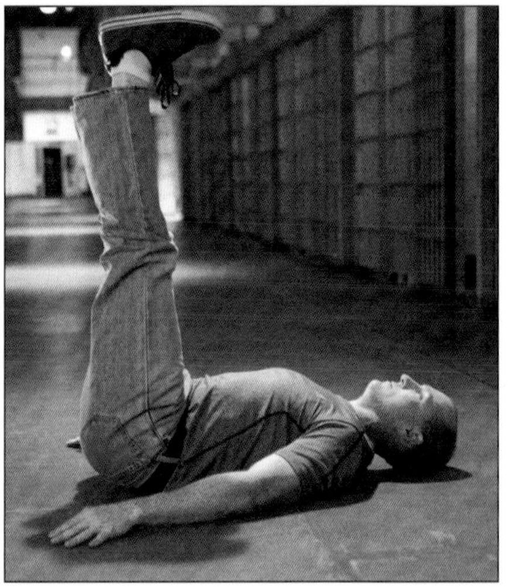

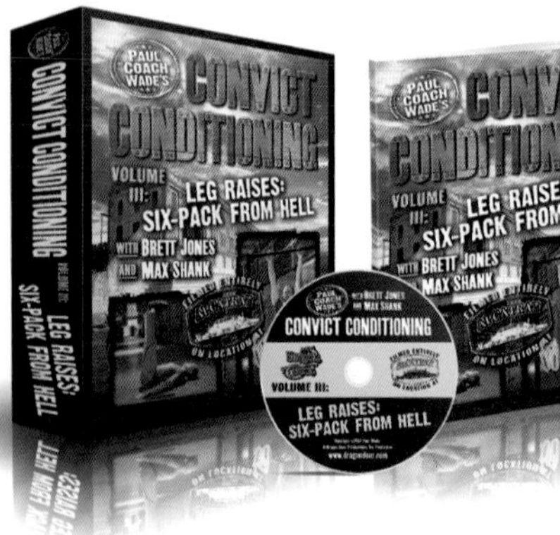

1 Beginner

2 Mid-Level

3 Advanced

Convict Conditioning
Volume 3: Leg Raises
Six Pack from Hell
By Paul "Coach" Wade featuring Brett Jones and Max Shank
#DV085 $59.95
DVD 57 minutes with full color Companion Manual, 82 pages

Erect Twin Pythons of Coiled Beef Up Your Spine and Develop Extreme, Explosive Resilience—With the Dynamic Power and Flexible Strength of

Advanced Bridging

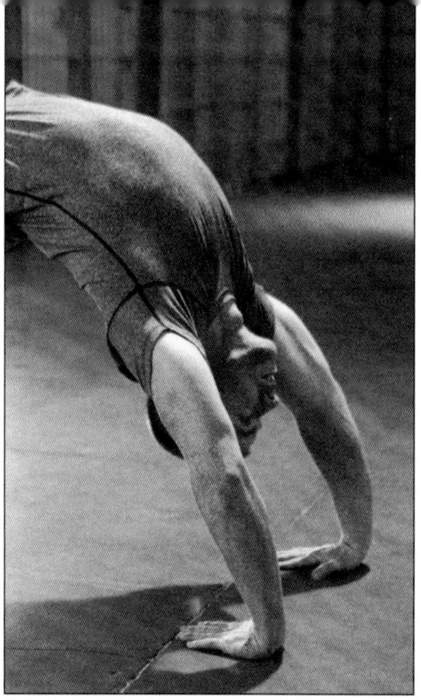

Paul Wade's *Convict Conditioning* system represents the ultimate distillation of hardcore prison bodyweight training's most powerful methods. What works was kept. What didn't, was slashed away. When your life is on the line, you're not going to mess with less than the absolute best. Many of these older, very potent solitary training systems have been on the verge of dying, as convicts begin to gain access to weights, and modern "bodybuilding thinking" floods into the prisons. Thanks to Paul Wade, these ultimate strength survival secrets have been saved for posterity. And for you...

Filmed entirely—and so appropriately— on **"The Rock"**, Wade's *Convict Conditioning Volume 4, Advanced Bridging: Forging an Iron Spine* explodes out of the cellblock to teach you in absolute detail how to progress from the relative ease of a Short Bridge—to the stunning, "1-in-1,000" achievement of the Stand-to-Stand Bridge. Ten progressive steps guide you to inevitable mastery of this ultimate exercise for an unbreakable back.

This home-study course in ultimate survival strength comes replete with bonus material not available in **Paul Wade's** original *Convict Conditioning* book—and numerous key training tips that refine and expand on the original program.

Prowl through the heavily and gorgeously-illustrated 80-plus-page manual and devour the entire film script at your animal leisure. Digest the brilliant, precise photographs and reinforce the raw benefits you absorbed from the DVD.

Paul Wade adds a bonus **Ten Commandments for Perfect Bridges**—which is worth the price of admission alone. And there's the additional bonus of **4 major Variant drills** to add explosivity, fun and super-strength to your core practice.

Whatever you are looking for from your pushups—be it supreme functional strength, monstrous muscle growth or explosive upper-body power—it's yours for the progressive taking with *Convict Conditioning Volume 4: Advanced Bridging: Forging an Iron Spine.*

Filmed Entirely On Location at Alcatraz

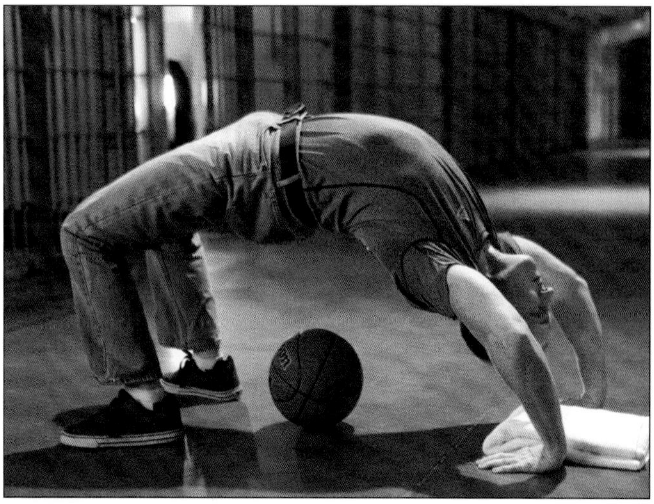

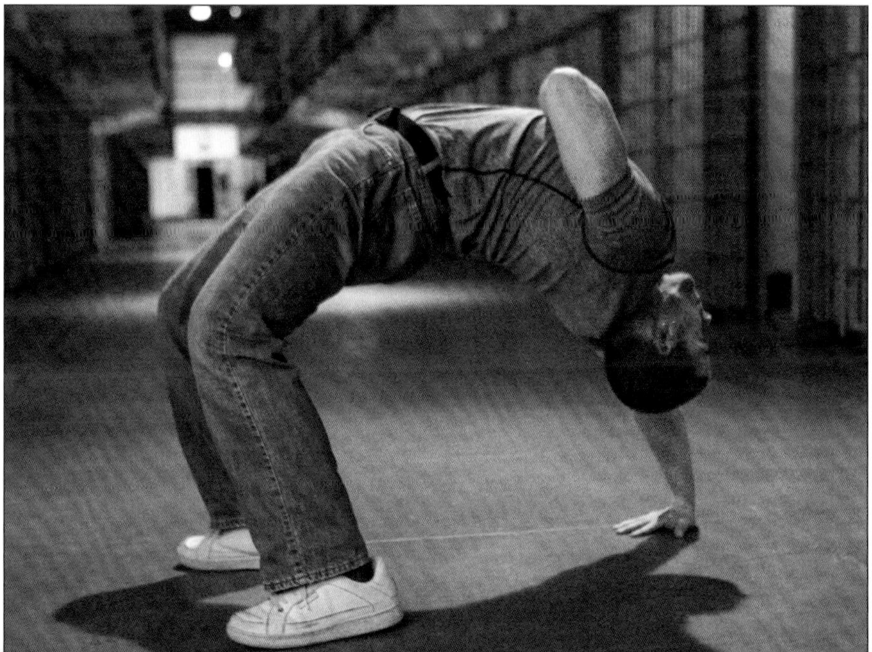

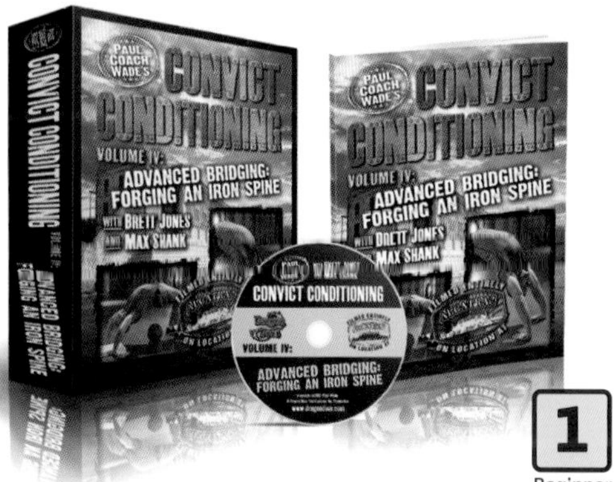

Convict Conditioning
Volume 4: Advanced Bridging: Forging an Iron Spine
By Paul "Coach" Wade featuring Brett Jones and Max Shank
#DV087 $59.95
DVD 59 minutes with full color Companion Manual, 88 pages

1 Beginner
2 Mid-Level
3 Advanced

DRAGON DOOR PUBLICATIONS PRESENTS
HARD-STYLE
HARD CORE TOOLS FOR HARD LIVING TYPES

1·800·899·5111
24 HOURS A DAY
FAX YOUR ORDER (866) 280-7619

VISA · MasterCard · American Express · Discover Novus

ORDERING INFORMATION

Customer Service Questions? Please call us between 9:00am– 11:00pm EST Monday to Friday at 1-800-899-5111. Local and foreign customers call 513-346-4160 for orders and customer service

100% One-Year Risk-Free Guarantee. If you are not completely satisfied with any product—we'll be happy to give you a prompt exchange, credit, or refund, as you wish. Simply return your purchase to us, and please let us know why you were dissatisfied—it will help us to provide better products and services in the future. *Shipping and handling fees are non-refundable.*

Telephone Orders For faster service you may place your orders by calling Toll Free 24 hours a day, 7 days a week, 365 days per year. When you call, please have your credit card ready.

Complete and mail with full payment to: Dragon Door Publications, 5 County Road B East, Suite 3, Little Canada, MN 55117

Please print clearly

Sold To: **A**

*Name*__________

Street __________

City __________

State __________ *Zip* ______

*Day phone**__________

** Important for clarifying questions on orders*

Please print clearly

SHIP TO: ***(Street address for delivery)*** **B**

*Name*__________

Street __________

City __________

State __________ *Zip* ______

Email __________

Warning to foreign customers:
The Customs in your country may or may not tax or otherwise charge you an additional fee for goods you receive. Dragon Door Publications is charging you only for U.S. handling and international shipping. Dragon Door Publications is in no way responsible for any additional fees levied by Customs, the carrier or any other entity.

ITEM #	QTY.	ITEM DESCRIPTION	ITEM PRICE	A OR B	TOTAL

HANDLING AND SHIPPING CHARGES • NO COD'S
Total Amount of Order Add (Excludes kettlebells and kettlebell kits):

\$00.00 to 29.99	**Add \$6.00**	**\$100.00 to 129.99**	**Add \$14.00**
\$30.00 to 49.99	**Add \$7.00**	**\$130.00 to 169.99**	**Add \$16.00**
\$50.00 to 69.99	**Add \$8.00**	**\$170.00 to 199.99**	**Add \$18.00**
\$70.00 to 99.99	**Add \$11.00**	**\$200.00 to 299.99**	**Add \$20.00**
		\$300.00 and up	**Add \$24.00**

Canada and Mexico add \$6.00 to US charges. All other countries, flat rate, double US Charges. See Kettlebell section for Kettlebell Shipping and handling charges.

Total of Goods	
Shipping Charges	
Rush Charges	
Kettlebell Shipping Charges	
OH residents add 6.5% sales tax	
MN residents add 6.5% sales tax	
TOTAL ENCLOSED	

METHOD OF PAYMENT ❒ CHECK ❒ M.O. ❒ MASTERCARD ❒ VISA ❒ DISCOVER ❒ AMEX

Account No. *(Please indicate all the numbers on your credit card)* EXPIRATION DATE

□□□□ □□□□ □□□□ □□□□ □□/□□

Day Phone: (___)__________
Signature: __________ **Date:** __________

NOTE: *We ship best method available for your delivery address. Foreign orders are sent by air. Credit card or International M.O. only. For* **RUSH** *processing of your order, add an additional \$10.00 per address. Available on money order & charge card orders only.*

Errors and omissions excepted. Prices subject to change without notice.

DRAGON DOOR PUBLICATIONS PRESENTS
HARD-STYLE
HARD CORE TOOLS FOR HARD LIVING TYPES

1·800·899·5111
24 HOURS A DAY
FAX YOUR ORDER (866) 280-7619

VISA · MasterCard · American Express · Discover Novus

ORDERING INFORMATION

Customer Service Questions? Please call us between 9:00am– 11:00pm EST Monday to Friday at 1-800-899-5111. Local and foreign customers call 513-346-4160 for orders and customer service

100% One-Year Risk-Free Guarantee. If you are not completely satisfied with any product—we'll be happy to give you a prompt exchange, credit, or refund, as you wish. Simply return your purchase to us, and please let us know why you were dissatisfied—it will help us to provide better products and services in the future. *Shipping and handling fees are non-refundable.*

Telephone Orders For faster service you may place your orders by calling Toll Free 24 hours a day, 7 days a week, 365 days per year. When you call, please have your credit card ready.

Complete and mail with full payment to: Dragon Door Publications, 5 County Road B East, Suite 3, Little Canada, MN 55117

Please print clearly

Sold To: **A**

Name ______________________

Street ______________________

City ______________________

State ____________ *Zip* ________

*Day phone** ______________________

* *Important for clarifying questions on orders*

Please print clearly

SHIP TO: ***(Street address for delivery)*** **B**

Name ______________________

Street ______________________

City ______________________

State ____________ *Zip* ________

Email ______________________

Warning to foreign customers:

The Customs in your country may or may not tax or otherwise charge you an additional fee for goods you receive. Dragon Door Publications is charging you only for U.S. handling and international shipping. Dragon Door Publications is in no way responsible for any additional fees levied by Customs, the carrier or any other entity.

ITEM #	QTY.	ITEM DESCRIPTION	ITEM PRICE	A OR B	TOTAL

HANDLING AND SHIPPING CHARGES • NO COD'S

Total Amount of Order Add (Excludes kettlebells and kettlebell kits):

$00.00 to 29.99	Add $6.00	$100.00 to 129.99	Add $14.00
$30.00 to 49.99	Add $7.00	$130.00 to 169.99	Add $16.00
$50.00 to 69.99	Add $8.00	$170.00 to 199.99	Add $18.00
$70.00 to 99.99	Add $11.00	$200.00 to 299.99	Add $20.00
		$300.00 and up	Add $24.00

Canada and Mexico add $6.00 to US charges. All other countries, flat rate, double US Charges. See Kettlebell section for Kettlebell Shipping and handling charges.

Total of Goods	
Shipping Charges	
Rush Charges	
Kettlebell Shipping Charges	
OH residents add 6.5% sales tax	
MN residents add 6.5% sales tax	
TOTAL ENCLOSED	

METHOD OF PAYMENT ❐ CHECK ❐ M.O. ❐ MASTERCARD ❐ VISA ❐ DISCOVER ❐ AMEX

Account No. *(Please indicate all the numbers on your credit card)* EXPIRATION DATE

□□□□ □□□□ □□□□ □□□□ □□/□□

Day Phone: (___) ____________

Signature: ______________________ **Date:** ____________

NOTE: *We ship best method available for your delivery address. Foreign orders are sent by air. Credit card or International M.O. only. For* **RUSH** *processing of your order, add an additional $10.00 per address. Available on money order & charge card orders only.*

Errors and omissions excepted. Prices subject to change without notice.